THE CENTER FOR MEDICAL CONSUMERS

ULTIMATE MEDICAL
ANSWERBOOK

———— ◆ ————

Also from the Center for Medical Consumers

Healthfacts

THE CENTER FOR MEDICAL CONSUMERS

ULTIMATE MEDICAL ANSWERBOOK

———— ◆ ————

MARYANN NAPOLI

Co-founder and Associate Director, Editor

and

CARL SHERMAN

Produced by The Philip Lief Group, Inc.

HEARST BOOKS

NEW YORK

Library of Congress Cataloging-in-Publication Data

The Center for Medical Consumers ultimate medical answerbook / Maryann Napoli, editor.
    p.   cm.
    Includes index.
    ISBN 0–688–12753–3
    1. Medicine, Popular—Miscellanea. I. Napoli, Maryann, 1940–
II. Center for Medical Consumers, Inc. III. Title: Ultimate medical
answerbook.
    RC81.C46   1995
    610—dc20   95–60
                                       CIP

Printed in the United States of America

First Edition

1   2   3   4   5   6   7   8   9   10

BOOK DESIGN BY MICHAEL MENDELSOHN OF MM DESIGN 2000, INC.

FOREWORD

———— ◆ ————

The current national preoccupation with reform of our health care system has brought into sharper focus some of the very basic flaws that "reforms" are not likely to address. The first of these appears to be a universal complaint: Many physicians do not really listen to what their patients are trying to tell them. A second common flaw is that many patients are not able to explain their problems clearly or to accurately convey their concerns—even when the physician is willing to listen. These failures of communication are a serious impediment in our current system of health care delivery. Medical training programs should assume responsibility for enhancing the physician's inclination and ability to "listen." Unfortunately, patients must educate themselves as to how they can interact with health care providers to obtain accurate evaluation and optimal management of their health problems.

Many individuals and organizations are aware of these fundamental flaws and the problems they create. Over the past eighteen years there has been a significant proliferation of programs and publications designed to help medical consumers improve their knowledge and understanding of the more common disorders and diseases encountered in our society. Now we are becoming more aware of the need for improving the consumer's ability to use health care systems—regardless of how they are organized and staffed—to obtain the care he or she seeks. The key to accomplishing this appears to involve two elements of self-education: (1) Learning appropriate techniques and skills in *talking with health care providers* to obtain accurate and comprehensive evaluation (diagnosis), and (2) Acquiring a basic understanding and insight into the disease or disorder to be managed. In other words, the consumer must know *what and how to tell* the health care professional when help is sought, and *what and how to ask* when advice and treatment are offered.

If a patient is to receive optimal attention and care from any health care systems, he or she must be able to make *informed decisions and choices* regarding health care providers and the services they offer. The Center for Medical Consumers' new publication *The Center for Medical Consumers Ultimate Medical Answerbook* by Maryann Napoli is clearly designed to provide assistance in this often perplexing undertaking. Patients soon learn the significance of the numerous controversies that exist within the medical community regarding the management of many serious conditions. Notable examples are breast cancer and prostate cancer. Although there are several treatment options currently available for both of these conditions, the paternalistic bent of many physicians is to decide which treatment the patient should have—without discussing the full ramifications of each option and then exploring the patient's opinions and wishes.

It is imperative that the patient and family educate themselves regarding the nature of the disorder and all available treatment options that have merit. Sources of relevant information include health information centers patterned after the Center for Medical Consumers in New York City, public libraries, health science libraries in community hospitals, bookstores, and primary physicians. A few hours of concentrated "homework" will enable the patient to ask the right questions and then decide which are the right answers.

—James W. Long, M.D.

CONTENTS

——— ◆ ———

INTRODUCTION

＿＿＿＿ ◆ ＿＿＿＿

We opened the Center for Medical Consumers in 1977 with this message in mind: People should know all they can before consenting to medical treatment. They cannot make a truly informed decision without knowing the risks as well as the benefits of the proposed treatment—and its alternatives. Believe it or not, this was still a new idea in 1977.

Our first move was the establishment of a medical library designed for the lay public. In the 1970s, people were hearing for the first time about unnecessary surgery, potentially fatal prescription drug interactions, and excessive X-ray examinations. There was a critical need for a neutral information source, quite apart from a hospital or doctor's office, where people can assess the quality of the information received from their physicians. At our library they can consult medical journals, textbooks, directories; in short, the same information sources used by doctors.

The next step for the Center for Medical Consumers was the publication of our monthly newsletter, *HealthFacts*, to help readers evaluate the most common medical decisions. *HealthFacts* summarizes the latest research findings to answer such questions as: Should I take postmenopausal hormones? How can I avoid unnecessary coronary bypass surgery? Is the new laparoscopic gallbladder surgery safer than the standard operation? What is the best treatment for an enlarged prostate? Is this vaccination safe and effective?

This book not only formulates the questions to be asked but also provides the answers. They are intended as a means of starting a dialogue with your doctor, to elicit additional information about your treatment, and to inspire you to do more research on your own. Why should you do your own homework? Simply put: your doctor doesn't know everything. The majority do not read medical journals regularly. Furthermore, several studies show that most doctors get the bulk of their postgraduate drug education from the promotional activities of the pharmaceutical industry.

A 1991 consensus conference on doctor-patient communication found that only a low percentage of the doctor visit includes any patient education, and a surprisingly high proportion of patients do not understand or remember what their physicians tell them about diagnosis and treatment. Studies reported at this conference show that doctors often misperceive the type and amount of information their patients want and use jargon in their explanations.

Instead of listening to their patients, many physicians want to control the interview. In fact, most people are interrupted by their doctors within the first eighteen seconds of beginning to explain their concerns. This finding came from a study of more than one thousand encounters between internists and their patients at a health maintenance organization in Michigan. It has been replicated by research teams in other countries, regardless of how long a doctor visit lasts. Dr. Richard Frankel, co-author of the Michigan study, was asked how people can control the inevitable interruptions. "Let's say that you are a patient who tells the doctor, 'I've got chest pain,' and the physician asks, ''Is that in the morning or afternoon?' You can say: 'I'm going to get to that, but I've got a couple of other concerns that I want to share with you.'' Physician interruption can prevent people from ever getting to the reason for their visit. Typically, people go to their physicians with about three concerns, and the most troubling complaint is not always presented first. Doctors aren't mind readers. Clarify for yourself the exact reason for the visit and state your problem concisely.

This book provides some examples of questions to ask your doctor, but it's up to you to control the visit in order to get the information you want. Experts suggest that people give serious thought to the questions they want answered well in advance of the visit, even rehearsing beforehand. It helps to be concise in explaining the purpose of the visit. Having someone accompany you as an ''extra pair of ears'' is also a good idea, especially when dealing with a life-threatening diagnosis like cancer.

In choosing a doctor, an assessment of her communication skills is essential to determining the quality of any future relationship. He can be the best doctor in the world, but this can be rendered meaningless, if he can't explain how to take your drugs properly. When preparing for your first visit to a primary care physician, think about the issues most important to you and then formulate the questions. If, for example, you have a living will prepared, discuss your wishes for withdrawing life support.

The need for a relationship with an open sharing of crucial information should be discussed at the first visit. Will you fax me the summary of my mammography, lab test, biopsy report, etc., so I can have a copy for my own file? I am likely to want a second or third opinion in the event of a recommendation for surgery or a lifelong drug regimen, would you support my desires and send on the necessary records?

During the initial encounter with a doctor, there are some questions to ask yourself: Is this doctor a good listener? Does this doctor allow me to have a sense of control over my own care? Is this doctor a good teacher? If you don't get satisfactory answers to your requests for more information, change doctors.

When choosing a specialist, questions are likely to be more specific. With a disease like cancer, you may want to ask: Will you treat my pain as aggressively as my cancer? Will you support my informed decision to reject chemotherapy? Can you help me make changes in my diet which may improve the quality of my life? The answers to such questions should give you an idea whether you can work with this doctor, whether you can be partners in the decision-making process. With chronic diseases like asthma or diabetes it is all the more crucial to have a doctor who will take the amount of time necessary to explain how to monitor your own condition and take medication accordingly.

In getting a second or third opinion, ask your family physician for a recommendation. Go outside of a group practice to avoid one doctor merely rubber-stamping a colleague's advice. In some cases, you're better off choosing an entirely different specialty in order to find a doctor who represents another school of thought. For example, if an orthopedic surgeon advises back surgery, consult a physiatrist (specialist in rehabilitation medicine) who is more likely to come up with a nonsurgical solution. If possible, find out as much as possible preferably from a nurse or other health care professional about the doctor you are considering for a second opinion consult.

Your desire for a second pathology opinion, on the other hand, usually requires the cooperation of the surgeon and is best discussed at first interview—before cancer surgery. In some parts of the country, women with breast cancer still have difficulties locating a surgeon who will offer breast-sparing treatment. In such cases, word of mouth may be the best way of learning the physician's bias prior to a second opinion consultation.

Find out about your treatment options first and then find the specialist who is skilled in your treatment of choice. For example, after reading about hemorrhoid treatment options, you may decide that rubber band ligation is the one for you. In the absence of a directory listing all doctors who perform this treatment, you are left with word of mouth as the means of finding a specialist, or calling the nearest teaching hospital for a list of gastroenterologists and then calling each one to learn whether he or she performs rubber band ligation.

Studies continue to show that people want information from their doctors, much more than their doctors realize. Questions and answers in *The Center for Medical Consumers Ultimate Medical Answerbook* demonstrate how to elicit information normally not volunteered by physicians. What do we know of the long-term effects of combining estrogen and progesterone? What will happen if I don't have this treatment? We've included a recurring theme in the answers we should expect from such questions: Has this treatment been subjected to a controlled clinical trial to prove safety and efficacy? Can you advise me about prevention?

Too often people get one-sided information about a recommended treatment: "You have mild hypertension, you must go on this drug regimen for the rest of your life in order to reduce your risk of having a stroke by forty-five percent." Sounds good; maybe even worth the risk of impotence and depression—two common side effects of antihypertensives. But here's the other side of the story: A person with mild hypertension has an infinitesimal chance of ever having a stroke; antihypertensive drug treatment will reduce those infinitesimal odds by 45 percent. (See Stroke.)

Much has changed in the years since the Center for Medical Consumers opened its doors to the public. People are less willing to leave treatment decisions entirely up to their doctors. They want to be part of the decision-making process. They are much more aware of options and the fact that unnecessary surgery and overtreatment are distressingly common. Going for a second opinion is no longer a revolutionary concept.

Information sources have increased enormously. Virtually all TV and radio news shows now have medical reporters. Toll-free hotlines like the National Cancer Institute's (800) 4-CANCER provide state-of-the-art treatment information from the computerized database of the National Library of Medicine (request the doctor's version). You can find out whether a doctor is a board-certified specialist by calling the American Medical Association's hotline at (800) 776-2378. Research services, many started by people who didn't get the information they needed from their own doctors, will—for a fee—search the medical literature for you. (Our favorites are Planetree in San Francisco, The Health Resource in Conway, Arkansas, and Medscan in Johnson City, New York.)

Community libraries are now more likely to carry prescription drug reference books, The Official ABMS Directory of Board Certified Medical Specialists, a four-volume set of textbooks for checking doctors' credentials, family medical guides, and sometimes even a medical journal or two. Consumer medical libraries similar to our own are now available in many areas of the country.

By all means, ask questions of your doctor. But don't leave it at that. Check the answer. This book is a good place to start.

—Maryann Napoli
Co-founder and Associate Director
Center for Medical Consumers
New York City

THE CENTER FOR MEDICAL CONSUMERS

ULTIMATE MEDICAL ANSWERBOOK

———— ◆ ————

✦ ACNE

Are you now, or have you ever been, an adolescent? If so, you probably know something about acne. The whiteheads, blackheads, and pimples are a rite of passage for an estimated 80 percent of teenagers. For a minority, acne lingers into adulthood. The problem may also develop in one's twenties, thirties, or later.

Increased production of androgens, the male hormones, stimulates the skin's secretion of an oily substance called sebum. When sebum and shed skin cells harden into a plug that blocks a pore, a comedo or blackhead develops. If the plug reaches the surface, skin pigment turns it into a blackhead.

Pimples appear when common bacteria, *Propionibacterium acnes,* digest sebum into fatty acids that cause inflammation in the surrounding skin. More extensive, boil-like infections produce "cystic" acne.

The sebaceous glands that produce sebum are especially abundant on the face, upper chest, and back, which is why acne is most common there.

WHY ME?

The extent and seriousness of acne varies widely from person to person. Because puberty starts earlier in girls, so does acne (typically at age eleven, as compared to thirteen in boys), but boys, who produce ten times as much androgen as girls, generally have worse cases. Some research suggests that girls and women with particularly bad acne have higher than average androgen levels.

Heredity plays a role. If you had severe acne in your youth, your children are likely to be similarly afflicted. Two parents with a blemished past load the dice heavily against their offspring.

The same factors—hormones and heredity—apparently influence adult acne. Men tend to have more severe cases, but women more often seek treatment. Many women find that pimples appear just before menstruation, or acne flares up as female hormones decrease with menopause. Lifestyle factors make a difference, too.

SHOULD I CHANGE MY DIET?

It makes sense that greasy foods, like french fries and potato chips, can cause or aggravate a condition that involves skin oils. And everyone knows that chocolate and soft drinks make acne worse. There's no scientific evidence, however, for either of these beliefs. In fact, no link has ever been proven between diet and acne.

Many people, however, do notice that particular foods, drinks, or spices seem to make their acne flare up. If you've had this experience, by all means see if changing your diet accordingly will improve your skin (it may take a month or more). Make sure that you don't compromise good nutrition, however.

Zinc supplements have been advocated, on the theory that they modify the inflammatory reaction that produces pimples. A real zinc deficiency can cause acne, but this is probably rare, and controlled studies of zinc supplementation for people who are basically well nourished have been inconsistent. Remember that megadoses of zinc, like other minerals, can be toxic. The recommended daily allowance (RDA) for zinc is 15 milligrams per day.

WILL SUNLIGHT HELP ACNE?

This is another "everybody knows" fact that hasn't been scientifically verified. Sunlight may well lessen acne for many people, not by drying out greasy skin, but by reducing inflammation. Frequently, the condition improves in summer; some people, however, find that excessive sunlight makes acne worse.

Remember, though, that whether you have acne or not, excessive sun (or sunlamp) exposure increases skin cancer risk and accelerates skin aging. Be especially careful if you use a sunlamp.

Certain medications make it essential to *avoid* sun exposure.

DO COSMETICS CAUSE ACNE?

The role of cosmetics in causing or worsening acne is debatable. Dermatological opinion in recent years has veered from indicting cosmetics as a principal villain in adult acne, to claiming that their role is minimal. Because most whitehead-causing ingredients have been removed from cosmetics, they are less likely to cause acne than they were.

You'll minimize the possibility that cosmetics will trigger or worsen acne by using light, hypoallergenic makeup and water, rather than oil-based products. Styling gels, creams, and sprays may provoke whiteheads and blackheads near the hairline.

SHOULD I USE FACIAL SCRUBS?

Good hygiene is important in controlling acne. Wash twice a day, with a mild, nonirritating soap, rinse thoroughly, and pat the skin dry.

While abrasive products are often used to remove oil and unplug blocked pores, their effectiveness against blemishes is uncertain. Sometimes they reduce their number at first, but seem to result in more later. If you have acne, your skin is unusually sensitive to injury and irritation, so scrubs should be used, if at all, with care.

DOES STRESS CAUSE ACNE?

Because stress affects hormones and the inflammatory process, both of which have a role in acne, it seems logical it can worsen outbreaks. Many people have had the experience of sprouting new pimples when the pressure is on to look their best. Although systematic studies are few, there have been reports of improvements with stress-control techniques, like relaxation, biofeedback, or psychotherapy, generally applied as an adjunct to medical treatment.

DO OTC REMEDIES WORK?

Some over-the-counter products are quite effective for mild to moderate acne. Benzoyl peroxide promotes peeling of the outer layer of skin, and kills bacteria by oxidation. It has been found effective in controlled trials.

The safety of this OTC drug has come into question, however. Several years ago, a Food and Drug Administration (FDA) review of research unearthed studies in which benzoyl peroxide promoted skin cancer in several strains of mice and other laboratory animals. Consequently, the FDA revoked the "safe" designation of the compound and ordered long-term studies to make sure it won't cause cancer in humans as well. At this writing, the FDA hasn't decided whether benzoyl peroxide should be taken off the market, pending the outcome of those studies.

Products containing benzoyl peroxide are still on the shelves (read ingredients lists), and whether to run the uncertain risk is your decision. If you do, start with the lowest concentration (2.5 percent) and work up to stronger preparations if that isn't effective. As with many other acne remedies, it takes six to eight weeks to know if the product works. Some reddening and peeling is normal, but more severe skin reactions suggest contact dermatitis (rash), which happens to about 1 percent of people who use benzoyl peroxide.

If you'd rather not use benzoyl peroxide, preparations containing salicylic acid, sulfur, or sulfur and resorcinol have been found to be safe and effective OTC treatments for acne. Salicylic acid, a chemical cousin of aspirin, promotes skin peeling. Controlled tests have found it more effective than a placebo, and in some cases more effective than benzoyl peroxide.

Salicylic acid also comes in different concentrations, and again, you're best off starting at the lowest level. In one test, there was little difference between results with .5 percent and 2 percent compounds.

Like benzoyl peroxide, sulfur apparently helps peel the dead outer layer of skin, and it also kills acne-promoting bacteria. It has been used for centuries for various skin disorders and has stood up to scientific trials. As noted, some products combine sulfur with resorcinol, another skin peeler.

ARE PRESCRIPTION DRUGS BETTER THAN OTC DRUGS?

Topical medications that require a prescription, notably tretinoin and antibiotic preparations, are usually prescribed when acne is more serious and doesn't respond to the above-mentioned OTC drugs.

Tretinoin (more familiar by its trade name, Retin-A), a chemical related to vitamin A, apparently helps push out sebum plugs and prevent new ones from forming. It's usually the first choice, often coupled with continued OTC treatment—applied to the skin in a cream (best for dry skin) and gel (more appropriate if skin is oily). Often, tretinoin dries and irritates the skin for a time, while the dose is adjusted. Acne may get worse before it gets better.

One invariable effect of tretinoin is photosensitivity (sensitivity to sunlight). Stay out of the sun (particularly in the hours between ten and three, when the sun is strongest) or use a sun block and protective clothing, or you may suffer painful irritation, even skin damage.

Topical antibiotics—tetracycline and erythromycin—usually aren't used unless Retin-A doesn't work, or when benzoyl peroxide can't be combined with Retin-A. Oral antibiotics are generally reserved for acne that doesn't respond to creams and lotions.

Wise physicians don't jump in with antibiotics, topical or oral, too quickly, because their overuse produces resistant strains of bacteria. According to a study in the *British Medical Journal* (February 27, 1993), antibiotic-resistant strains of *P. acnes,* once almost virtually nonexistent, have become widespread. Cultures from the skin of 239 people with acne, about two thirds of whom had not responded to antibiotic treatment, showed antibiotic-resistant strains in 178 cases. Women taking antibiotics are susceptible to vaginal yeast infections.

IS ACCUTANE SAFE?

Isotretinoin (Accutane), another derivative of vitamin A, is an oral drug meant for use only against severe nodular and inflammatory acne that hasn't responded to any other treatment. Several months of isotretinoin can frequently resolve cystic lesions that nothing else can touch.

But it's a drug with a lot of side effects, both major and minor. The most serious danger is fetal malformations. Before the magnitude of the risk was recognized, it was estimated that sixteen thousand women became pregnant while taking the drug; twelve thousand had abortions, and nearly one thousand gave birth to babies with birth defects, including fatal and severe cardiac and nervous-system abnormalities. Babies who seem anatomically intact may develop abnormally.

For this reason, Accutane must be used with extreme caution by women of child-bearing age. A physician must see a negative pregnancy test before prescribing the drug and make sure it's understood that effective contraception must be used throughout the treatment. Because isotretinoin remains in the body, you shouldn't become pregnant for at least a month— possibly three—after discontinuing the drug.

Whether topical tretinoin (Retin-A) can also cause birth defects is not clear, but the manufacturer warns women not to use the drug during pregnancy unless absolutely necessary. At least one case of birth defect (an ear malformation) has been reported in the baby of a woman who used Retin-A during a critical period—the first eleven weeks—of her pregnancy (*The Lancet,* March 14, 1992).

Accutane also causes the triglyceride (a lipid) level to rise in 25 percent of people who take the drug; cholesterol rises in 7 percent of users. Pancreatitis and liver damage are a danger. Headaches, muscle pain, and joint pain may occur. Night vision may abruptly decline. Dryness of the skin and mucus membranes is common, sometimes causing nosebleeds and peeling of the nose and mouth.

You're best off taking Accutane under the supervision of a specialist experienced in its use, who monitors your blood and liver function every few weeks, at least at the start.

Resources

James E. Fulton, M.D.
Acne Research Institute
1617 Westcliff
Suite 100
Newport Beach, CA 92660
(714) 631-3376
(800) 94-NUFACE

A nonprofit institute started by Dr. Fulton dedicated to acne research and treatment.

Call or write for more information.

◆ ACUTE OTITIS MEDIA (Middle Ear Infection) and

◆ OTITIS MEDIA WITH EFFUSION
(Middle Ear Effusion)

Although otitis media (OM)—infection of the middle ear—can afflict adolescents and adults, the chief sufferers are small children. Just about everyone has at least one ear infection during childhood, and many children have them regularly.

A widely cited study in the *Journal of Infectious Diseases* (1989, no. 160) found that nearly two thirds of children in the Greater Boston area had had at least one episode of otitis media by the end of their first year, and 83 percent by age three. Nearly one fifth had had three infections or more by their first birthday; by the time they were three, almost half had had that number of infections.

This and other studies show that ear infections reach their peak in the second half of the first year; before that, infants are protected by antibodies they received while in utero, and as time goes on, their own disease resistance increases.

Besides being painful and distressing, ear infection can lead to complications, particularly middle ear effusion (MEE). Fluid builds up in the ear and, even after repeated treatment, can remain for weeks to months. This may temporarily impair hearing, which in turn could have negative effects on speech and learning. While this is a very real possibility for some children, most are unlikely to suffer permanent disability from hearing loss that is transient. An even greater concern for parents is the excessive and inappropriate use of antibiotics and other drugs commonly prescribed for otitis media. There is evidence that ear tube placement surgery is also overused in the treatment of children with MEE. New government-

sponsored guidelines, based on all available studies, will help parents identify appropriate medical treatment.

WHY DOES OTITIS RECUR?

A number of risk factors for recurrent ear infections have been identified.
About some, little can be done: boys are more likely to be afflicted than
girls; Native Americans more often than whites, who are affected more
often than blacks. There seems to be a family factor: if older siblings have
had recurrent OM, the risk rises about threefold, according to a paper in
Pediatric Annals (November 1991).

Infants who attend day care are at similarly heightened risk of recurrent
ear infection, probably because of increased exposure.

One risk factor that can be eliminated is exposure to cigarette smoke.
Children of smoking parents are nearly three times more likely to develop
OM, and the more the parents smoke, the greater the risk. One researcher
suggests that one third of recurrent OM would be eliminated if such exposures were prevented. If you must smoke, don't do it around young
children, and, in particular, avoid subjecting them to smoke in enclosed
places, such as the car.

A number of studies have found less OM among breast-fed children.
Whether this reflects immunological protection by breast milk, or a risk
associated with commercial formulas, isn't clear. Although it isn't conclu-
sive, there's some evidence that propping up the formula bottle in bed
leads to more OM, possibly because fluid can back up into the ear while
the infant is lying flat. "Prudence suggests this practice should be avoided,"
the Pediatric Annals article says.

Ironically, antibiotics, the standard treatment for recurrent ear infection, have been implicated in chronic ear infection.

DO ANTIBIOTICS DO ANY GOOD?

Although the preventive prescription of antibiotics is almost always the first
step for recurrent OM, questions have arisen about its effectiveness. A
meta-analysis of twenty-seven studies, which appeared in the Journal of the
American Medical Association (September 15, 1993), gave "mixed support"
to the practice, concluding that the prophylactic approach significantly re-

duces recurrences, compared with placebo, at least in the short term. "The magnitude of the effect is limited, though, requiring treatment of nine children to show an improved outcome in one," the authors wrote.

Typically, the child is given an antibiotic daily (usually about half the dose used for active infection) for a period that may vary from three weeks to more than three months. (Some doctors believe that relapses are less likely after longer courses of treatment.) If the infections have occurred during the cold months (a common pattern in much of the United States), prophylaxis is generally scheduled accordingly.

Some experts believe that antibiotics are overused for chronic middle ear infection and, worse, may actually cause the problem. One study showed that six weeks after completing amoxicillin therapy (the most commonly prescribed antibiotic), the recurrence rate was two to six times higher in the treated group of children than in those given a placebo (*Journal of the American Medical Association*, December 18, 1991). The safety and effectiveness of antibiotics for acute ear infection are also in doubt. Some doctors believe that the common practice of giving antibiotics to children in the first three years of life will impair their immunity.

WHAT CAN I DO TO PROTECT MY CHILD FROM INAPPROPRIATE ANTIBIOTIC THERAPY?

Keep in mind that acute ear infection is a self-limiting disease, which means that the body will rid itself of this infection without treatment. This includes cases in which bacteria can be found in the ear fluid. In most children, acute ear infection is merely one of several symptoms of a cold.

Children can be made comfortable with an ear drop solution containing benzocaine (a local anesthetic) and a painkiller, such as acetaminophen. This has become the standard treatment in Switzerland, Holland, the United Kingdom, and Scandinavian countries where overuse of antibiotics in children has become a major concern.

To learn more about home treatment and when to call a doctor, read "Childhood Ear Infections: What Every Parent and Physician Should Know About Prevention, Home Care, and Alternative Treatment," available from Homeopathic Educational Services. Call (800) 359–9051.

WHAT CAN BE DONE TO PREVENT THE CHRONIC ACCUMULATION OF FLUID IN THE EARS?

Avoiding inappropriate antibiotic use is the first step. If you follow the home treatment described above, your child will not go from one antibiotic prescription to another. There is evidence that the overuse of antibiotics actually causes the buildup of fluid in the ears.

An example of a situation likely to prompt an inappropriate antibiotic prescription is this: The baby has a cold, and the doctor judges him or her to be prone to otitis media merely on the basis of finding that the eardrum is red.

HOW CAN I AVOID INAPPROPRIATE TREATMENT?

Follow the practice guidelines proposed by the U.S. Agency for Health Care Policy Research (AHCPR), which drew upon the expertise of a panel of physicians, representing the American Academy of Pediatrics, the American Academy of Family Physicians, and the American Academy of Otolaryngology (head and neck surgeons).

First, the AHCPR panel found evidence to suggest that MEE "usually follows a benign course without treatment." It advised against the use of antihistamines and/or decongestants. Though these drugs are commonly prescribed separately or in combination, four randomized controlled studies failed to show a significant benefit.

Antibiotics do provide a modest benefit (14 percent increase in the probability that MEE will resolve), according to the AHCPR. This must be weighed against the adverse effects of antibiotics, which were described as "from common to rare and from nuisance to life-threatening." The most common effects are gastrointestinal, primarily diarrhea; others include vomiting, nausea, and skin rashes. A potentially serious adverse reaction would be an allergic response.

HOW SERIOUS IS THE HEARING-LOSS CONCERN?

It should be underscored here that the hearing loss is temporary. Because it occurs at the time in life when a child is learning to speak, there is a concern that this temporary hearing impairment will have long-range effects on speech and language development.

Since hearing loss is the motivation for treatment, this question was thoroughly explored by the AHCPR panel of experts who agreed that untreated hearing loss that is long-term and significant could lead to serious disability. Yet little is known about the long-term consequences of fluctuating hearing loss in otherwise healthy children.

HOW WILL I KNOW WHETHER SURGERY IS APPROPRIATE?

Here, too, the AHCPR guidelines are extremely helpful: "Myringotomy (excision of the tympanic membrane) with or without tympanostomy tubes [ear tube placement surgery] should NOT be performed for initial management of MEE in an otherwise healthy child." The surgery should not be considered until the MEE has lasted four to six months. In this circumstance, the child should have a hearing deficit in both ears (defined as twenty-decibels hearing threshold or worse in the better-hearing ear). The panel also advised against adenoidectomy as a treatment for MEE in children one to three years old and tonsillectomy as a treatment for MEE in children of any age.

Resources

Call the U.S. Agency for Health Care Policy and Research at (800) 358-9295. Request a free copy of the July 1994 "Clinical Practice Guidelines for Otitis Media with Effusion in Young Children." Make sure you request the physicians' version, because it contains more in-depth information about research supporting the new recommendations.

◆ AIDS (HIV Infection)

In the decade and a half since it appeared, AIDS (Acquired Immune Deficiency Syndrome) has become a health problem of stunning dimensions, here and throughout the world. Over three hundred thousand Americans have developed the disease since 1981, and an estimated one million are currently infected with HIV, the virus thought by most experts to be responsible. Worldwide, fourteen million people are infected, a number which is expected to rise to between thirty and forty million by the turn of the millennium.

HIV infects cells of the immune system that normally protect the body, leaving its victims open to malignancies and infections by organisms that are normally kept easily under control. People infected with HIV commonly remain healthy and essentially symptom-free for five to ten years, before the consequences of a weakened immune system begin to emerge. One study of gay men in San Francisco has reported that a small percentage of those infected with HIV did not progress to AIDS or major symptoms within fifteen years. An English study of HIV positive male hemophiliacs projects some will remain AIDS-free from twenty to twenty-five years after infection. Overall, the few existing studies show that 5 to 10 percent do not develop full-blown AIDS.

Although research in the field is intense (in 1990, $1.6 billion was spent on AIDS research, more than for cancer, and one and a half times as much as on heart disease), the foreseeable future seems unlikely to produce a vaccine to prevent AIDS or a drug to cure it. What seemed like significant breakthroughs in slowing the progression of the illness or forestalling its most serious consequences have proven disappointing.

Still, because of better treatment of some of the more serious opportunistic infections that occur in people with HIV, many can remain relatively healthy and active over a longer period of time.

ARE THERE DRUGS THAT WORK AGAINST HIV?

There remains controversy as to the benefits and risks of antiviral drug therapy for people with HIV and AIDS. The drugs are very toxic and are particularly risky for people with compromised immune systems. When diagnosed with HIV, a person should seek care from a doctor who specializes in the treatment of HIV and AIDS and who is more likely to be up-to-date about the benefits and risks of various drug treatments. As of the end of 1994 there were four approved antiviral drugs. They are commonly known by their abbreviations: AZT, ddc, ddi, and d4t. These drugs are usually given to people whose CD4 counts have fallen to very low levels (CD4 cells are the cells that fight infections). A low CD4 level is generally considered the best predictor of being at high risk of opportunistic infection.

Antivirals, especially AZT, have been used also for HIV positive persons who had no symptoms and whose CD4 cell counts were not very low. Because of information from the initial test of AZT versus no AZT, which involved a very few patients over a short span of time, it was thought that antivirals might work to delay the progression from HIV infection to symptoms and opportunistic disease. However, more recent research from a large, longer-term, French-English collaborative trial reported in 1993 that such prophylactic use produces no significant benefit.

Some doctors who treat many people with HIV and AIDS, along with a number of patients and advocates, believe that toxic antivirals can cause an HIV-positive person to become sicker, quicker. In general, the newer antiviral drugs, ddc, ddi, and d4t, have been disappointing whether used alone or in combination with AZT. The use of antivirals, therefore, continues to be controversial.

HOW CAN I PROTECT MYSELF AGAINST PNEUMONIA AND TB?

Recurrent *Pneumocystis carinii* pneumonia (PCP) is the leading cause of AIDS-related death, but some substantial progress has been made in prevention. It was established several years ago that prophylaxis with aerosolized pentamidine can help prevent PCP, but special equipment is required to administer the treatment, making it expensive and inconvenient to use. A 1992 study reported in the *New England Journal of Medicine* (December 24, 1992) found that trimethoprim-sulfamethoxazole (TMP-SMX) is a more effective prophylaxis against PCP than aerosolized pentamidine. Because it is taken orally, trimethoprim-sulfamethoxazole is also easier to use and as much as one quarter less expensive. However, adverse drug reactions such as fever and nausea are more frequent with trimethoprim-sulfamethoxazole.

In its 1994 "Clinical Practice Guidelines on the Evaluation and Management of Early HIV Infection," the U.S. Agency for Health Care Policy and Research recommended TMP-SMX as the PCP prophylaxis of choice. They advise beginning prophylaxis when CD4 lymphocytes drop below 200/microliter, after a first episode of PCP, or when other symptoms show the immune system is weakened.

The HIV-weakened immune system often allows *Mycobacterium tuberculosis,* the TB organism, to become active. People with AIDS have been hard hit by the recent resurgence in TB (see Tuberculosis). The AHCPR guidelines recommend TB testing when HIV infection is first detected, and at least yearly thereafter, with X rays taken when indicated. If the test shows exposure to TB, even if there are no signs of active disease, a year of prophylactic medication may be advisable.

HOW WILL I MONITOR FOR CONDITIONS THAT NEED TREATMENT?

Even before HIV infection becomes full-blown AIDS, close, careful surveillance is necessary to detect and treat viral, fungal, and bacterial infections as they emerge. Doctors who are experienced in treating people with HIV and AIDS are more likely to recognize and appropriately treat opportunistic infections. As a result people are living longer and having a better quality of life.

Eye disorders can be sight threatening if undetected. An eye examination should be part of routine doctor visits, the AHCPR guidelines recommend, and a full workup by an ophthalmologist should be done regularly. Make sure your doctor explains how to look for the early signs of cytomegalovirus (CMV) retinitis, a viral infection that can rob you of vision if it's not treated promptly.

Women with HIV infection are particularly prone to cervical disease, including premalignant lesions and invasive cancer. One study of 414 women found positive Pap tests in 5 percent of uninfected women and in 63 percent of those who had been exposed to HIV. In fact, the Centers for Disease Control included invasive cervical cancer in its expanded 1993 criteria for AIDS. Because HIV and AIDS in women present unique gynecological problems, it is very important that, if at all possible, the doctor selected has experience in treating women with HIV and AIDS.

Pap tests should be done at least yearly and followed up carefully when findings are suspicious, the AHCPR report says.

WILL I FIND SUPPORT FOR MY EFFORTS TO FIND THE BEST TREATMENT?

Medical information about AIDS has proliferated to the point where no one can keep on top of everything. And in the absence of a cure or truly satisfactory treatment, many alternative healing approaches have their advocates. The possible benefits of diet, exercise, and such modalities as acupuncture and homeopathy are not likely to be explored in the average clinic.

This is one area where being your own researcher and an active part of your treatment is an option that can't be ignored. Not only is it an antidote to the sense of helplessness that makes any serious illness more difficult to endure, it may well keep you alive and healthier longer. A study of fifty-three longtime survivors of AIDS, presented at the 1991 annual meeting of the American Psychological Association, found that virtually all were actively involved in their own care, aware of recent medical developments, and full partners, with their doctors, in medical decision-making. They had no qualms about changing doctors when they were dissatisfied.

There are various advocacy groups and treatment centers that publish newsletters discussing established and alternative treatments for HIV and AIDS. There are centers established to provide access to nonmedical, nontoxic therapies that others have found helpful. Some groups will help you do you own search of the scientific literature.

People with HIV and AIDS have struggled to force the medical establishment to confront the issue of sharing power and information. One result is that more doctors, especially among those who specialize in treating people with AIDS, have come to respect the autonomy of their patients and their right to make decisions about their own treatment.

Many doctors have difficulty with the sharing of power and expertise that this approach assumes, but not all do. The founder of Medic Aware, Tom Holte, said in an interview that two physicians are on the organization's board of directors, and a number of others regularly refer their patients to the service. Finding a doctor who will encourage and facilitate a real working relationship should be a high priority.

HOW EXPERIENCED IS THIS HOSPITAL IN TREATING AIDS?

If you're having surgery, it's well known that you're better off at a hospital where the procedure is done often, than a place that has little experience with it. The same principle can apparently make a life-or-death difference in AIDS.

A 1992 study reported in *Journal of Acquired Immune Deficiency Syndrome* followed over three thousand people with AIDS-related PCP, cared for in seventy-three different New York City area hospitals, and found that those admitted to "low-volume" hospitals (less than fifty PCP cases a year) were twice as likely to die as those treated at "high volume" (over one hundred and sixty patients a year) institutions.

Another study of 806 AIDS-related admissions to forty Boston-area hospitals found that the risk of death was nearly tripled in the institutions with little experience treating AIDS, after differences in age, sex, severity, and other factors were controlled for. The patients at the more experienced hospitals didn't stay any longer, didn't pay any more, and weren't subjected to more intensive care. They were just more likely to survive (*Journal of the American Medical Association*, November 18, 1992).

HOW CAN I DEAL WITH THE PSYCHOLOGICAL CONSEQUENCES OF AIDS?

Living with HIV infection can exact a heavy psychological toll. Depression and anxiety are common and may require treatment. According to an article in the *Journal of the American Medical Association* (October 21, 1992), the risk of suicide among men with AIDS (in the period between 1987 and 1989) was more than seven times higher than in the general population—although this seems to be declining.

Given the gravity of the diagnosis, the stigma attached to AIDS, and the trauma of recurrent illness and its treatment, some form of psychotherapy, counseling, or other means of support (as well as medication when needed) can be essential.

AIDS itself, or the infections it leads to, can affect the nervous system, physically causing psychiatric problems like depression and even dementia. Your doctor, or a specialist to whom he or she can refer you, must be able to tell the difference between organic and psychological symptoms, and treat them accordingly.

On a more positive note, relaxation techniques like meditation and physical exercise can be invaluable in coping with the stress that is an inevitable consequence of being HIV positive. These practices may even be therapeutic.

In a study of eighty-six homosexual men, reported at the 1992 meeting of the American Psychosomatic Society, thirty-three learned they were HIV positive while the research was going on. Among twenty-one of these men followed for two years, four had died, one had AIDS, and five had symptoms that suggested that AIDS was imminent. The group who had gotten sick or died, the researchers found, were least committed to regular exercise and relaxation. Those who practiced exercise and relaxation also had higher levels of CD4 lymphocytes.

Both moderate aerobic exercise and relaxation techniques can boost immune function, other research has shown; this may help the body resist the ravages of the virus.

IF I'M AN HIV-POSITIVE MOTHER, HOW CAN I PROTECT MY BABY?

According to the AHCPR guidelines, there's no consistent evidence that HIV infection, at least in its early stages, has an adverse effect on pregnancy (such as increased prematurity, stillbirth, or low birthweight), or that pregnancy accelerates the progression of the infection.

The infection appears to be transmitted to the newborn, however, in 13 to 39 percent of cases. One recent study suggested a way to protect the baby. It found that giving the mother AZT during pregnancy could sharply reduce the risk of transmission.

If you're HIV positive, breast-feeding is probably a poor idea. It appears to be another route of transmission, and mortality is higher among breast-fed than bottle-fed infants of HIV-positive mothers.

HOW CAN I KEEP FROM GETTING—OR SPREADING—HIV?

Preventing the spread of HIV infection should be a priority for everyone. If you're HIV-positive, informing yourself fully about the risks of contagion can help deal with the anxiety, stigma, and paranoia that often surround the disease.

In the United States AIDS is spread primarily by sexual contact and through sharing of needles by intravenous drug users. Because of better screening of the blood and blood product supply, these are much less likely to be a source of transmission than when the epidemic began in the 1980s.

Evidence cited in a report by the Surgeon General (*Journal of the American Medical Association,* June 9, 1993) suggests that conscientious condom use, while not foolproof, is an effective means of protection. The report projected that among couples in which one partner is HIV-positive, the risk of exposure for the other is four in one hundred per year. Other studies have shown no virus spread among couples who used condoms consistently.

The risk of exposure in the condom-using general population is estimated at two to four per hundred thousand; if everyone used condoms consistently and correctly, the report projects, the rate of HIV spread would be slashed by 80 percent.

Other barrier contraceptives, such as the diaphragm or sponge with a spermicide, may interfere somewhat with viral spread (the spermicide nonoxynol-9 has been shown to inactivate HIV), but their efficacy is unproven. In fact, a study of women who used a contraceptive sponge with nonoxynol-9 found they were more likely to become HIV-positive, possibly because the sponge caused genital irritation and ulcers that made it easier for the virus to invade.

A factor in the transmission of HIV that has had particular attention recently is the presence of other sexually transmitted diseases. One study cited at the 1993 international AIDS conference found that the risk of female-to-male transmission was five times greater if the woman had a genital ulcer.

A lot of anxiety—much of it unwarranted—has surrounded the spread of AIDS by less intimate contact. A paper in *The New England Journal of Medicine* (December 16, 1993) cited seventeen studies showing that the risk of transmission through household contact was extremely low—no infections in more than eleven hundred people, followed for more than seventeen hundred person-years.

Even so, the report said, "Precautions are warranted to prevent contact with blood in households and similar settings." If you or someone in your household is HIV-positive, learn what steps you can take to minimize risk and anxiety.

Resources

HEAL (Health Education AIDS Liaison) connects AIDS activists who pool information on alternative, nontoxic therapies. They'll share their information and experience with members of the public, and refer you to alternative practitioners in the New York area and elsewhere.

HEAL
16 East 16th Street
New York, NY 10003
(212) 674-HOPE (4673)

The National Association of People With AIDS offers information and referrals for HIV-positive people. It can put you in touch with helpful groups in your own community.

National Association for People with AIDS
1413 K Street, NW
Washington, DC 20005
(202) 898-0414

AIDS Treatment Data Network can be contacted by telephone, fax, and E-mail. The network provides approved and experimental (including clinical trials) AIDS and HIV treatment information, advice, and referrals.

AIDS Treatment Data Network
259 West 30th Street
New York, NY 10001-2809
Outside NY State: (800) 734-7104
NY State (800) 858-2111
New York City (212) 268-4196
Fax (212) 260-8869
E-mail AIDStreatD@aol.com

✦ ALZHEIMER'S DISEASE

Other diseases can rob people of their independence, vigor, or mobility. Alzheimer's disease strikes at the very heart of selfhood. The estimated four million Americans who have this condition suffer profound memory loss, disorientation, impairment in reasoning ability, and marked personality change.

In Alzheimer's, brain tissue progressively deteriorates, eventually affecting vital body functions. The average victim lives for seven to ten years after diagnosis, and most often dies of pneumonia.

Alzheimer's is predominantly a disease of aging: most people who have it are over sixty-five, and it is most common after age eighty. But about 5 percent are under retirement age, and an early-onset form can strike in the forties or fifties.

The number of people with Alzheimer's has noticeably increased in recent years, not because the disease is becoming more common, but as a reflection of the "graying" of America. People live longer today; those over eighty—at highest risk for Alzheimer's—represent the fastest-growing segment of the population.

WHAT CAUSES ALZHEIMER'S?

It is well documented that the brains of people with Alzheimer's have abnormal structures called plaques, composed of a protein called beta-amyloid, and tangles of nerves similar to unwound string. A number of researchers believe that this accumulation is responsible for the nerve-cell degeneration at the heart of the disease; a gene that greatly increases production of beta-amyloid has been linked to some cases. Other studies have found that some people with Alzheimer's produce a mutant form of the protein that is turned into beta-amyloid.

Not all are convinced that beta-amyloid plaques cause Alzheimer's disease; some experts believe they are actually a consequence of nerve degeneration. One rather radical theory proposes that Alzheimer's is a chronic inflammatory disease, something like arthritis.

As research delves more deeply, it appears that there may be not one, but a number of disease processes, and that nerve-cell degeneration and its tragic symptoms are a final common pathway of several "Alzheimer's diseases."

HOW CAN I BE SURE IT'S ALZHEIMER'S?

Right now, the only way to diagnose Alzheimer's definitively is by biopsy of brain tissue, which, for obvious reasons, is rarely done except as a postmortem. In practice, the diagnosis is made by weighing symptoms, appearance, history, and family background; when the evaluation is done by experts in specialized centers, it appears to be correct about 90 percent of the time.

Dementia, impairment of reasoning severe enough to interfere with normal life, is due to Alzheimer's about half the time. Some 15 percent of dementia is caused by potentially reversible factors, such as tumor, depression, hypothyroidism, or reactions to medication, so a full physical and psychiatric examination is vital before the diagnosis is made.

DO MEMORY LAPSES MEAN I HAVE ALZHEIMER'S?

Any number of things can cause loss of memory—anxiety and depression, to name two. "Benign forgetfulness," a familiar concomitant of normal aging, may be inconvenient, but shouldn't interfere with work or personal relationships. Noticeable decline in memory that comes on suddenly is unlikely to herald Alzheimer's.

Memory loss in Alzheimer's is typically quite severe. Instead of forgetting what level of the parking garage you left the car on, you may repeatedly forget that you took the car at all; instead of forgetting your keys, you can't remember what a key is for. It is usually part of a more general decline in brain function, reflected as well in speech, emotions, and appearance.

IF MY MOTHER OR FATHER HAD ALZHEIMER'S, WILL I GET IT TOO?

About half of people with Alzheimer's have a family history of the disease, but it is estimated that only 5 to 10 percent of cases clearly represent the effect of a single defective gene.

Thus far, three different genes have been associated with Alzheimer's. Two of them have been linked to relatively uncommon early-onset forms of the disease. The third, which has aroused great recent interest, may be involved in the far greater number of cases of Alzheimer's that develop later in life.

That gene produces a protein, ApoE, that carries cholesterol through the bloodstream. There are four types of ApoE: most people have genes that produce one variant, ApoE3; another, ApoE4, has been associated with greater risk of Alzheimer's. A study of people with Alzheimer's found that nearly two thirds carried one or two genes for ApoE4, compared with one third of healthy people.

What this research suggests is that ApoE4 (or, possibly, the absence of ApoE3), increases the *likelihood* of Alzheimer's, or lowers the age at which it appears. Other factors clearly come into play, some of which may be environmental.

DOES ALUMINUM CAUSE ALZHEIMER'S?

Aluminum, to which we are exposed in food, drinking water, antacids, and cooking utensils, has long been a suspect in Alzheimer's. The metal can be neurotoxic, and concentrations five to fifty times higher than normal have been found in the plaques and neurofibrillary tangles of the brains of people who have died of Alzheimer's disease.

But does aluminum cause the damage? We don't yet know. It's possible that dying brain cells simply soak up the metal. And a British research team showed that some of the excess aluminum was actually put there as a result of the testing process.

Drugs to relieve Alzheimer's symptoms by removing aluminum from the brain have been tested, but results have been inconsistent. Right now, the majority of researchers doubt that the metal is a real threat. But the question is still open.

DOES SMOKING PREVENT ALZHEIMER'S?

One of the few nice things anyone has said about cigarette smoking lately is that it reduces the likelihood of Alzheimer's. Indeed, case-control studies have suggested that smokers have between one third to three quarters the chance of having the disease.

There may be a less appealing explanation, however. As an article in *The Lancet* (September 25, 1993) observed, smokers are more likely to die at any age (more than twice as many nonsmokers survive to age seventy-seven and a half). Those who have *survived* their cigarette habit may be genetically endowed with cells that efficiently repair DNA damage, or may be genetically programmed to age more slowly. In other words, smoking selects out people who for some reason are better able to fight off cellular attacks responsible for chronic diseases, including Alzheimer's.

WHEN ARE DRUGS PRESCRIBED?

No drug known can slow the progression of Alzheimer's disease. For the most part, medications are prescribed to alleviate some of the problems that arise. Antipsychotics like haloperidol (Haldol) and tranquilizers like lorazepam (Ativan) can calm people with the disease when they become agitated, or help them to sleep. These drugs should be used carefully. Older people react more strongly to lower doses, and overuse can compound confusion and disorientation.

In 1993, tacrine became the first drug approved for Alzheimer's disease by the FDA. Tacrine apparently doesn't influence the actual disease process, but it increases the availability of acetylcholine, a brain chemical that declines in people who have Alzheimer's.

If the drug represents a breakthrough, it's a modest one. Large-scale multicenter trials show that tacrine brings about a significant, but undramatic, improvement in symptoms for about 40 percent of people with mild to moderate disease. And it has drawbacks. Side effects are common—especially nausea, vomiting, diarrhea, abdominal pain, and headache—and can be hazardous; liver function must be watched closely for signs of damage to that organ.

It's also expensive. The wholesale cost of tacrine, in 1993, was about

$1,135 per year, and this doesn't include the cost of frequent doctor visits and lab tests.

Another drug that has been used for Alzheimer's disease, ergoloid mesylates (Hydergine), has been generally disappointing, and some studies suggest it may do more harm than good. A number of new compounds are under investigation which, like tacrine, aim to raise levels of brain chemicals. As the actual mechanism of the disease is better understood, there's hope for pharmacology that will halt or even reverse the degeneration itself.

HOW CAN I HELP SOMEONE WITH ALZHEIMER'S?

Common sense, compassion, and intelligent planning can make life easier for a relative with Alzheimer's. Try to create a safe, structured, stable environment. It may be necessary to remove dangerous objects (take the knobs off the stove when you're at work, if he or she turns on the stove, for example). Try to augment and compensate for lost function—make charts and lists to aid a failing memory, for example. Reinforce and encourage the activity he or she is still capable of. Many people with the disease become agitated in the evening. Schedule whatever you can for times when your relative can function best.

Eventually, a person with Alzheimer's will need hospitalization and nursing care. Prepare for this eventuality by making financial and legal arrangements in advance.

Resources

Care for a person with Alzheimer's is draining and depressing. Don't do it alone. Community agencies can provide support, education, and respite care that will allow you to take time for yourself. There are often day-care centers where your relative can stay while still living at home.

One of the best sources of information and support is the local chapter of the National Alzheimer's Association. Call (800) 272-3900.

◆ ANXIETY (and Panic)

No one is a stranger to anxiety. The combination of psychological distress (nervousness, restlessness, fear) and physical discomfort (racing heart, tense muscles) is an inborn reflex, a kind of alarm system that readies us for fight or flight in the face of danger.

The anxiety reaction is essential in a real crisis, but all too easily, it's triggered by daily situations where neither fight nor flight are useful options—in which the "threat" is to self-esteem, for example.

When anxiety is frequent and severe enough to interfere with normal life, it's called *anxiety disorder,* and represents the most widespread class of psychiatric problem in the United States. Nearly 15 percent of the population, it is estimated, have anxiety disorders in the course of their lives, about twice as many women as men.

The most common kinds of anxiety include *phobias,* which are focused on particular objects (like snakes) or situations (like high places), and *obsessive-compulsive disorder,* whose victims can't turn off distressing thoughts and are driven by anxiety to repeatedly check the stove to be sure it's turned off or wash their hands.

Panic attacks, which are experienced by an estimated 3.4 percent of the population, are devastating episodes of runaway anxiety, severe enough to feel life-threatening, that may occur spontaneously. *Generalized anxiety disorder* is an uncontrollable exaggeration of normal worry to the point where it blankets nearly all of life.

Although we often think of anxiety as a nuisance, if it is severe, it can make normal life impossible. And panic disorder may be fatal. In a random sample of 18,011 adults, 12 percent of those with a history of panic attacks had attempted suicide (*The New England Journal of Medicine,* November 2, 1989).

IS IT AN ANXIETY DISORDER OR JUST STRESS?

Anxiety symptoms are a common consequence of stress; you may feel unusually edgy and fearful when your life is full of demands and changes. In addition, periods of excessive stress often trigger anxiety disorders that had previously been dormant.

The key question is whether the anxiety lessens once the pressure is off. This isn't to say that stress-related anxiety should be ignored. If it interferes with your ability to enjoy life or function, it deserves attention. But the treatment, if any, will be different and shorter-term than when a true anxiety disorder is to blame.

DO I HAVE AN ANXIETY DISORDER OR A PHYSICAL ILLNESS?

The average person suffers with an anxiety disorder for nine years before he or she seeks help—a victim of the stigma surrounding emotional disturbance and unawareness of the effective treatment that's available. Less than half of anxiety sufferers seek help at all, according to an article in the *British Medical Journal* (May 4, 1991). What's more, not every doctor recognizes anxiety for what it is.

While many people learn to live with their emotional distress, what often brings them to the doctor are the physical symptoms of anxiety, which closely mimic those of medical illness.

In a way, it's misleading to differentiate between anxiety and "physical" disorders, insofar as the nervous system arousal triggered by anxiety has a very real physical impact throughout the body. Stomach cramps, diarrhea, and nausea can be the consequence for the digestive system; back spasms and headaches can occur when muscles tighten up. By promoting inflammation, anxiety can cause maladies as physical as hives and eczema.

The physical effects of panic are so catastrophic that people very often are terrified that they're dying. In addition to sweating, choking, trembling, and dizziness, palpitations and chest pain are common, and can easily be mistaken for heart disease. This often leads to expensive, invasive diagnostic procedures. According to an article in *American Family Physician* (September 1992), 33 to 43 percent of people who have chest pain and whose coronary arteries are normal on arteriography suffer from panic disorder.

COULD MY ANXIETY HAVE OTHER CAUSES?

Thyroid and other endocrine disorders, breathing problems, and hypoglycemia are among the conditions that may contribute to or cause the same
symptoms as anxiety. On the other hand, anxiety can *amplify* symptoms of
a physical disease that shouldn't be overlooked.

Anxiety symptoms can also be a reaction to medication, including
asthma drugs like theophylline, and OTC decongestants like pseudoephedrine or phenylpropanolamine. Caffeine consumption is an anxiety factor
that should be explored before making decisions about treatment.

The connection between anxiety and alcohol is complex. On the one
hand, many people apparently self-medicate their anxiety with this drug
in the years before they seek medical help. (It's been suggested that the
tendency to drown anxiety is one reason why relatively few men come in
for treatment.) On the other hand, anxiety is a consequence of alcohol
abuse. The emotional disorder can't be effectively treated until the abuse
is addressed.

Anxiety is itself often the result, or a partner of, other psychiatric
disorders. It can be a symptom—or a cause—of depression. Whichever
came first, treatment must take both into account. The failure to appreciate
the complexity of anxiety is often responsible for unsuccessful treatment.

HOW CAN I CHOOSE BETWEEN ALTERNATIVE TREATMENTS?

There's good evidence that anxiety disorders have their roots in nervous-
system dysfunction; it's like a car alarm that goes off whenever someone
touches the car, or even spontaneously. Consequently, anxiety can often
be treated successfully with medications that "turn down" the part of the
brain that gives the arousal signal, or make the body less reactive to the
signal.

At the same time, much anxiety is psychological. The perception of
being threatened comes too readily out of ordinary experiences (like social
interactions), and therapy that changes how you feel about these situations
can often relieve it. Another psychotherapy approach—training to keep
the beginnings of anxiety from escalating unmanageably—is also successful
for some people.

Which approach is best for you depends on your particular symptoms, and your feelings about medication and psychotherapy. Often, the choice is a matter of personal preference.

WHAT MEDICATION THERAPY IS RIGHT FOR ME?

Different kinds of anxiety respond to different drugs. Generalized anxiety disorder, which turns everyday concerns and situations into an endless trial of relentless worry, is often treated with benzodiazepines like diazepam (Valium), alprazolam (Xanax), or lorazepam (Ativan). They reduce anxiety about twice as effectively as a placebo, but their side effects can include sleepiness and memory lapses. They can also interact dangerously with alcohol or other drugs.

Benzodiazepines are rarely abused by people for whom they're prescribed—few take more than the recommended dose—but the body develops a dependence on them after just a few weeks. If you've been taking these drugs, you must go off them gradually, or else severe withdrawal symptoms—including anxiety much worse than before—is a danger.

How long benzodiazepines should be used is a question for which there is little data. Some studies have shown that relatively short-term use is effective: in one, 50 percent of chronically anxious people got better after six weeks on Valium (*Journal of the American Medical Association* (August 12, 1983); in another, 70 percent were largely relieved of symptoms after four weeks on Tranxene or Ativan (*American Journal of Psychiatry,* March 1988).

A relatively new antianxiety drug, BuSpar (buspirone) has the advantage of not causing drowsiness or, apparently, physical dependency. It appears to be as effective as the benzodiazepines, but takes a week or longer to work.

Antidepressants, both the older tricyclics and newer drugs like Prozac and Zoloft, also work more slowly, and their effectiveness in general anxiety is not as well established. (For a fuller discussion of antidepressants, see Depression.)

Obsessive-compulsive disorder was resistant to drug therapy until a decade ago. Now a number of medications, including Anafranil (clomipramine), Prozac, and Zoloft have been shown effective in double-blind trials. Overall, Anafranil has the highest success rate—about 60 percent—but in any individual one might work better than the others.

Panic disorder can be treated with antidepressants, or high-potency benzodiazepines like Xanax. These drugs generally work well, but relapses are not uncommon when they are withdrawn, according to a 1991 consensus statement of the National Institutes of Health.

Beta-blockers, which dampen the body's response to arousal signals from the brain, are often effective for performance anxiety, such as stage fright. Placebo-controlled studies have shown these drugs to benefit musicians suffering from stage fright. In several instances, they even played better, according to judges who didn't know who had taken the drug.

WHAT KIND OF PSYCHOTHERAPY WOULD BE HELPFUL TO ME?

Psychotherapy can aim to change the way you think about things to make life less threatening (cognitive therapy), alter your conditioned responses (behavior therapy), or uncover and resolve unconscious conflicts (psychodynamic therapy). It may involve exercises to help you relax and short-circuit the anxiety process. For certain kinds of anxiety in particular, the scientific support for behavioral and cognitive therapy is strongest.

In the case of phobias—anxiety focused on specific objects or situations—behavior therapy is most effective. You're exposed to whatever triggers your anxiety (whether it's being on a plane or just leaving the house) gradually to get desensitized, or in a way that allows you to be "flooded" with the anxiety and thus overcome it. Behavior therapy usually begins to help quickly, often within a week, and is generally complete in weeks or months. Benefits have been observed for six years or longer after a course of therapy (*British Medical Journal,* May 4, 1991).

A similar approach has been used with some success for obsessive-compulsive disorder. In one study of more than two hundred people, half had 70 percent or greater reduction in symptoms; 39 percent had reductions of 31 to 69 percent. The process is quite demanding, however, and about 25 percent of people offered refuse it. When drug therapy is combined with psychotherapy, the success rate rises to 90 percent.

Psychotherapy that combines elements of behavioral and cognitive therapy is often effective for panic attacks. Improvement often begins three to six weeks into the treatment, which typically lasts eight to twelve weeks. There appears to be little relapse, according to the NIH consensus statement. Controlled data on the effectiveness of other kinds of psychotherapy are lacking.

Drug therapy and psychotherapy are often combined in treating panic disorder, but whether the combination works any better than either alone "is not a settled issue," the NIH statement says.

A principal advantage of psychotherapy is the absence of side effects. In some people with panic disorder, however, the relaxation techniques used in behavioral therapy can actually trigger attacks.

Resources

This clearinghouse of information will refer you to practitioners in your area who are knowledgeable about panic and anxiety disorders:

Anxiety Disorders Association of America
6000 Executive Boulevard
Rockville, MD 20852
(301) 231-9350

◆ ASTHMA

No one should die of asthma. Yet deaths from asthma in this country have more than doubled (to nearly five thousand per year) since 1978. The incidence of asthma is also on the rise, both worldwide (it is the only chronic disease, other than tuberculosis and AIDS, to show such an increase) and in the United States, where it currently affects more than fifteen million people.

In asthma, the air passages in the lung are prone to constrict, become inflamed, and fill with mucus, causing shortness of breath, wheezing, coughing, and even collapse. The length and severity of attacks vary greatly from person to person.

Our understanding of asthma has been radically transformed in the past decade, and the treatment strategies recommended by experts have changed accordingly. Yet the word has apparently been slow getting out to the medical community. In a 1993 press conference sponsored by the American Medical Association, Michael Kaliner, M.D., chief of the allergic diseases section at the National Institute of Allergy and Infectious Diseases, faulted primary care physicians for failing to provide up-to-date therapy that would eliminate most hospitalizations and deaths.

If you have asthma, it's especially important that you take an active role in securing effective medical care.

WHICH DRUGS DO I USE FIRST?

Since 1990, there has been a revolution in how asthma is understood and treated. Major reports by groups like the National Asthma Education Program, the International Asthma Management Project, and the British government have endorsed the idea that while bronchoconstriction may be a key process in acute attacks, asthma is at bottom an inflammatory disease. And while drugs to open the airways may have their use, the first line of defense should be inhaled steroids to treat the inflammation.

For years, bronchodilators like beta-agonists (albuterol is commonly prescribed) and theophylline (available in OTC as well as prescription products) have been prescribed in oral or inhaled form as a first-line treatment to reduce the frequency and severity of attacks. Nowadays, virtually all experts would limit their use, for the most part, to occasional inhaled doses to abort actual attacks or for pretreatment before exercise.

Instead of bronchodilators, current guidelines recommend inhaled anti-inflammatory drugs, such as corticosteroids and cromolyn, as the first choice for virtually anyone whose asthma is severe enough to require regular medication. Bronchodilators just treat the symptom, not the actual disease process. Anti-inflammatory drugs appear to reduce the airway sensitivity at the heart of asthma, and may prevent the gradual scarring that adds an element of irreversible lung damage to long-term illness.

To an alarming degree, however, the practice of medicine hasn't followed the shift in scientific consensus. According to an article in the *Journal of the American Medical Association* (April 22/29, 1992), only one out of ten American doctors who treat asthma prescribes inhaled steroids for the disease.

SHOULD I USE BRONCHODILATORS AT ALL?

In recent years, significant safety questions have surrounded these drugs. The widespread use of more powerful beta-agonist bronchodilators, some suggest, may be partly responsible for the rise in asthma-linked deaths. But other experts disagree: A review of data in the *Journal of the American Medical Association* (October 20, 1993) concluded that only an "extremely small" association between beta-agonists and asthma deaths could be documented.

One theory is that because such drugs address symptoms without touching their cause, people with severe disease may be lulled into a false sense of security as the condition of their lungs silently deteriorates. A British study in *The Lancet* (December 8, 1990) suggested that long-term use of beta-agonists could lead to heart damage.

That overreliance on beta-agonists can lead to a dangerous delay when care is urgently needed was suggested by a study at Albert Einstein College of Medicine, Bronx, New York. When surveyed, two thirds of 125 patients hospitalized for asthma said they'd waited at least two days to get the oral steroid treatment needed for severe exacerbations, and nearly half waited three days or more. In the interim, they increased their beta-agonist use ninefold, on average, to nearly thirty-eight puffs per day (*Journal of the American Medical Association,* July 21, 1993).

The main problem with theophylline is that blood levels not far above the therapeutic range can be toxic, causing hyperactivity in children, learning problems, and even seizures. Any number of factors, including other medication, viral illness, and smoking, can substantially raise or lower the blood level. Several years ago, the Association of Trial Lawyers of America issued a "legal consumer alert" calling theophylline hazardous, and citing twenty-six cases where theophylline was blamed for serious injury and death.

While the role of inhaled bronchodilators to abort or (in specific circumstances, such as exercise) prevent acute attacks remains well accepted, more regular use is highly questionable.

BUT AREN'T STEROIDS DANGEROUS?

Corticosteroids are powerful drugs, with a host of adverse effects that may affect the heart, brain, and skeletal system. However, these are almost always associated with *oral* medication; the inhaled form recommended for most asthma is unlikely to produce systemic problems. And precautions (like using a device to increase the distance between the inhaler and the back of the throat—called a spacer—and rinsing out your mouth after using the steroid) should reduce the risk of hoarseness and candida infection associated with corticosteriod use.

A study of fifteen severely asthmatic children who used inhaled corticosteriods daily for three to five years found that growth and gland function (two areas of concern with steroids) were normal, and that there was no sign of cataract formation, another concern (*The New England Journal of Medicine,* December 2, 1993).

Cromolyn, the other anti-inflammatory often used for asthma, is quite a safe drug that poses little risk of serious side effects.

HOW CAN I AVOID ASTHMA ATTACKS?

The basic problem in asthma is that the airways are overreactive—any number of things can make them constrict and fill with mucus. Avoiding these triggers, rather than waiting for attacks and then treating them, should be the first goal of asthma management.

Most, but not all, asthmatics have allergies. You should find out what you're allergic to and eliminate exposure to the extent possible. If you're allergic to certain pollens, curtail your outdoor activities accordingly during the season when they're in the air, and use air conditioning, especially where you sleep. Allergy to dust mites is common in asthma; take precautions, like keeping rugs, carpets, and drapes to a minimum. People who are allergic to cats and dogs must avoid them.

Desensitization therapy—allergy shots—are available for many common allergens, including pollens, dust mites, and molds. They can be very successful for the allergic component of asthma, but are expensive and lengthy, and carry some risks.

Some people have food allergies that can trigger asthma. Eggs, milk, and shellfish are the most common culprits. Sulfites (widely used as preservatives) and certain food dyes can bring on attacks, although what's involved isn't an allergy but something like a drug reaction. Tougher labeling laws have made it easier to avoid them.

Viral respiratory infections like colds and flu are a significant cause of attacks. In a *British Medical Journal* study (October 16, 1993), 89 percent of colds were associated with asthma symptoms. Avoid exposure to colds and flu, and consider flu vaccinations. Sinusitis has been shown to chronically worsen asthma, so if you have sinus problems, they should be treated.

Lung irritants, including air pollution, cigarette smoke, paint fumes, insect sprays, and household cleaners may trigger serious reactions in the sensitive airways of asthmatics, and may in part explain the increase in incidence and deaths from the disease.

The impact of air pollution, in particular, has probably been underestimated. According to an Environmental Protection Agency study, concentrations of airborne particles considered safe under federal air quality laws are responsible for one emergency visit in eight, among asthmatics.

The role of salt in asthma remains controversial. A study reported in the *British Medical Journal* (November 6, 1993) found more asthma among people who adopted the high-salt Western diet, and a correlation between table salt sales and deaths from asthma in men and children. Lab experiments also showed an increase in bronchial reactivity when dietary salt was increased—for male, but not for female asthmatics.

CAN DRUGS WORSEN ASTHMA?

Any number of medications, including some of the most common OTC ones, can cause trouble. Aspirin and drugs containing it (like some cold remedies) are frequent offenders. Another likely source of difficulty are nonsteroidal anti-inflammatory drugs (NSAIDs), which are chemically similar to aspirin. These are available over the counter (Nuprin, Advil, and Motrin are popular brands) and in more potent prescription drugs.

Antihypertensive drugs, particularly beta blockers (Inderal and Tenormin, for example) cause respiratory difficulties, including asthma attacks, in susceptible people. And some preparations (including, remarkably, some asthma medications), contain sulfites.

Make sure any doctor you see knows you have asthma. If you have doubts about the safety of any drug (prescription or OTC), get medical advice before you take it.

DOES STRESS CAUSE ASTHMA?

Stress can't give you asthma, but if you have it, emotional turmoil is one of the things that may trigger attacks or increase their frequency or seriousness. The nervous system arousal produced by stress, anger, or anxiety can make hyperreactive airways constrict, initiating an episode (the same way stress may worsen irritable bowel syndrome or migraine in someone predisposed to those maladies). During a time of sustained depression or upset, the disease may take a general turn for the worse.

Stress control can be quite helpful in asthma. Techniques like meditation, muscle relaxation, or hypnotherapy can generally soften your body's reaction to day-to-day hassles and major confrontations, and may specifically moderate the chain of physiological events that lead to an attack. Psychotherapy to help depression or resolve deep-seated emotional conflicts makes life in general less stressful and often brings improvement in asthma. For children in particular, family therapy can be helpful.

CAN I EXERCISE WITH ASTHMA?

Exercise is a two-edged sword for asthmatics. Clearly, the potential benefits of regular, aerobic exercise are even greater for asthmatics than for people in general. It trains the body to use oxygen more efficiently, reduces stress, and can help the lungs clear mucus. Asthma need not be the barrier to real athletic accomplishment, as the careers of track-and-field champion Jackie Joyner-Kersee, star basketball player Danny Manning, and others attest.

But exercise can also induce asthma attacks—in about 80 percent of people with asthma, and 12 to 15 percent of the population as a whole. Typically, wheezing, coughing, or shortness of breath occur during or just after five minutes or more of exertion.

Exercised-induced asthma is most likely to occur in cold, dry air, which is one reason why swimming is an ideal sport for asthmatics, and also a good argument for indoor exercise in the winter. Air pollution or allergens in the air also increase the risk.

Timing workouts appropriately, allowing adequate warmup and time for rest, also can help you get the benefits of exercise without the downside. Some research indicates that a well-designed training program gradually increases the ability to exercise without asthma.

Pretreatment with drugs to keep the airways open can significantly increase tolerance for exercise. This should be discussed with your doctor.

HOW CAN I MAXIMIZE THE EFFECTIVENESS OF ASTHMA TREATMENT?

The self-help allergen- and stress-reducing steps outlined above can aid the general management of your illness. If you use inhaled medications, make sure you've been taught how to administer them properly. Metered dose inhalers and spacers to ensure proper technique can be most helpful.

If you've been instructed how to use a twenty-dollar device called a peak flow meter, you can assess how well your lungs are functioning each day, tell when an attack is imminent before you begin to feel symptoms, and adjust your medication accordingly. In a study at New York City's Bellevue Hospital, the peak flow meter was part of an "aggressive self-management" program that reduced hospital admissions by two thirds in a group of people with severe asthma.

DO CHILDREN OUTGROW ASTHMA?

This comforting belief has, regrettably, not stood up to closer examination. Attacks continue in about half of those who first manifest the illness before the age of sixteen. Among the others, the period of remission frequently ends by the mid-twenties. About half of children who develop asthma before the age of eight will stop having attacks during their teenage years, but half of them will resume by the time they reach their thirties.

Asthma can appear at any age. The cause of adult-onset asthma may be occupational exposure to irritants like chemical fumes or dusts, which activate the predisposition. Recent research suggests that pneumonia caused by chlamydia, an increasingly widespread bacterium, may be responsible for a fair number of cases (*Journal of the American Medical Association,* July 10, 1991).

CAN ASTHMA ITSELF BE PREVENTED?

It used to be thought that asthma resulted from particularly toxic parenting, and removal from the "asthmatogenic family" was sometimes prescribed. This theory has been discarded, but it's true that asthma is a family disease. The predisposition is clearly hereditary, and children of asthmatic parents are at risk.

Some research suggests that the environment in the earliest years, under age two, may determine whether an at-risk child goes on to develop asthma. Infants should be protected from colds and flu and not exposed to irritants like cigarette smoke. Common allergens (like cat dander) and foods that are known to be allergenic (eggs and dairy) should be avoided.

A more conjectural aspect is the psychological environment. There is evidence to associate high levels of family stress in early infancy (and even in the months before birth) with a greater likelihood of asthma. A study now under way will test whether assistance in coping and resolving family conflicts can reduce the risk.

Resources

Asthma Update: A Newsletter for People with Asthma is published quarterly (one year $12; two years $20).

Asthma Update
123 Monticello Avenue
Annapolis, MD 21401
(410) 267-8329

◆ BREAST CANCER

When Cleveland Clinic surgeon George Crile, Jr., M.D., an outspoken critic of overly radical cancer surgery, was asked to name the key advances in the treatment of breast cancer, he said, "The major advances have actually been retreats. Physicians are performing less aggressive surgical treatments and finding the survival rates unaltered or sometimes improved."

That was at a 1980 cancer conference, held in New York City. It's now firmly established that, for most women, the radical surgery once standard for breast cancer offers no advantage over less mutilating procedures.

Today, the issue of overly aggressive treatments for breast cancer is still a concern, but one that has now shifted to include the use of chemotherapy and radiation. What's more, the value of mammography screening and early detection as it relates to women under age fifty has been oversold to the public.

WHAT EXACTLY IS MY DIAGNOSIS?

Not all tumors are equal. If you've been told you have early breast cancer, find out whether it's invasive cancer, or carcinoma in situ (CIS). In fact, request a written report stating your exact diagnosis. CIS, which shows up on mammogram or biopsy, has tripled in incidence over the last decade, as mammography screening has become more widespread. Today, nearly one third of new breast-cancer cases are CIS.

CIS (Latin for "cancer in place") is actually not cancer but a microscopic lesion that *may* become cancer at a later time. One form of CIS, lobular carcinoma in situ (LCIS), is regarded by most researchers as no more than a risk factor for future cancer—roughly equivalent to having a strong family history of breast cancer. LCIS is always found incidentally in a breast cancer biopsy of a woman under fifty, whereas DCIS usually shows up as microcalcifications on a mammogram of an older woman.

About one quarter of women with LCIS will develop an invasive tumor in one or both breasts sometime within the next twenty-five years. LCIS is no longer treated with double mastectomy because that is too drastic. Since it is merely a risk factor for breast cancer, LCIS is not treated but followed up.

The other type is ductal (also known as "intraductal") carcinoma in situ (DCIS), a multiplication of cells within the milk duct which may grow into cancer without forming a lump. A woman with this kind of lesion also has a 33 percent risk of developing breast cancer in the next ten to eighteen years (British Medical Journal, January 7, 1995).

DCIS was a rare diagnosis until the introduction of mammography screening. These microscopic lesions had never been seen beyond the autopsy table, and doctors are not sure how they should be treated. For over two decades, the standard treatment has been mastectomy, that is, surgical removal of the breast. While this treatment cures 98 to 99 percent of women with DCIS, it is believed to be too aggressive for all cases of DCIS, because most would never progress to invasive cancer even if left untreated. Strangely, DCIS is currently treated more aggressively than stages I and II breast cancer, for which breast-sparing options are valid considerations. In some cases, the excision of the lesion alone can provide a cure. An ongoing nationwide clinical trial is exploring the question of how conservatively DCIS can be treated without compromising survival. Half the participants were given excision alone and the other half received further treatment with radiation.

Preliminary results of this trial by the National Surgical Adjuvant Breast Project suggest that excision plus radiation is more effective in reducing recurrences than excision alone. In nearly four years of follow-up of more than eight hundred women with DCIS, 15.6 percent of those treated with excision and radiation had recurrences, compared with 26.2 percent of women treated with excision alone. More follow-up is necessary to determine whether radiation therapy will also reduce the rate of death.

HOW CAN I AVOID OVERTREATMENT OF DCIS?

Get a second pathology opinion once a microscopic lesion is diagnosed. (Pathologists are MDs who specialize in diagnosing disease in biopsied tissue and cells.) Sometimes DCIS is referred to as stage O breast cancer, a precancer, or a noninvasive lesion. Medical journals report that even seasoned pathologists can confuse DCIS with atypical hyperplasia (a benign lesion that requires no treatment) and with invasive cancer. An article in *Cancer* (February 1, 1990) cited three major studies that found over half of the lesions originally identified as early invasive cancer were actually only CIS.

In recent years, pathologists have made progress in distinguishing among different subtypes of DCIS, which include comedo, micropapillary, papillary, solid, and cribriform. Some pathologists have begun looking beyond these conventional subtype classifications and refining their diagnosis, according to Michael D. Lagios, M.D., medical director of the Breast Cancer Consultation Service at St. Mary's Medical Center, San Francisco.

Dr. Lagios described a nuclear grading system for assessing the components, the individual nuclei of the cells. For example, one type of DCIS called comedo has been singled out in the last few years as particularly aggressive, thus meriting aggressive treatment. But, Dr. Lagios explained, not all comedocarcinoma are equal. What is important to know, according to this new nuclear grading system, is whether the comedo is high grade or low grade. The former is high risk, the latter is not. "Every study that looked at subtyping of DCIS has found that low-grade lesions progress very slowly and infrequently," said Dr. Lagios. "In fact, low-grade DCIS is not a cancer; like LCIS, it is just a risk marker for cancer (cancer *may* develop in this breast within the next ten to twenty years)." Dr. Lagios said that this nuclear grading system was not used in the National Surgical Breast Project, whose preliminary results favored follow-up radiation therapy. "They failed to make further distinctions according to the nuclear grading system."

HOW CAN I GET A SECOND PATHOLOGY OPINION?

Call Dr. Lagios's WomanKind Breast Cancer Consultation Service at St. Mary's Medical Center, San Francisco, (415) 750-5848. This is an unusually consumer-friendly second-opinion service because it is willing to deal directly with women diagnosed with breast cancer, precancer, or atypia. (Other services will deal only with physicians.) The service will have the slides containing the biopsied tissue and mammography films picked up from the hospital by Federal Express. In about four or five days, the woman—and all physicians she lists—receives a copy of her report in lay terms for $350. For $650, she can meet with the pathologists and other members of the tumor board of St. Mary's Medical Center, who will discuss her case with her. Out-of-town women can receive this consultation by phone.

Another, much less expensive, consultation service is the Armed Forces Institute of Pathology in Washington, D.C., which has been described as the repository of expertise in this field. The AFIP performs about forty-eight thousand second-opinion consultations per year. Cases are accepted only from pathologists or surgeons, so you'll have to ask one or the other to request a consultation on your behalf. The cost is about one hundred dollars. Call Leo Bell, coordinator of the Civilian Consultation Program, (202) 782-2110.

IF I HAVE A TRUE MALIGNANCY, IS THE CHOICE OF TREATMENT UP TO ME?

Yes. Since a landmark NCI-sponsored national trial in 1985, it has been clear that women with stage I or stage II cancer (cancer confined to the breast or that has spread to nearby lymph nodes), have the same survival rates whether they are treated with mastectomy, lumpectomy plus radiation, or lumpectomy alone. This includes quite large cancers, up to one and a half inches in diameter. (In 1994, the public learned for the first time that some of the data from this trial had been falsified, but the principal investigators reported their yet-to-be published reanalysis indicating that the exclusion of these "tainted" results did not change the study's original conclusion.)

There are exceptions. Lumpectomy has little to recommend it in women with small breasts and large tumors, multicentric disease (evidence of more than one focus of malignancy), or a tumor near the nipple. Today, doctors take a wide margin of tissue near the tumor, so many prefer to use the word *quadrantectomy* or *segmental mastectomy,* rather than *lumpectomy.*

The decision of which treatment route to take isn't always easy. Mastectomy is a disfiguring procedure. On the other hand, the weeks of radiation following lumpectomy carry side effects. The skin of the affected breast can become hardened after radiation therapy, and lung injury has been reported. Women with large breasts may not have as good a cosmetic result with radiation. Furthermore, there is some indication that radiation therapy contributes to lymphedema (permanent fluid retention in the arm). And a study of more than forty-one thousand women under forty-five found an increase in cancer of the other breast after radiation treatment (*The New England Journal of Medicine,* March 19, 1992). This risk can presumably be reduced or eliminated by careful shielding of the opposite breast during radiation treatment. The decision is up to you, if the above exceptions do not apply.

WHY ISN'T THE OPTION OF LUMPECTOMY ALONE USUALLY OFFERED?

While all three treatment groups in the NCI trial had the same survival rate, the women in the group given lumpectomy alone showed a 40 percent rate of recurrence. In other words, the addition of radiation therapy does not improve survival; it merely reduces the rate of recurrence.

Most doctors do not offer lumpectomy alone, because the NCI trial has yet to publish follow-up results longer than eight years. It remains a valid option, however, that should be offered to women, especially women over age fifty-five. An Italian study of 567 women with small breast cancers (less than 2.5 centimeters) were randomly assigned to receive either quadrantectomy followed by radiotherapy or quadrantectomy without radiotherapy. (Quadrantectomy is a larger excision than lumpectomy.) At four-year follow-up, there was no difference in survival between the two groups. Significantly, the women over age fifty-five who had not received radiotherapy had an extremely low recurrence rate of 3.8 percent (*The New England Journal of Medicine,* June 3, 1993).

HOW IS BREAST CANCER TREATED MOST OFTEN?

You want a doctor who acknowledges that all three treatment options have the same survival rate. A doctor who performs only mastectomies is not paying attention to the results of the NCI-sponsored clinical trial.

Unfortunately, this trial has not had sufficient impact on actual treatment of breast cancer. Despite the well-documented and well-publicized findings that breast-sparing procedures are equally effective, 65 percent of all newly diagnosed breast cancers continue to be treated by mastectomy.

Doctors, like the rest of us, have their individual values, preconceptions, and biases, which they often unwittingly impose on those they treat. If your doctor does nothing but mastectomies or presents it as the superior choice ("'better to be safe''), look elsewhere.

IS THERE ANY REASON TO REMOVE MY LYMPH NODES?

If you have decided not to undergo chemotherapy, no matter what the stage of your disease, then the answer is no. The main reason to undergo axillary node dissection (removal of some lymph nodes near the armpit) is to determine the chemotherapy regimen. There is no point in risking the infection, numbness, and lymphedema (permanent fluid retention in the arm) that occurs in a minority of cases, if you wish no further treatment beyond the standard three options. If you have a microscopic lesion (less than 5 millimeters), this is another reason to forgo axillary node dissection, because you are not a candidate for chemotherapy. Another situation in which lymph node dissection would be useless is the diagnosis of breast cancer in a woman so young that chemotherapy is clearly advisable.

Before the mid-1980s, lymph node dissection was thought to be a treatment. It was firmly believed that cancer spread from a primary tumor in the breast to nearby lymph nodes, and then to the rest of the body. We now know that this is not true. It takes eight to ten years for most breast cancers to become palpable, and for much of that time, malignant cells may have traveled throughout the body. Removal of lymph nodes, whether they test positive or negative for cancer, hasn't been shown to improve survival.

Today, lymph node dissection is performed in order to determine the stage of the cancer and to plan further treatment. In the recent past, women who were node negative (stage I, no evidence of cancer in the nodes) did not get further treatment with chemotherapy. The reason for lymph node dissection was the elimination from chemotherapy of such women, who were not seen as candidates for chemotherapy. Some have argued that removal of cancerous nodes has the value of keeping the chest wall free of disease but even they concede that this has no effect on survival.

In 1988, preliminary results of clinical trials showed a modest benefit to giving chemotherapy to node-negative women following mastectomy or breast-sparing treatment. Now, virtually all women with breast cancer are viewed as candidates for chemotherapy whether they have evidence of cancer in their lymph nodes or not. Thus, some doctors have argued that the condition of the lymph nodes is largely irrelevant. In a 1992 conference on breast cancer surgery, several prominent surgeons questioned the rationale for lymph node removal. ''I must affirm that there is no reason to do an axillary dissection at all in 1992," said Peter J. Deckers, M.D., Murray Heilig Professor and Chair of Surgery at University of Connecticut School of Medicine, Farmington. "I'm persuaded . . . that within the next decade this operation . . . which is today threatened with extinction, will, in fact, be extinct."

WHAT ARE THE ADVANTAGES OF CHEMOTHERAPY FOR MY TYPE OF BREAST CANCER?

The current tendency to view all women with breast cancer as candidates for chemotherapy should be scrutinized carefully. Too often, women are given chemotherapy without an explanation of how truly modest its benefit can be. Always ask for the data to support the recommended chemotherapy regimen, and make a point of asking for the definition of success. Frequently, success may be three months extended survival or a lower recurrence rate for a minority.

Most women with stage I breast cancer (tumor confined to the breast) are cured by the initial treatment, be it mastectomy, lumpectomy plus radiation, or lumpectomy alone. In 30 percent of cases, however, the malignancy recurs and progresses to a fatal outcome within ten years. Unfortunately, it is impossible to say at the time of diagnosis whether the tumor is of a type that is likely to recur and progress.

Because a breast tumor has been growing and possibly spreading malignant cells for years by the time it is diagnosed, removing the growth is no guarantee of cure. "Systemic chemotherapy at the time of diagnosis can get rid of some of these cells and can slow the growth of others," according to Susan Love, M.D., chairperson of the Research Task Force of the Breast Cancer Coalition. "This adds disease-free years to women's lives but does not necessarily cure them."

Of all women with stage I breast cancer who are given chemotherapy, only four to fifteen of that 30 percent—the ones whose disease is likely to progress—are likely to benefit; the other 70 to 96 percent will suffer the side effects of treatment and derive no benefit. It's impossible to know ahead of time who in that 30 percent group will be most likely to gain from chemotherapy.

The effectiveness of chemotherapy depends in part on the type of tumor, the extent to which it has already spread, your age, and some other factors. Ask your doctor to detail what published studies say about your individual situation. Also, check with CancerFax (see Resources).

If you look into relevant research papers yourself, keep in mind that "response rate" cited by researchers may mean nothing but a slight reduction in size of the tumor, and that reducing the risk of recurrence isn't the same thing as increasing long-term survival.

HOW WOULD I BENEFIT FROM MAMMOGRAPHY?

The importance of mammography as a protection against breast cancer has been accepted uncritically for years and has been the subject of advertising drives and political pressure. More recently, however, the dogma of early detection has come under rational scrutiny, and it has not held up well.

In women between the ages of fifty and sixty-nine, mammography screening and early treatment of detected tumors has indeed been documented to reduce breast cancer deaths (by nearly one third, according to a summary of all clinical trials published in the *Journal of the National Cancer Institute,* October 20, 1993).

For younger women, though, the story is a lot less clear. Although repeated studies found little or no advantage to screening in women under fifty, most medical organizations (including the NCI, the American Cancer Society, and the American College of Radiology) persist in recommending annual mammography for women in their forties.

In 1992, the Canadian National Breast Screening Study reported findings of a study that followed fifty thousand women in their forties for eight years. It found no reduction in breast cancer mortality among the women who underwent mammography screening, compared with those who had not.

A meta-analysis of many studies, the following year, confirmed these findings: women in their forties whose breast cancer is found early due to mammography screening die of the disease at the same rate as women who were not screened.

As a result of these analyses, the National Cancer Institute finally dropped its recommendation of mammography screening for women under fifty—even those with close relatives who have breast cancer.

An important thing to remember is that breast cancer (like many malignancies) increases dramatically with age. "More than 75 percent of breast cancers occur in women who are older than fifty," according to a

1993 NCI report. Ironically, younger women have apparently been most influenced by mammography campaigns, yet this group has nothing to gain from the procedure. Perhaps advertising drives, which invariably show younger women, have something to do with this disturbing fact.

IS MAMMOGRAPHY WORTH THE RISK?

The breast is particularly sensitive to radiation's carcinogenic effects, making radiation-induced cancer a small but real possibility. Over the last decade, new equipment and low-dose techniques have dramatically reduced radiation exposure with mammography. But there is wide variation in the quality of equipment and technique—and radiation exposure—from one clinic to another. Image quality is an even greater concern: a 1992 FDA survey of mammography facilities showed that 14 percent were substandard. If you get screened, make sure it's at an American College of Radiology-accredited facility (see Resources).

A much more likely risk is unnecessary treatment. A study of thirty-two thousand California women who underwent mammography screening found that for those over age fifty, there were twenty-five biopsies for every ten cancers found (2.5 of which weren't actual cancers, but DCIS). For women under fifty, there were thirteen biopsies for every two cancers found (one of them being DCIS). The firm, dense breast tissue of younger women, combined with their low rate of actual cancer, make false-positive mammography results especially common in this age group.

Unnecessary biopsy (a portion or all of the tumor is removed surgically or by needle aspiration) is unpleasant, but the real risk is unnecessary surgery. If mammography detects CIS, remember the difference between this and invasive cancer before you make a decision on treatment. Also, be sure to get a second pathology opinion.

IF I AM IN A HIGH-RISK GROUP, DO I NEED MORE SCREENING?

The idea of increased breast cancer risk has scared many women into mammography. Most women are familiar with the list of risk factors: having a mother or sister with breast cancer; being over age fifty; never having borne a child; having your first child after thirty; early menarche; and menopause after fifty-five.

The importance of risk factors shouldn't be overestimated. A study that followed nearly eighteen thousand women for twelve years found that among the 2,389 who developed breast cancer, only 2.5 percent could be attributed to a family history. In particular, those whose mothers developed the disease after age seventy had only a 1.5 percent increased risk (*Journal of the American Medical Association*, July 21, 1993).

On the other hand, most women with a close relative who has breast cancer will themselves never get the disease. Age, again, is a far more important issue: in its new guidelines, the NCI no longer recommends mammography screening for women under fifty—even those with a mother or sister who had breast cancer. This is because such women are still at a lower risk than women in their sixties with no relatives who had breast cancer.

Resources

Call the local chapter of the American Cancer Society; or the National Cancer Institute at (800) 4-CANCER (422-6237) for the names of several facilities in your area that have passed the American College of Radiology's accreditation program that requires special mammography training for both radiologists and technicians.

Use CancerFax to receive a printout on breast cancer from the computerized data base of the National Cancer Institute. You will need access to a fax machine with an attached telephone. Dial (301) 402-5874 on a touch-tone phone and receive a faxed report on state-of-the-art treatments for breast cancer. Request the physicians' version.

Contact (800) 221-2141, or (708) 799-8228, Y-Me National Organization for Breast Cancer Information and Support: emotional support, free literature, and support groups.

Call (800) 875-4837 or (202) 686-2210, the Breast Cancer Hotline, sponsored by the Physicians Committee for Responsible Medicine in Washington, D.C., for free information about the links between diet and breast cancer.

◆ CARPAL TUNNEL SYNDROME

Tingling, burning, or aching pain (especially at night) in the fingers, and perhaps the wrist as well; these are the basic symptoms of carpal tunnel syndrome (CTS). If untreated, nerve damage and muscle wasting can occur, perhaps irreversibly.

Carpal tunnel syndrome has become increasingly common in recent years, thanks to technology. One cause of the disorder (involved in nearly half of cases, according to the Centers for Disease Control) is work that demands repetitive hand motions. Long hours at the computer keyboard is the classic scenario, but repetitive motion is actually common in many work situations and can lead to CTS in individuals as diverse as assembly-line workers, bricklayers, and violinists.

The cause of CTS symptoms is pressure on the nerve—specifically, the median nerve that runs through the carpal tunnel, a narrow channel of tendons and bones in the wrist, to the thumb and first three fingers. The tendons flex the fingers; the friction of repeated movement can make them swell, and in the crowded conditions of the tunnel, exert pressure on the nerve, causing pain. Usually, symptoms occur in both hands.

WHY DO SOME PEOPLE GET CARPAL TUNNEL SYNDROME?

Occupational overuse isn't the only risk factor. In one study, diabetes and pregnancy were each roughly two and a half times as common in people with CTS as in the general population, and rheumatoid arthritis, more than three and a half times as common (*Mayo Clinic Proceedings,* 1992, no. 67, pp. 541–48). Hypothyroidism and infections may also be underlying causes. Such conditions may make tendons more easily inflamed or may predispose a person to edema (water retention in tissues) that increases pressure on the nerve.

More women than men develop CTS. One explanation may be that women are particularly likely to find themselves performing the kind of repetitive motion work that brings on CTS. Furthermore, certain situations unique to women, such as pregnancy, use of oral contraceptives, and gynecological surgery are all associated with an increased incidence of CTS. Although the association has never been explained, the prevailing hypothesis centers upon the role of estrogen. Pregnancy, oral contraceptives, hysterectomy, and oophorectomy (surgical removal of the ovaries) can alter the levels of estrogen, which in turn increases fluid retention in the carpal tunnel. The swelling causes pressure on the median nerve.

WHAT TREATMENT IS BEST FOR CTS?

The first treatment is simple and conservative: rest. Often, the wrist is splinted in a neutral position, full-time for as long as three weeks, and then at night only for three more weeks. If an underlying illness is involved, it must be treated.

If CTS is associated with your job, you'll have to make some changes or the problem will never go away and will probably get worse. Switching careers is not an option for most of us, but many jobs can be made less stressful to the wrist. Moving the computer screen and keyboard, adjusting the height of your seat, and having a place to rest your wrist and avoid repeated flexing may minimize the strain. Take brief, frequent breaks to relieve the stress. The guidance of an expert like an occupational therapist can be very helpful.

Anti-inflammatory drugs are often used, sometimes in addition to splinting, to reduce the pain and inflammation of CTS. Aspirin and ibuprofen are less expensive and may work as well as prescription anti-inflammatories. Diuretics may relieve pressure by reducing swelling.

Corticosteroids, which are extremely potent weapons against inflammation, may be injected directly into the wrist. This is likely to cause greater discomfort for a short time, but then may dramatically reduce symptoms. Relief is rarely permanent, however, and these injections cannot be repeated more than several times before they start to damage soft tissue.

Medical management is most likely to be effective in people who are under fifty years old, and whose symptoms are intermittent and have lasted less than ten months.

DO VITAMINS HELP?

For over a decade, researchers have reported positive results by treating CTS with large doses of pyridoxine—vitamin B$_6$. According to Dr. Karl Folkers, who received the Priestly Medal, the highest award of the American Chemical Society, for his work in the area, many people with the syndrome are severely deficient in this vitamin, and redressing the deficiency makes symptoms go away.

Although some investigators have gotten similarly encouraging results, others have failed to corroborate Folkers's findings in controlled studies. The vitamin B$_6$ treatment is still, in other words, questionable.

Even according to those who claim that B$_6$ is effective against CTS, it's no quick cure. It may take twelve weeks or longer to take effect.

More important, when vitamin B$_6$ is taken in the large doses used in these tests (up to 150 milligrams daily—seventy-five times the recommended daily allowance for adults), it is no longer a vitamin, but a drug. The point at which severe toxicity (including, paradoxically, nerve damage) has been reported is higher—500 milligrams daily—but the bottom line is that megadoses of vitamin B$_6$ are not to be used carelessly.

WHAT ABOUT SURGERY?

The most direct way to relieve pressure on the nerve is surgery. This must be considered a last resort, to be used when pain persists despite more conservative measures, or when signs of muscle wastage or laboratory tests suggest that permanent nerve damage is taking place.

In the classic procedure, the surgeon cuts the ligament that forms the carpal tunnel, releasing pressure on the nerve. Pain is relieved and you regain use of your hand in two to three weeks, although you may have to avoid strenuous activities for several months, until full function returns.

Among the possible complications of the surgery are damage to blood vessels or to the nerve: in one series of 186 cases, the complication rate was 12 percent.

Although the immediate results of carpal tunnel release are usually good, a retrospective review of sixty cases (*Journal of the American Medical Association,* April 17, 1991) suggests a less attractive long-term picture. Michael P. Nancollas, M.D., a fellow in hand surgery at the State University of New York, Buffalo, followed these cases for an average of five and a half years. He found a return of some symptoms, usually pain, in half the cases. Almost one third of the people had significant pain and weakness two years after the surgery, and 30 percent rated the results of the procedure as "poor to fair."

A refinement of the surgical procedure developed in recent years claims to improve results and reduce complications. Here, a thin tubelike instrument called an endoscope makes it possible to cut the carpal tunnel ligament without actually opening the wrist. In theory, this will cause less scarring and muscle damage, so postoperative pain will be reduced, and recovery will be quicker.

In one multicenter trial that compared eighty-two endoscopic procedures with sixty-five conventional ("open") surgeries, those who had the endoscopic procedure recovered hand strength sooner, had less postoperative pain, and returned to work in half the time. The rate of serious complications was similar in the two groups.

According to a Diagnostic and Therapeutic Technology Assessment issued by the American Medical Association late in 1992, a panel of thirty-two experts considered the procedure "investigational" but "promising" as a safe and effective way to minimize postsurgical tenderness and weakness.

Whether long-term results will be better with endoscopic surgery is as yet impossible to say.

Resources

If you believe your job poses a risk of CTS (or any other health hazard), you can arrange an expert evaluation of your workplace by NIOSH. Request an HHE Form for a health hazard evaluation by a visiting NIOSH expert.

National Institute of Occupational Safety and Health (NIOSH)
Hazard Evaluation and Technical Assistance Branch
4676 Columbia Parkway
Cincinnati, OH 45226
(513) 841-4382

If you're a woman, call 9 to 5, National Association of Working Women, Cleveland, (800) 522-0925, and request a list of fact sheets on such topics as office injuries and office design. The hotline will also provide callers—you don't have to be a member, but you do have to be a woman—with job-related advice to minimize the risk of CTS, and offer suggestions on finding a doctor who knows about occupational injuries.

◆ CATARACTS

With age, the lens of the eye—the only transparent organ of the body—begins to cloud. Its proteins clump together and (if the process continues) eventually become opaque, and a cataract develops. More than half of all people over age sixty-five have cataracts to some degree.

The process that creates cataracts is irreversible, and the only effective treatment is surgery to remove them. This is a big-ticket item for the American health-care system: more than 1.3 million such operations are performed yearly, at an estimated cost to Medicare of $3.4 billion.

HOW SAFE IS CATARACT SURGERY?

The modern procedure is a vast improvement over cataract surgery of a generation ago. Instead of a long hospital stay and immobilization while the lens heals, people now have cataracts removed under local anesthesia in an outpatient procedure that in most cases takes less than an hour. The cloudy part of the lens is removed through a small incision in the cornea and replaced by a tiny artificial lens made of plastic. Serious complications are uncommon.

According to a study at Johns Hopkins University, this procedure (extra-capsular cataract extraction, or ECCE) cuts by 75 percent the risk of retinal detachment, compared with the next most popular procedure, intra-capsular cataract extraction, in which the entire lens capsule is removed. Retinal detachment is a serious complication, wherein the retina separates from the choroid, the layer of blood vessels that provides the retina with nutrients and oxygen. Detachment causes visual abnormalities which—if left untreated—may lead to permanent blindness. Retinal detachment can be corrected by a surgical procedure in which the hole causing the detachment is closed.

With a more recent innovation, phaco-emulsification (PE), the lens is broken up by ultrasound and then sucked out. This procedure requires a much smaller incision than either extra- or intra-capsular extraction; as a result, healing is more rapid. However, according to the Johns Hopkins study, the risk of retinal detachment with PE is 17 percent higher than with ECCE.

With any of these procedures, hemorrhage and infection are possible complications, in addition to retinal damage. Younger people are more likely to suffer retinal detachment, and whites more likely than blacks.

WHEN IS SURGERY NECESSARY?

Just because you have cataracts doesn't mean they should be removed. An estimated 40 percent of people ages fifty to sixty-four and 75 percent of those sixty-five to seventy-four have some lens clouding, but vision is unaffected or is only slightly affected in the vast majority of cases.

Strictly speaking, surgery is necessary when *you* decide you need it. According to guidelines recently issued by the U.S. Agency for Health Care Policy and Research, it's only appropriate when the cataract interferes with your daily life. There is no evidence that postponing the surgery increases risks or leads to a poorer outcome.

A report by the Government Accounting Office (GAO) suggests that the procedure is often performed unnecessarily. In a random survey of nearly two thousand Medicare recipients who had had cataracts removed, only three quarters reported substantial impairment in their ability to drive, read, or watch television before the surgery. If the presence of symptoms like blurred vision and sensitivity to glare was included, the proportion of procedures that were justified was 84 percent.

"Surgery may have been more questionable for the remaining 16 percent of patients, depending on the weight given to 'slight' symptoms and functional limitations relative to the risk of the surgery itself," the report said.

The U.S. Agency for Health Care Policy and Research concluded that people should undergo surgery when cataracts interfere with their daily life activities. By this standard, *one quarter* of all the procedures were questionable. Amazingly, 6 percent of the respondents said they had had *no* difficulty in reading, driving, or watching TV before surgery, and another 18 percent reported only slight impairment.

HOW GOOD ARE THE RESULTS OF SURGERY?

The GAO survey reported generally favorable outcomes: 74 percent of people said their visual functions had improved; 71.4 percent reported reduction in symptoms; and 65.9 percent said both had gotten better. On the other hand, 30 percent had mixed results—some functions, or some symptoms, had failed to improve or had gotten worse. And 4.6 percent of the people said their overall visual function had deteriorated; 5 percent said their symptoms were worse; and 2.4 percent reported worsening of both.

In the GAO sample, most surgery recipients had little postoperative bleeding, pain, or swelling, although 1 to 2 percent reported severe pain or swelling and 7 to 8 percent reported moderate pain or swelling, which generally lasted one or two days. Five percent of patients developed infections, 13 percent needed some sort of follow-up procedure, and 1.5 percent needed to be hospitalized because of complications.

SHOULD I HAVE CATARACT SURGERY?

Again, this is your decision to make. If your vision is not substantially impaired, changing your eyeglass prescription frequently may be enough to allow you to function normally, at least for a while.

Well-financed outpatient procedures seem to tempt some health-care providers to perform unnecessary surgery. You are best off seeking help from an ophthalmologist who is experienced in cataract removal, but doesn't do this only. Second opinions are, as ever, a good idea.

CAN CATARACTS BE PREVENTED?

In recent years, research has given us a better idea of the factors that increase or reduce the risk of cataracts. A landmark study at Johns Hopkins (*The New England Journal of Medicine,* December 1, 1988) found that exposure to sunlight promotes their formation. When researchers surveyed 838 boatmen who worked on Chesapeake Bay (and who were thus regularly exposed to strong, reflected sunlight), they found the rate of cataracts tripled in those who didn't protect their eyes with sunglasses or a broad-brimmed hat.

Apparently, it is UVB light (the band primarily responsible for sun tanning and burning) that promotes cataracts. Other studies, however, suggest that the entire ultraviolet spectrum may cause other eye damage, including severe corneal disease.

You can best protect your eyes by wearing large-framed, close-fitting, wraparound sunglasses whenever there's enough sun to risk sunburn (from ten in the morning to four in the afternoon, May to September). Look for sunglasses that say "blocks 100 percent UVB and UVA" or "blocks 100 percent UV light up to 400 nanometers").

Other findings from the same study indicate that smokers are at increased risk of certain kinds of cataracts. The conclusion to be drawn from this is obvious.

Such precautions may be particularly important if you have dark brown or hazel eyes. A study (*American Journal of Public Health,* November 1988) found a higher risk of cataracts among dark-eyed people. This finding confirms population studies that reported high prevalence in areas like Nepal and India, where people are dark-eyed. The same pigment, melanin, that protects the skin against sun damage, apparently makes the eye more vulnerable by absorbing ultraviolet light.

DOES DIET MAKE A DIFFERENCE?

Repeated recent studies have suggested that antioxidant nutrients—vitamin C, vitamin E, and carotenoids (vitamin A precursors)—protect the eye against the process that produces cataracts.

In a study that followed over fifty thousand American female nurses (*British Medical Journal,* August 8, 1992) the women in the highest fifth of total vitamin A intake had a 39 percent lower risk of cataracts than those with the lowest intake. Cataracts were nearly 50 percent less likely among the women who used vitamin C supplements for ten or more years. In a Finnish study of forty-seven people who had cataracts and ninety-four people who did not (*British Medical Journal,* December 5, 1992), those in the lowest third in serum levels of vitamin E and beta carotene had 2.6 times the risk of cataracts of the others.

Animal studies confirm the protective effect of these nutrients. The theory is that the cataracts develop as the protein in the lens is damaged by oxidation—a normal part of the aging process that may be accelerated by sunlight or smoking—and that antioxidants slow down the process.

These same nutrients may also play a role in protecting against diverse illnesses, including cancer and heart disease. Whether or not you take supplements is up to you, but a diet rich in the fruits and green and yellow vegetables that provide antioxidants (kale, collard greens, sweet potatoes, cantaloupe, nectarines) can be recommended for any number of reasons.

IS IT TOO LATE?

Since the development of cataracts is a gradual process, the sooner you take protective lifestyle measures, the better. Will they slow down deterioration enough to make a difference, if you already have some lens clouding? Research on this hasn't been done, but no one suggests that preventive measures will hurt. Sunglasses and a diet rich in antioxidants are important at any age.

Resources

You can get your own free copy of the government guidelines for cataract surgery by writing:

Agency for Health Care Policy and Research
Publications Clearinghouse
P.O. Box 8547,
Silver Spring, MD 20907
(800) 358-9295

The guidelines come in separate versions for physicians and "patients." In such situations, the doctor's version tends to be more straightforward and informative.

◆ CERVICAL CANCER (Pap Test)

An estimated 6 percent of malignancies in women are cervical cancers. Each year, sixteen thousand new cases are diagnosed, and five thousand women die. Cervical cancer is typically slow to develop, and in its early stage, it should be detectable by one of the most widely used screening procedures—the Pap test. For the test, a familiar ritual for millions of women, a smear of vaginal fluid is searched, microscopically, for abnormal cells that have been shed from the cervix.

But the test's use hasn't had as great an impact as might be hoped. The rate of cervical cancer has in fact increased in one population group—white women under the age of fifty—by 3 percent per year since 1986. Changes in the way screening results are reported could explain some of the increase, but not the 1-percent-per-year rise in *deaths* from cervical cancer in the same population, according to the *Journal of the National Cancer Institute* (January 5, 1994). The relatively new standardization of Pap test results has contributed to the overtreatment of so-called precancerous lesions of the cervix, most of which would never have become malignant even if left untreated.

HOW GOOD IS THE LAB THAT WILL READ MY PAP TEST?

As lab work goes, the Pap test is pretty low-tech. While other tests use automated or semiautomated equipment and techniques, reading Pap smears relies on the lab technician's ability to spot abnormal cells. The test is no better than the anonymous eye that scans it, which in some cases is none too good. While in theory the Pap test should catch 90 percent of cancers, its false negative rate (missed cancers) in practice can run as high as 40 percent. Half of the errors are attributed to how the physician takes the smear, and half to lab personnel.

Diane Solomon, M.D., chief of the National Cancer Institute's cytopathology section, advises using a lab accredited by the College of American Pathologists or the American Society of Cytology. The only way to find this out is to ask your gynecologist about the lab he or she uses before making the appointment for a Pap test. Some experts believe that a large teaching hospital lab is a safe choice.

HOW CAN THE ACCURACY OF THE TEST BE MAXIMIZED?

When the smear is taken makes a difference. To increase accuracy odds, schedule the test for mid-menstrual cycle. Don't douche before the test.

It's inadvisable to have the test repeated too soon, as is often done to confirm a positive finding or to clarify things when the first test was uncertain. If a second smear is taken just a few days or weeks later, 60 percent of abnormal tissue samples (neoplasia) will be reported as negative. It may be that the abnormal cells scraped off the first time haven't had a chance to grow back.

WHAT SHOULD I DO AFTER HAVING A PAP TEST?

Don't assume that no news is good news. If you haven't learned the results in two to three weeks, call the doctor's office and request the written description of the test findings.

WHAT ARE THE ODDS THAT A LESION WILL ACTUALLY BECOME MALIGNANT?

Cellular abnormalities requiring attention can take a number of different forms: the relatively new Bethesda classification system, introduced in 1989, grades smears from ''normal'' to ''cancer;'' with three grades in between.

Just one premalignant lesion in ten will progress to invasive cancer, without treatment. Among certain types of abnormal cell growths, the chances of later cancer are just one in a hundred.

The next step after a positive Pap test is an examination called colposcopy, which allows the doctor to inspect the cervix under magnification. If a premalignant lesion is found, it is usually removed by Loop Electrosurgical Excision Procedure (LEEP), laser surgery, or cryosurgery (freezing). These procedures carry a risk of infection or bleeding. One type of biopsy, called cone biopsy because it removes a cone-shapes wedge of tissue from the cervix, can adversely affect future pregnancies.

It wasn't that long ago that hysterectomy was a common treatment for cervical "premalignancies." Nowadays, it shouldn't be an option in any but a few situations, but in practice, an unknown number of unnecessary hysterectomies are still being done. Many of these so-called premalignancies are simply abnormalities that would never progress to cancer even if left untreated.

When they do progress to cancer, most of these lesions do so slowly, but some are more aggressive. Discuss with your doctor the specific diagnosis if your Pap test was positive, and the relative merits of a removal procedure, versus watchful waiting with close surveillance for signs of progression. If you plan to become pregnant in the future, ask about the amount of tissue that will be removed during a biopsy. There is some evidence that fertility can be compromised by a cervix weakened from multiple or overly aggressive biopsy techniques.

HOW IS HPV INFECTION TREATED?

There is no effective treatment for the human papilloma virus (HPV), which can cause genital warts—an extremely common sexually transmitted disease. And the virus is a significant risk factor for cervical cancer: evidence of HPV infection in the cervix will mean a positive Pap test. But there are over sixty strains of HPV, and only six of them are associated with cervical cancer. The majority of genital warts are caused by other strains. Typing procedures to identify whether the virus found on the Pap test increases the risk of cancer haven't yet undergone a clinical trial. Doctors disagree on how to proceed when HPV infection is present.

HOW CAN I REDUCE MY RISK OF CERVICAL CANCER?

Sexual activity is an identified risk factor. Women who have had multiple sexual partners are more likely to develop cervical cancer; the sexual experience of their partners raises the risk, too. A 1988 National Cancer

Institute study found that monogamous women whose husbands had had more than twenty-five sex partners had twice the risk of cervical cancers of those whose husbands had six or fewer sex partners.

Women who become sexually active at an early age are at even greater risk, possibly because the youthful cervix is particularly vulnerable to HPV infection. Using a barrier method of contraception, such as a diaphragm, condom, or a cervical cap, will protect the cervix.

Other factors that increase the risk are cigarette smoking (or exposure to the smoke of others for three or more hours a day), poverty, and the use of oral contraceptives.

Good nutrition is important. The antioxidants vitamin E, vitamin C, and beta carotene apparently protect against this and other cancers. Studies have associated a high intake and high blood levels of these nutrients with lower cervical cancer rates. Low levels of folate, a B vitamin, have been found to increase the odds that HPV will lead to cellular abnormalities.

All of these nutrients are abundant in green, red, and yellow vegetables (*folate* comes from a Latin word meaning leaf). Vitamin supplements can ensure that you're getting enough, but can't take the place of a healthful diet.

AT WHAT AGE CAN I STOP HAVING PAP TESTS?

The U.S. Preventive Services Task Force, which bases its recommendations on reviews of all related studies, says screening may be stopped at age sixty-five if all previous smears have been normal.

DO I NEED REGULAR PAP TESTS IF I'VE HAD A HYSTERECTOMY?

Many gynecologists would probably say yes to this question, but there is no scientific evidence to support the advice. A woman who has no cervix is unlikely to develop cervical cancer. Many doctors argue that the Pap smear is advised in hysterectomized women as a means of finding vaginal cancer. But screening women for vaginal cancer makes no sense. It is an extremely rare form of cancer; there is no evidence that the Pap test has any accuracy in detecting vaginal cancer; and there's no evidence that finding vaginal cancer at an early stage will alter the course of the disease. A spokesman for the U.S. Preventive Services Task Force said it did not address this question in its 1989 report because Pap testing has no role in the health care of women who have had a hysterectomy.

♦ CHLAMYDIA

Chlamydia infection may not have the sinister reputation of syphilis or gonorrhea, but it's the most common bacterial sexually transmitted disease (STD) in the United States, with an estimated four million episodes each year.

Because chlamydia is often without symptoms (in 80 percent of cases in women and 10 to 20 percent of those in men), it frequently goes untreated. Even these subclinical infections, however, can cause serious consequences, including arthritis, infertility, and ectopic pregnancy. Transmitted to a newborn infant, it can result in pneumonia or severe eye disease.

Although it hasn't become a household word, growing recognition of the toll taken by chlamydia, and simpler, less expensive tests have been important advances. Chlamydia's importance wasn't really appreciated until the mid-1970s, and from 1987 to 1991, the number of states requiring doctors to report cases of chlamydia (as is done for other STDs like syphilis and gonorrhea) doubled, from eighteen to thirty-six.

The reported cases of chlamydia also doubled in this time period, but the Centers for Disease Control assumes this simply reflects extended legal reporting requirements, according to an article in the *Journal of the American Medical Association* (October 13, 1993).

AM I AT RISK FOR CHLAMYDIA?

The prevalence of chlamydia infection varies widely from one group of people to another. Among sexually active women, the rate is 5 to 10 percent of college students, and 35 percent of pregnant women screened in some lower socioeconomic-status urban communities. There were nearly six times as many infections reported in women as in men in 1993, which may reflect a high proportion of male infection that is never diagnosed.

The factors that increase risk are like those of other STDs: young women are more likely to have chlamydia than older women; blacks more likely than whites; unmarried more than married. Having multiple sex partners raises the risk, as does the use of oral contraceptives or an IUD rather than barrier contraceptives like condoms or a diaphragm and spermicide, according to an article in *Obstetrical and Gynecological Survey* (July 1992).

As with other STDs, using condoms and limiting the number of your sex partners is the best protection.

HOW ACCURATE IS THE TEST FOR DIAGNOSING CHLAMYDIA?

In men, the most common manifestation of chlamydia is nongonococcal urethritis—typically painful urination, possibly with a light discharge. In women, an inflammation of the cervix is most common, and this often produces slight symptoms, such as a discharge, or (fully half the time) no symptoms at all. Untreated chlamydia is liable to become chronic.

The fact that the chlamydia organism can grow only inside living cells means that the usual bacterial culture techniques will miss it. The most accurate test is a special culture that requires obtaining cells from the cervix or urethra. It is complicated and expensive, and takes up to a week to get results.

Because they are simpler, faster, and less expensive, enzyme immunoassay and direct immunofluorescence have come into wide use. They are not, however, as sensitive as cell culture, and their accuracy may depend on the skill and experience of the person reading them. With both tests, false positive results are particularly likely in low-risk groups, and some experts recommend confirming positive findings by cell culture (*Postgraduate Medicine*, January 1992).

HOW CAN I PROTECT MY FERTILITY?

Chlamydia infection in the cervix spreads to the upper genital tract about 25 percent of the time, causing pelvic inflammatory disease (PID); a single attack of PID leaves one fifth of women infertile (see Pelvic Inflammatory Disease). As much as half the infertility in some populations is due to chlamydia, according to an article in *Hospital Practice* (February 15, 1992).

Scarring of fallopian tubes caused by PID also greatly increases the risk of ectopic pregnancy.

PID caused by chlamydia is often far more subtle than when other organisms, like gonococci, are involved. But it can cause just as much reproductive damage. A key to protection is treating chlamydia before it becomes PID.

Here, of course, the problem is the asymptomatic nature of chlamydia infection, which may smolder chronically for years. For this reason, many public health officials recommend screening of women at risk. According to one set of criteria, proposed by the Centers for Disease Control, this includes all sexually active women under age twenty, and those under thirty-five who have had a new partner in the last two months, more than one current partner, or a partner who is not monogamous.

Anyone with another STD should also be tested for chlamydia. If you're sexually active, routine testing is worth the trouble and expense.

Although it hasn't gotten nearly as much publicity, there's reason to believe that chlamydia infection can cause infertility in men as well. In one study reported in the *American Journal of Public Health* (July 1993), male partners in couples with unexplained infertility were significantly more likely to have high levels of antibodies against chlamydia, suggesting infection. Half of these men had no history of symptoms.

How chlamydia might impair male fertility is uncertain. One well-known complication of the infection is epididymitis, an inflammation of part of the testicle that plays a critical role in the growth and delivery of sperm, the authors of the above study note. Whatever the link, it argues for greater efforts to detect chlamydia infection in men, and to treat it promptly.

HOW CAN I PROTECT MY BABY?

Between 2 percent and 35 percent of pregnant women have evidence of chlamydia infection. Its effects on the pregnancy can be severe. Researchers have reported a tenfold increase in stillbirth and neonatal death, and a greater risk of premature labor, rupture of membranes, and early delivery, according to the 1992 *Hospital Practice* article.

More than half of newborns exposed to chlamydia during childbirth show evidence of infection. The most common consequences are eye inflammations and pneumonia, which may not appear for as long as four months.

To prevent newborn infections, screening for chlamydia is usually part of the first prenatal visit, along with tests for other STDs. If you're at high risk, it may be advisable to repeat the test in your third trimester. If an infection is found and treated at that time, it should protect your baby.

WILL TREATMENT ERADICATE CHLAMYDIA?

Chlamydia can be wiped out quite effectively with antibiotics, and the ones most often used are tetracycline or related compounds (except in special cases, like pregnancy, where tetracyclines are inadvisable). More established infections, like PID, may require the addition of other drugs.

What's sometimes overlooked is the necessity for a full course of antibiotics—generally a week—at an adequate dose. Treatment that is too light or too short may relieve the immediate infection, but leave enough organisms to regroup and cause a recurrence. Some high-powered, expensive new antibiotics (such as azithromycin) appear to be effective with a single large dose.

Even using antibiotics as directed isn't foolproof, however. A paper in the *Journal of the American Medical Association* (November 3, 1993) suggested that chronic, longstanding infections may be harder to eradicate, for example, than those of recent origin. Whether or not to follow up treatment with another culture to make sure of cure is a matter of debate. It's something to discuss with your doctor.

More than half of the sexual partners of people with chlamydia are also infected with the disease, and leaving them untreated is a recipe for recurrence. Some doctors will simply write a prescription to give to your partner, but this isn't the best way to do things for a number of reasons. Your partner should make a visit to his or her own doctor and undergo appropriate tests.

Resources

Call the National STD Hotline (800) 227-8922 M-F 8 A.M.–11 P.M. eastern time. The hotline, sponsored by the American Social Health Association, will answer questions on common STDs, provide referrals to clinics and health centers, and mail free literature on STDs and prevention.

✦ CHRONIC FATIGUE SYNDROME

Fatigue is so common that it's easy to take lightly. One survey found it a major problem for one quarter of people attending general medical clinics. Chronic fatigue syndrome (CFS) is something else: relentless exhaustion profound enough to cut in half capacity for work, play, and life in general, accompanied by a host of aches, pains, and mental difficulties.

CFS affects roughly three times as many women as men. Its prominence in the 1980s, among thirtyish, white, middle-class people led inexorably to the nickname "yuppie flu." But a look back finds that what appears to be the same disorder has a long history under a series of labels: *neurasthenia* was popular at the turn of the century; more recently came *Icelandic disease, chronic mononucleosis,* and *postviral fatigue syndrome.*

IS MY DOCTOR EXPERIENCED IN TREATING CFS?

You want a doctor with extensive experience in the treatment of people with CFS, one who keeps up with the latest research and is open to trying nonmedical treatments. Ask about all these issues. The idea is to detect whether the doctor takes a dismissive attitude toward CFS.

Like many disorders with common symptoms, no objective test, and uncertain cause, CFS has inspired more skepticism than compassion in many medical people. In recent years, however, a consensus has emerged that CFS is a real disease; people who suffer from it appear to have certain immunological, neurological, and biochemical abnormalities in common.

In 1991, the Centers for Disease Control set forth criteria to define CFS. Under their definition, the disease involves chronic or recurrent fatigue that can't be explained by any other physical or emotional condition, severe enough to reduce activity by 50 percent for at least six months. In addition, eight of eleven other features must be present, including moderate fever, swollen or tender lymph nodes, aches and pains in the head, throat, muscles, joints or elsewhere, sleep disturbance, and generalized muscle weakness.

Still, there is disagreement whether CFS is a single disease or a group of disorders that have disabling fatigue and other symptoms as a common consequence.

WHAT CAUSES CFS?

Originally, it was believed that CFS was a kind of chronic infection. The first candidate examined as a possible cause was the Epstein-Barr virus, which causes mononucleosis (another illness in which fatigue is prominent) as well as some malignancies. Most people with CFS show signs of exposure to Epstein-Barr, but so do most people who don't have CFS.

Other organisms suspected of a role in CFS have included a type of herpesvirus (HHV6), human T-cell lymphotropic virus, and a class of viruses called Spumavirus.

A currently favored explanation is that CFS is caused not by a single virus, but by an abnormal immune response to any of several viruses. In other words, lots of people may be exposed to Epstein-Barr or HHV6, but only someone whose immune system has a specific defect will develop CFS. It may be the immune reaction, not the viral infection itself, that produces the symptoms.

Another important discovery is a hormonal abnormality in many people with CFS, involving the complex process through which the body responds to stress. Ordinarily, the hypothalamus, a part of the brain, produces a hormone called corticotropin-releasing hormone (CRH). This stimulates the pituitary gland to secrete corticotropin, which leads to production of cortisol, the stress hormone, by the adrenals.

In a study that measured this group of hormones in eighteen women and twelve men with CFS, researchers found levels that were within the normal range, but significantly lower than those of a healthy comparison group. Further tests showed that the key deficiency was in the secretion of CRH by the hypothalamus (*Journal of Clinical Endocrinology and Metabolism*, December 1991).

IS CFS RELATED TO AIDS?

Noting that an abnormality of the immune system seems associated with CFS, some advocates and patient groups believe the disease should be renamed chronic fatigue immune dysfunction syndrome (CFIDS). Immune disorders have a frightening ring in the age of AIDS, and the suggestion by one researcher that a retrovirus (the same class of virus as the HIV that causes AIDS) plays a role in CFS wasn't reassuring.

Actually, the diseases have little in common. In AIDS, a virus decimates the immune system, killing helper T-cells necessary for defense against cancer and infection. The abnormality in CFS, on the other hand, appears to be *activation:* the subtle checks-and-balances system that govern the body's reaction to infection goes awry, and doesn't turn off naturally.

If anything, it seems that CFS resembles autoimmune disorders like inflammatory bowel disease. One study found that helper T-cells in people with CFS changed in ways that took them out of the bloodstream and into the tissues. In tissues like lymph nodes, muscles, and joints, messenger chemicals normally secreted by the T-cells to regulate immune function may cause inflammation and pain. A similar process is known to occur in inflammatory bowel disease (*Journal of Clinical Immunology,* January 1993).

ARE MY SYMPTOMS ALL IN MY HEAD?

The observation, in some studies, that people with CFS have higher rates of emotional symptoms, particularly depression, than the population as a whole has led many sufferers to feel their complaints were being dismissed as psychosomatic, and they as hypochondriacs or hysterics. The behavior of some doctors has done little to allay these fears.

Whenever psychiatric symptoms and chronic illness seem associated, the question of cause and effect becomes complex. CFS advocacy groups insist that depression is a consequence of the disease, not a cause.

Some researchers have agreed. A study reported in the British Journal of Psychiatry (1990, no. 156) found a high rate of major depression among CFS sufferers: twenty-two of forty-eight had had at least one episode since their illness began, and seven were clinically depressed at the time of the study. Before they got sick, however, just 12.5 percent of the group had a history of depression, and 24.5 percent a history of any psychiatric disorder. This, the authors note, is no more than in the community at large.

"We conclude that psychological disturbance is likely to be a consequence of, rather than an antecedent risk factor to the syndrome," they write.

On the other hand, there is reason to speculate that the connection between CFS and depression may go deeper. Fatigue, after all, is one of the principal symptoms of depression. And depression can have many forms. Sometimes, physical pain—of the sort common in CFS—is more prominent than emotional suffering. The thinking problems that are part of the definition of CFS—memory loss, confusion, difficulty concentrating—are frequent in depression, too. Sleep problems are common to both disorders.

Like CFS, depression is often associated with disruptions of immune function. And the hormonal abnormalities of chronic fatigue resemble closely those of the mood disorder.

Perhaps what needs closer scrutiny is the distinction—made by a good part of the medical profession as well as the public—between "physical" and "mental" illness, and the implication that anything related to a psychiatric disorder is "all in the mind." Depression has a physical basis, too—but it also has an unfair and unnecessary stigma that adds emotional resonance to what should be a scientific question.

IS THERE AN EFFECTIVE TREATMENT FOR CFS?

Studies of drugs for CFS have ranged from inconclusive to disappointing. Acyclovir, an antiviral drug that has been effective against genital herpes, shingles, and chicken pox, appears no more effective than a placebo in CFS. A single issue of the *American Journal of Medicine* (1990, no. 89) contained two articles about intravenous immune globulin for CFS: one found it significantly more effective than placebo, the other did not.

A highly publicized report suggested that Ampligen, an antiviral drug, could improve symptoms in people severely ill with CFS. The drug is still in clinical trials, and may cause serious side effects.

A study reported in *The Lancet* (March 30, 1991) found that levels of magnesium in red blood cells were slightly but significantly lower in twenty people with CFS than in healthy matched controls. In a clinical trial, twelve of fifteen people with CFS reported more energy, better mood, and less pain after six weeks of magnesium sulfate injections (compared with three of seventeen who had injections of water). This study was small, preliminary, and brief, its authors cautioned. Unsupervised megadoses of magnesium can be dangerous.

Low doses of antidepressants may improve the sleep disturbances that accompany CFS and may relieve pain, as they do in other kinds of chronic pain. Be cautious with antidepressants. The best-designed studies of their efficacy in the treatment of depression shows they are not much better than placebos. When used in the treatment of chronic pain, they are theoretically raising the pain threshold. Antidepressants usually take several weeks to take effect; if they don't, then discontinue usage.

CAN I DO ANYTHING TO FEEL BETTER?

In the absence of specific therapy, you're left with general lifestyle recommendations. Stress is both a consequence of any chronic, disruptive illness and a cause of magnified distress, so whatever relaxation or distraction techniques work for you are well worth the effort. Whether depression is the chicken or the egg, it deserves to be taken seriously. Get counseling or therapy.

Although no special diet has much effect on CFS, good nutrition, with limitations on caffeine and alcohol, is vital if you're sick.

Exercise is a two-edged sword. It may boost your energy and raise your mood, or lead to exhaustion and pain. Let your body be your guide, and if you want to increase your exercise output, do it gradually.

Resources

Call (800) 442-3437, the information hotline of the Chronic Fatigue and Immune Dysfunction Syndrome.

◆ CHRONIC OBSTRUCTIVE PULMONARY DISEASE (Bronchitis and Emphysema)

As its name suggests, chronic obstructive pulmonary disease (COPD) is a persistent condition that interferes with normal breathing. Emphysema, probably the most familiar type, is a progressive, irreversible destruction of the air sacs in the lung where the blood receives oxygen from the air and delivers carbon dioxide to be expelled from the body. The other aspect of COPD is chronic bronchitis: inflammation and swelling of air passages in the lung, which is often related to asthma. Usually, emphysema and bronchitis are both present at the same time.

If allowed to progress, COPD can be highly disabling. It can lead to heart failure, permanent changes in the heart, life-threatening infections, and death.

While other factors, such as occupational exposure and heredity, may be involved, what's clearly responsible for most COPD is cigarette smoking. A current smoker is ten times more likely to die of COPD than a nonsmoker.

CAN COPD BE CURED?

No. How effectively COPD can be treated symptomatically depends in large part on the stage at which it is detected. Small studies suggest that lung function returns quite rapidly if young smokers quit while still in the earliest stages of the disease. Lungs damaged by emphysema can never be restored, however, and changes in the heart and other organs are generally irreversible.

At virtually any stage, however, giving up smoking can apparently keep the damage from progressing further, and treatment may help make it possible to live more comfortably.

HOW CAN COPD BE SPOTTED IN ITS EARLY STAGES?

Rather than seeking a test to detect COPD early, change your lifestyle to protect your lungs. In addition to giving up smoking, avoid toxic chemicals, fumes, and dusts at home and in the workplace.

Shortness of breath (at first, after exertion, but later, at rest), fatigue, and persistent cough are the most frequent symptoms of COPD. But by the time they appear, the disease is already well advanced, irreversible damage has taken place, and lung function is compromised.

IS MY COPD HEREDITARY?

About 2 percent of people with emphysema have an inherited deficiency of alpha-1-antitrypsin (AAT), an enzyme that normally protects the lung. Regular intravenous infusions of a replacement enzyme are believed to prevent further lung damage, although this hasn't been proven in large clinical trials. There's no question of the importance of giving up smoking: the lungs of AAT-deficient people are exquisitely sensitive to the destructive effects of tobacco.

The blood test for AAT deficiency is relatively inexpensive: some experts recommend it for relatives of anyone known to have the disorder, nonsmokers with emphysema, and smokers younger than forty who already have airflow obstruction.

WHY SHOULD I STOP SMOKING IF MY LUNGS ARE ALREADY DAMAGED?

Giving up smoking is one of only two things documented to prolong life for people with COPD (the other is oxygen therapy).

Lung function normally declines gradually throughout life, as lungs lose their elasticity. One way to think of COPD is as a drastic acceleration of this process. As long as you smoke, you'll continue to lose lung tissue at a faster rate; once you stop, you'll lose it at the same rate as everyone else. The longer you wait before quitting, the less lung power you'll have to spare, and the faster you'll reach a point where breathing difficulties have a major effect on your life.

HOW MUCH HELP CAN I EXPECT FROM DRUGS?

The role that drugs play in COPD depends to a great extent on the relative contributions of emphysema and chronic bronchitis. Medications to open up the breathing passages (bronchodilators) are often helpful for the bronchitis component of COPD, but not for the emphysema.

Theophylline, a drug commonly prescribed for COPD, has some serious risks. It appears to improve the mechanics of breathing, as well as opening up airways. But theophylline becomes toxic at concentrations not much higher than the therapeutic range, particularly among older people with chronic lung disease. Other drugs can raise or lower the amount of theophylline in the blood. To be used safely, serum levels of theophylline must be checked regularly.

Corticosteroids apparently help 10 to 20 percent of people with COPD; some respond well, others not at all. These drugs are usually tried when bronchodilators fail. Taken orally, corticosteroids have serious systemic effects and should be used only when no infection is present, because they hide the signs of infection. Steroid inhalers cause fewer side effects than oral medication.

Not prescribed as widely, but potentially helpful, are drugs to control mucus production in the lungs, which often makes breathing more difficult. Iodated glycerol and guaifenesin (a familiar component of nonprescription cough syrups) can be effective aids in thinning mucus.

WHAT SYMPTOMS MERIT AN IMMEDIATE CALL TO A DOCTOR?

COPD can become dramatically worse very quickly, and effective treatment depends on knowing what causes the flare. Acute inflammation can be treated with steroids, but not if infection is causing it; in that case, antibiotics—and sometimes hospitalization—may be lifesaving. Any substantial worsening in breathing symptoms, and any fever, should be looked into promptly.

Lungs damaged by COPD are highly vulnerable to infection, particularly in the cold months. Flu shots are generally recommended. November is the best time. If you take the shot later, you won't be protected when the season starts; earlier, and protection will fade before flu season is over.

Some doctors also advocate vaccination against pneumococcus and *Hae-mophilus influenzae b,* but their effectiveness in COPD hasn't been shown.

CAN I LIVE AN ACTIVE LIFE WITH COPD?

A fear of the shortness of breath that accompanies COPD can lead to increasing inactivity, and this in turn causes deconditioning that worsens the symptoms and makes day-to-day activities more difficult. In the last two decades, the recognition that exercise can make a real difference in quality of life has led to more active rehabilitation efforts.

According to a review article in the *Mayo Clinic Proceedings* (February 1992), pulmonary rehabilitation programs focusing on exercise have been shown to produce real improvements in tolerance for activity. While pulmonary function itself rarely changes, people in such programs improve their aerobic capacity, their motivation, and their ability to take shortness of breath in stride. With time, they learn to walk and move more efficiently, so they can do more with their limited breathing capacity.

The kind of exercise that's best depends on the specifics of you and your illness. A person with relatively mild COPD can work out at levels of aerobic intensity not much lower than healthier folk. If the disease is more severe, exercise can be tailored to capacity.

Walking—on a treadmill, in the street, or in a shopping mall—is a safe, practical, and acceptable exercise for most people, and trains one specifically for activities essential for daily life. Workouts with a stationary bike or arm exercises can be useful for some people. Whatever you do, do it regularly—at least three times a week and preferably daily.

Particularly if your illness is at all severe or if you have become deconditioned from extended inactivity, a supervised program with a physical therapist can help you get through initial difficulties and anxieties.

If COPD is quite severe, exercise can be made easier—and its benefits brought within reach—with supplemental oxygen. In various trials, people with COPD could exercise longer and suffered less shortness of breath when they received oxygen.

Other aids for activities that might otherwise be taxing are some extra puffs on a bronchodilator, if you use one, or special breathing techniques, in which you breathe through pursed lips or use your diaphragm (most people breathe shallowly from the chest). These techniques have been shown to reduce shortness of breath in one half to three quarters of patients with severe disease.

SHOULD I BE ON A SPECIAL DIET?

Adequate nutrition is important in COPD, as in any chronic disease. Your body is already under stress, so make sure you get enough of all the essential vitamins, minerals, and protein. Obesity gives your breathing apparatus extra work to do. On the other hand, inadequate calories also affect respiration badly. Weight lost is difficult to put back on if you have COPD, so low-calorie diets are a poor idea.

As in any chronic disease, drug therapy may affect your nutritional needs: a person taking steroids, for example, should make sure to get adequate calcium and vitamin D. Discuss this with a nutritionist.

◆ COLORECTAL CANCER

Cancer of the rectum and large intestine is the second most common malignancy in the United States, and the second leading cause of cancer death. There are about 150,000 new cases diagnosed, and 60,000 deaths from colorectal cancer each year. More men die of the disease, but the toll on women is also high. According to the *Journal of the National Cancer Institute* (August 4, 1993), a sixty-five-year-old woman is as likely to die of colorectal cancer over the next twenty years as of breast cancer.

The rate of colorectal cancer, which had been on the rise for decades, is decreasing. Since 1973, deaths from the disease have declined by nearly 1 percent per year. According to the article referred to, much of the credit for this decline goes to healthier lifestyle and earlier detection.

Colorectal cancer is largely a disease of the later years. More than half of the people diagnosed with the disease are over seventy, and many deaths in subsequent years are due to other causes.

HOW SHOULD I BE CHECKED FOR COLORECTAL CANCER?

It is not clear whether early detection of colon cancer will reduce your chances of dying of this disease. Though screening tests have been advised for years, their value is unproven.

The National Cancer Institute has begun recruitment for a randomized clinical trial to determine whether screening—the testing of symptomless people—for colon cancer with frequent checkups and various tests will save lives. The trial will compare the colon cancer death rates of older people who received regular screening tests with those who did not. Unfortunately, the results of this trial will not be ready before 2005.

The simplest screening test is for occult (hidden) blood in the stool. Stool samples are applied to specially treated paper, and examined in the laboratory. Occult blood is an early sign of cancer (as well as many other things) and, when detected, should be followed up by further investigation. Research into the effectiveness of this approach has been inconsistent.

Occult blood screening is quick, easy, and inexpensive, but far from perfect: it misses some cancers and precancerous growths, and thus suggests the need for further testing in a substantial number of people who actually have no tumors. A study in the *Journal of the American Medical Association* (March 10, 1993) called fecal occult blood "at best a flawed screening marker for colorectal neoplasia."

Like all screening tests, this one identifies only something worthy of further evaluation. In that event, the next step is usually a sigmoidoscopy. This is an office procedure, which involves the insertion of either a rigid or flexible endoscope (viewing tube) through rectum and into the colon. It provides a visual examination of the lining of the rectum and the lower portion of the colon. According to the 1993 *Journal of the National Cancer Institute* editorial, some case-control studies suggest that regular sigmoidoscopy (the sigmoid is the last part of the colon, where half of colorectal cancers occur) may cut the rate of death from colorectal cancer by as much as half. The National Cancer Institute's screening trial is designed to answer questions about the role of sigmoidoscopy.

Sigmoidoscopy is considerably more expensive than the occult blood test. Colonoscopy, which inspects the full length of the large intestine, will detect still more cancers. But because of the cost and invasiveness of this procedure, it is generally reserved for follow-up when the occult blood test points to the need for further investigation.

Of all colon cancers, 90 percent are diagnosed in people older than age fifty-five. The U.S. Preventive Health Services Task Force recommends either the occult blood test annually for all people over age fifty or sigmoidoscopy or both. The Task Force did not determine the appropriate interval for a sigmoidoscopy. There is some evidence that people with a family history of colon cancer should start screening earlier.

IF I HAVE COLORECTAL POLYPS, WILL I GET CANCER?

The assumption has been that colorectal cancer begins as a benign polyp or adenoma—a growth on the colon wall—which becomes malignant. But the picture may actually be more complicated. According to an analysis in *Annals of Internal Medicine* (January 1, 1993), an estimated 725,000 Americans harbor a malignant polyp. Some of these, the author proposes, remain latent for many years. And in many cases of actual cancer, the polyp was malignant from the beginning.

It is estimated that one in three persons over age fifty has colon polyps, and almost all of them never develop into cancer. According to an editorial in the same issue of *Annals,* just 8 percent of larger polyps become malignant in the course of a decade, and "people with small (under 1 centimeter) tubular adenomas discovered at sigmoidoscopy have a very low long-term risk for developing colorectal cancer."

The presence of polyps should be regarded as a risk factor, to be taken into account in planning and scheduling screening procedures. According to an article in the *British Medical Journal* (June 26, 1993), a consensus panel recommended that polyps over five millimeters be removed if they are causing symptoms, and that colonoscopy be repeated every three to five years subsequently.

IF THERE'S CANCER IN MY FAMILY, WILL I GET IT?

The susceptibility to colorectal cancer clearly can run in families: an estimated 15 percent of cases occur in families where the disease is widespread. If you have a close relative with the disease, your risk of getting colorectal cancer is twice that of someone without a family history. If you have two relatives with colorectal cancer, your risk is even higher, particularly if the relatives were diagnosed with the disease before age forty-five, according to *Annals of Internal Medicine* (May 15, 1993).

Mutations in a number of different genes have been identified as causes of colon cancer. Recently, researchers located a gene on chromosome 2 that appears to be involved in a large number of familial cancers, and perhaps in some apparently isolated cases as well. In time, it should be possible to screen members of high-risk families—and, when the gene is located more exactly, the general population—to see who carries the mutation (*Science,* May 7, 1993).

Having the gene doesn't mean you're destined for colorectal cancer, but it does mean that you should have more frequent tests to catch cancer at an early stage, should it develop. It should also motivate you to take seriously some of the preventive measures suggested here.

WHAT ELSE CAN PUT ME AT RISK?

Certain bowel diseases, particularly the inflammatory disorder called ulcerative colitis, carry a substantially increased risk of colorectal cancer, and careful surveillance should be part of their management. In addition, anyone who has had one colorectal cancer is at heightened risk of another.

Apparently, the susceptibility to cancers in the colon and to cancers elsewhere in the body are sometimes linked. A study in *Cancer* (May 1, 1991) found increased rates of breast, prostate, uterine, ovary, and bladder malignancies in people who have had colorectal cancer, suggesting that these diseases may have some common causes. Overall, the study concluded, the risk of other cancers increased by 30 to 40 percent.

Conversely, having had a malignancy elsewhere may increase your chances of colorectal cancer. Several studies, for example, have suggested that a woman with breast cancer is 1.5 to 2.5 times more likely to develop colorectal cancer (*Cancer,* February 1, 1989).

HOW CAN I LOWER MY RISK?

There is substantial evidence that connects diet to the risk of colorectal cancer. Fats, particularly saturated fats, appear to increase incidence; fruits, vegetables, and whole grains seem to bring it down.

A meta-analysis of thirteen studies, which compared 5,287 people with colorectal and 10,470 controls, found that those who consumed the most fiber (a component of fruits, vegetables, and grains, but not meat or dairy products) had about half the cancer risk of those who had consumed the least amounts. The authors estimated that if everyone in the country increased their fiber intake by 70 percent, the cancer rate would fall by nearly one third (*Journal of the National Cancer Institute,* December 16, 1992).

Another study (*Journal of the National Cancer Institute,* October 7, 1992), which followed nearly seven thousand people for six years, found that the risk of dying from colorectal cancer was about one quarter lower in men and one third lower in women who had the highest fiber intake.

Other researchers have examined the association between diet and possibly precancerous polyps. They have found significantly lower incidence of these lesions in people who consumed more fruits, vegetables, grains, and fiber, and a higher incidence in those who ate more red meat.

A diet high in fiber, lower in fat, and where fruits, vegetables, and grains largely replace meat, has been widely advocated to reduce risk of other diseases, too, such as coronary heart disease.

There's evidence that taking aspirin, which has also been recommended as a heart protection strategy, may reduce colorectal cancer risk, too. A six-year prospective study of 662,424 men and women found that death rates from colorectal cancer were about 40 percent lower in those who took aspirin sixteen or more times per month, for at least one year (*The New England Journal of Medicine,* December 5, 1991).

Other epidemiological studies have found similar reductions in people who often take nonsteroidal anti-inflammatory drugs (NSAIDs), which, like aspirin, inhibit the production of chemical messengers called prostaglandins.

It may be that aspirin and diet can work together, synergistically, to lower risk still further. In one study, men and women who consumed the most fruits, vegetables, and whole grains, and took sixteen or more aspirins monthly were more than two and a half times less likely to die of colorectal cancer than those who ate least of those healthful foods and took no aspirin.

Physical activity may also be protective. In a study reported in the *Journal of the National Cancer Institute* (September 18, 1991), 17,148 Harvard male alumni were followed for twenty-three years. Those who were highly active (more than 2,500 calories per week expended in stair climbing, walking, and sports) and those who were moderately active (more than 1,000 calories expended per week), when questioned on two occasions, ten or more years apart, had half the risk of colon cancer of those who were inactive. Activity seemed to offer no protection against rectal cancer, however. (Rectal cancer refers to cancer in the six to eight-inch terminal portion of the large intestine as it connects to the anus.)

IF I HAVE CANCER, HOW EFFECTIVE IS SURGERY?

Resection—removal of the cancer and the part of the colon or rectum to which it has spread—is the standard treatment for colorectal cancer. About 60 percent of people are considered curable by this operation at the time their cancers are detected, according to a study reported in the *British*

Medical Journal (September 18, 1993). Among 421 people considered to have curable cancer, three quarters were alive, or had died without recurrence, seven years later.

The *British Medical Journal* study also indicated that improved surgery has reduced the mortality of the procedure itself significantly: 9 percent of patients operated on in 1968–1969 died, compared with 5 percent in 1980–1982. Deaths during surgery are far more frequent in older people (the average age of those dying in the study was seventy-seven), and are almost always due to cardiovascular complications.

The extent of the operation depends on how far cancer has progressed. If it hasn't spread to the bowel wall, just the tumor itself may be excised; in more advanced cases, parts of the colon or rectum, lymph nodes in the area, or affected portions of the liver may also need to be removed. In recent decades, surgical techniques have progressed to the point that the rectal sphincter can be preserved most of the time, making it easier to live normally after surgery as a colostomy is not necessary.

When cancer has spread to the point where it's no longer considered curable, "palliative" surgery may be offered to extend life and relieve symptoms. In the *British Medical Journal* study, 24 of 133 people who had such surgery for advanced cancer lived two years or longer, and many more reported symptom relief until near the time of death. Among the twenty-four with advanced cancer who declined surgery, none survived more than eleven months.

WILL CHEMOTHERAPY HELP IN MY CASE?

The effectiveness of chemotherapy is uncertain. The support for this approach is stronger for stage III disease, when the malignancy has spread to regional lymph nodes. In a randomized trial, 49 percent of people with this stage of cancer who received combination chemotherapy starting within five weeks after surgery survived for five years, compared with 37 percent who had surgery alone. Other studies confirm that chemotherapy improves both disease-free survival and total survival. The 12 percent advantage shown for the treated group should be weighed against the potential adverse effects of chemotherapy. Check for possible effects in the *Physicians' Desk Reference,* a popular textbook on prescription drugs, available at most local libraries and at major bookstores. Preliminary results from a randomized, controlled study in the Netherlands found no benefit to chemotherapy for people with colon cancer that has spread to the lymph nodes (*Journal of the National Cancer Institute*, April 5, 1995).

For less-advanced cancer, the argument for chemotherapy is on shakier ground. Even without it, 70 to 80 percent of people with stage II cancer (the tumor has spread through the bowel wall, but apparently no further) will survive for five years, and about half of those who don't, have died of other causes. The National Cancer Institute recommends that, in general, people with this stage of cancer be offered chemotherapy only as part of a clinical trial, if at all. This recommendation indicates that chemotherapy for stage II cancer would be experimental. Some specific types of tumors, however, may more clearly benefit from chemotherapy or radiation.

People with even earlier stages of cancer are not candidates for chemotherapy; those with more advanced cancer have not been shown to live longer.

In weighing outcome studies, keep in mind that "five-year survival" is the same as cure. When doctors quote a five-year survival rate for a proposed chemotherapy regimen, it simply refers to the number of cancer patients alive five years after diagnosis. It does not mean they are in remission, nor does it take into account quality of life.

Resources

Use CancerFax to receive a printout on breast cancer from the computerized data base of the National Cancer Institute. You will need access to a fax machine with an attached telephone. Dial (301) 402-5874 on a touchtone phone and receive a faxed report on state-of-the-art treatments for breast cancer. Request the physicians' version.

◆ COMMON COLD

Just because the common cold isn't serious doesn't mean it can't make you miserable. The sneezing, congestion, runny nose, and fever are responsible for more illness-related days lost from school and work than any other disease.

A cold is a viral infection of the mucous membranes lining the nose and throat. As so often is the case, it's not the virus itself that causes the suffering, but the body's self-defense maneuvers: sneezing, coughing, and runny nose are the body's way of getting the virus out; inflammation, a part of the immune response, is responsible for nasal congestion; and fever (which is more common in children's colds) is intended to kill the virus.

A cold can be caused by any of two hundred different viruses, but about one third are caused by one family, the "rhinoviruses." This accounts for the fact that children and adolescents generally get so many more colds than adults (nine or so per year, versus two to three). The older you are, the more viruses you've already met up with, and your immune system is prepared to fight off. The diversity of cold-causing viruses also means little hope for a vaccine to prevent colds.

DO I NEED A DOCTOR'S TREATMENT FOR A COLD?

No. The vast majority of colds are self-limited; for example, they go away by themselves (generally within a week) no matter what you do for them. There's no drug—OTC or prescription—that has been shown to kill cold-causing viruses or shorten the duration of the illness. For most colds, a doctor visit is hardly worth the trouble or expense.

If, however, you have a chronic disease (like bronchitis) that lends itself to complications, a visit, or at least a call to your doctor is justified.

In addition, you should call the doctor if deep breathing is painful (it could be a chest infection like pleurisy). If throat soreness is severe (or if you've been exposed to someone with the disease), you could have a strep throat, which may need antibiotics. A continued fever (especially in an adult) suggests that the cold may have led to bacterial infection like sinusitis.

ARE ANTIBIOTICS EVER PRESCRIBED FOR A COLD?

No. Colds, being viral diseases, are unaffected by antibiotics. Some doctors may prescribe them prophylactically to reduce the possibility of complications, but this is a bad idea. For one thing, it's never been shown that prophylactic antibiotics (given either to cold sufferers or their family members) actually prevent bacterial infections on top of the cold. It makes more sense to wait until there's some sign that such an infection has developed, like an earache or sinus pain, and then to treat it.

What's more, if you're taking antibiotics prophylactically, and *then* develop a bacterial infection, the chances are good that the organism will be resistant and harder to treat. In addition, antibiotics can cause irritating side effects—stomach upset, diarrhea, yeast infections—which aren't likely to make your cold any easier to tolerate.

WHAT OTC DRUGS ARE RECOMMENDED?

A review of twenty-seven well-designed controlled clinical trials of cold remedies was published in the *Journal of the American Medical Association* (May 5, 1993). Overall, the researchers reported, no studies found that such remedies improved symptoms in preschool children. In older children, adolescents, and adults, some appeared effective, but many did not.

For example, three studies found that the antihistamine chlorpheniramine reduced sneezing, nasal mucus, and general symptoms, but one study did not. And other studies of two other antihistamines, diphenhydramine and triprolidine hydrochloride, found no more benefit than a placebo.

The decongestants pseudoephedrine and phenylpropanolamine reduced nasal congestion, as did the nasal spray oxymetazoline, while another nasal spray, tramazoline, did not.

There were virtually no studies of cough medicines that met quality criteria for the article, the authors wrote. One trial of guaifenesin, an expectorant, found that it thinned mucus in some people, but didn't reduce the amount of coughing.

ARE OTC MEDICATIONS HARMFUL?

Many common cold remedies have side effects. With antihistamines, drowsiness, dry mouth, and constipation are common. About 30 percent of people using decongestants experienced side effects in the studies reviewed in the article referred to: these tended to be insomnia, nervousness, and irritability. Children are likely to suffer side effects like hyperexcitability with both antihistamines and decongestants.

Antihistamine side effects aren't apt to be dangerous, unless you unwisely drive when the drug has made you sleepy. Not everyone realizes that antihistamines can greatly magnify the effects of alcohol. Don't take a cold pill, drink (even a little) and then drive.

The side effects of decongestant pills are potentially more of a problem. Even the standard dose can greatly elevate blood pressure, and strokes have been reported as a result. If you have heart disease, thyroid disease, or diabetes, or are taking prescription medication, check with the doctor before using a decongestant.

Decongestants in nasal spray form cause fewer side effects and, because they're delivered right to where they're needed, are more effective. But they're particularly likely to bring about "rebound congestion"—as the cells in your nose adapt to them, you'll be even more congested than before—if you use them for more than two to three days.

Many cold remedies come in combination pills that include an antihistamine, a decongestant, and possibly something for fever, aches, and pains. There's no advantage to this arrangement, except for people who find taking pills an intolerable chore. The disadvantage is that you'll be taking drugs you probably don't need, and run the risk of extra side effects you *certainly* don't need. Try to match the drug to your symptoms and buy it generically or as a store brand product. You will save money.

If you do take a number of remedies, keep track of the ingredients in each one. Some cough syrups contain an antihistamine, for example; if you add a cold pill, you may easily exceed the recommended dose.

CAN COLD REMEDIES MAKE SYMPTOMS WORSE OR LAST LONGER?

A runny nose is the body's attempt to flush out cold viruses, so there's logic in letting it run (as long as you can stand it). Antihistamines could conceivably lengthen the cold by undermining this self-defense mechanism, but since these drugs aren't terribly effective for colds, the risk is minimal. Some doctors are concerned that antihistamines can increase the risk of ear infection by drying out mucous membranes.

Questions have been raised for years about the possibly counterproductive effect of taking aspirin or other fever-reducing medications for a cold. In a study reported in the *Journal of Infectious Diseases* (December 1990), fifty-six people were intentionally given colds, and randomized to groups that took aspirin, acetaminophen, ibuprofen, or placebo.

Antibody levels were reduced in both the aspirin and acetaminophen group, and these people also had more severe symptoms, including nasal membrane swelling and congestion, than those who took placebo. People who took aspirin or acetaminophen continued to shed virus longer, too, but the difference wasn't significant.

One study in *Annals of Internal Medicine* (July 1, 1992), suggested that naproxen, a drug that like aspirin reduces pain, fever, and inflammation, may not have this drawback. In a randomized, double-blind, controlled trial, seventy-nine people were infected with colds and given naproxen or placebo. A 29 percent reduction in overall symptoms was seen in the drug-receiving group—in particular, improvements in headache, muscle pain, and cough—but no change in viral shedding or immune responses. (Naproxen was recently approved for OTC use by the FDA.)

CAN HOME REMEDIES HELP?

Often, nondrug remedies offer as much relief as medications. The traditional advice of drinking a lot of fluids—eight to ten glasses a day—can thin mucus and reduce congestion.

Even the old standby, chicken soup, has some research support. One study found that it speeded the flow of mucus, theoretically aiding the removal of virus from the body. Another demonstrated, in the laboratory, that samples of chicken soup reduced part of the immune response that causes inflammation. In theory, these effects would reduce cold symptoms and shorten their duration, but this bottom-line benefit hasn't been documented.

HOW CAN I KEEP FROM CATCHING A COLD?

Nasty weather, changes in temperature, even wet feet won't give you a cold. You catch a cold by exposure to a cold virus that you haven't encountered before. Although this could be in droplets sprayed your way by an inconsiderate sneezer, more often, it's by hand-to-hand contact with nasal secretions. A person with a cold touches his eyes, mouth, or the inside of the nose. You shake hands with that person, or touch an object he has touched, and bring the virus home when you rub your nose or eyes. The best defense is frequent hand washing. And, if you can remember (few people can), keep your hands away from your face.

Because colds are contagious for a day before symptoms appear (as well as two to three days after), it's impossible to know for sure who can give it to you.

A factor that seems to reduce our ability to fight off colds is stress. In one study, nearly four hundred people were intentionally exposed to cold viruses. Those who had scored high in tests of psychosocial stress (they were asked about distressing events of the past year, their ability to cope, and their current feelings) were nearly twice as likely to develop cold symptoms as those who scored low (*The New England Journal of Medicine*, August 29, 1991).

WILL VITAMIN C PREVENT COLDS?

Although this belief has held on tenaciously for decades, there's little scientific reason to believe it. Controlled trials of up to 2,000 milligrams daily haven't reduced the frequency of colds.

On the other hand, a better case can be made for the ability of vitamin C to lessen cold symptoms and hasten their departure. Many people feel that taking 1,000 milligrams or more of vitamin C daily, as soon as they feel the first cold symptoms, means shorter, less miserable colds. Short-term use of vitamin C in daily doses up to 4,000 milligrams is safe.

WHAT ELSE CAN I TRY?

Echinacea, an herb that can be taken as a tincture or a tea, is said to have antiviral properties. Zinc gluconate, which can also be purchased at most health food stores, has been shown in a clinical trial to reduce the duration of a cold by seven days. The problem here is the zinc supplements containing 23 milligrams of zinc gluconate must be sucked for ten minutes every two hours. The taste is bad, and efforts to disguise it with citrus or other flavorings will interfere with efficacy.

Don't bother buying one of those steam machines to raise the intranasal temperature ("hair dryer for the nose"). Two controlled clinical trials proved this method to be useless (*Journal of the American Medical Association,* April 13, 1994).

✦ CONGESTIVE HEART FAILURE

Congestive heart failure (CHF) isn't as catastrophic as the name implies. The heart doesn't stop beating (that's cardiac arrest); what it fails to do is maintain adequate circulation throughout the body.

The consequences of CHF can be severe enough to be disabling, however, and eventually fatal. It affects an estimated two to three million Americans, about one third of whom must be hospitalized each year—the most common reason for hospitalization among people over sixty-five. More than half of people with severe CHF die within a year of their diagnosis.

Not long ago, CHF was regarded as inevitably progressive; the disease could only get worse, you'd get more disabled, and eventually, you'd die of it. The last fifteen years have changed that. Research has sharpened our understanding of CHF, and drug therapy has made it possible not only to halt the deterioration of CHF, but to reverse it.

Centers that have put modern findings into practice (such as the one at Columbia-Presbyterian Medical Center, New York) report mortality rates as much as 25 percent lower than elsewhere.

HOW CAN I TELL IF I HAVE HEART FAILURE?

The earliest symptoms of CHF are typically shortness of breath during exercise and sometimes at night, and general fatigue. A lingering cold or cough aren't uncommon. The change may be subtle: you have more trouble climbing stairs than you used to; you avoid strenuous activity; you may have swelling caused by retained fluid (edema).

A physical examination may point to CHF, but the most effective way to diagnose it is with echocardiography, a modern imaging technique that uses ultrasound to reveal the size, shape, and condition of the heart. Exercise testing can clarify the diagnosis.

More than half the time, CHF is caused by coronary heart disease: damage caused by a heart attack leaves the heart unable to pump adequately, or severe heart disease without an acute attack might have weak-ened the left ventricle (the main pumping chamber of the heart) gradually.

Hypertension is also common in people who eventually get CHF. Im-proper functioning of the heart valves is sometimes responsible, and pro-longed, heavy alcohol consumption may be the cause of some cases. Between 20 and 30 percent of the time, no cause can be identified, ac-cording to an article in *Patient Care* (April 15, 1991).

WHAT DRUGS ARE PRESCRIBED FOR CHF?

Ten or twenty years ago, the aim of CHF treatment was to ease symp-toms—it was all doctors thought they could do. Today, however, it's been shown that drug treatment can do more: improve quality of life, reduce mortality, lessen the need for hospitalization, slow the progression of the disease, and even reverse it.

One important discovery was that some drugs that help symptoms and seem to improve heart function in the short run have poor long-term effects, while others that seem to do little immediate good have positive long-range benefits. Chosen wisely, drugs can improve symptoms *and* get at the basic disease. The goal of treatment, according to an article in *The American Journal of Cardiology* (June 4, 1992), should be "to improve both the quality and the quantity of life."

The drugs that seem to offer most in both these areas are the angio-tensin converting enzyme inhibitors (ACE inhibitors). These drugs (the most familiar are captopril and enalapril), were originally used to treat high blood pressure. In addition to easing the symptoms of CHF, they apparently reduce the enzymes that the body oversecretes in compensation for failing circulation, that make the situation progressively worse.

One major study was halted early when it was found that enalapril reduced mortality in severe CHF by more than 40 percent, compared to placebo. Another study found a 16 percent reduction of mortality among people with mild to moderate heart failure; the drug also slowed the worsening of symptoms and led to less hospitalization. A meta-analysis of twenty-eight trials found that only ACE inhibitors, among drugs tested, both reduced deaths and improved the ability to function (*Journal of the American Medical Association,* April 8, 1994).

As a result of these positive findings, the combination of ACE inhibitors, digoxin (which makes the heart pump more strongly), and diuretics (to get rid of retained fluid) has become the standard therapy for CHF in a number of medical centers.

Beta-blockers, drugs that are used primarily for high blood pressure and angina, were long avoided for people with CHF; they reduce the heart's response to stimulatory chemicals like adrenalin, which is part of the body's compensation for the heart's diminished pumping capacity. At usual doses, they can make CHF symptoms worse.

A number of studies have found, however, that a lower dose of beta-blockers can be helpful for some people with CHF. A Swedish trial, for example, reported that adding beta-blockers to standard therapy improved quality of life, reduced the need for hospitalization, and made fewer heart transplants necessary.

Here, too, the drug apparently acts paradoxically. By making the heart less responsive to increased adrenalin, it short-circuits a cycle that ordinarily makes heart function worse and worse (*Patient Care,* August 15, 1993). Research supporting the use of beta-blockers is far less compelling than that for ACE inhibitors, and they appear to be appropriate only for some people with CHF.

The latest addition is flosequinan, which was recently approved by the FDA as a treatment for heart failure. It dilates both arteries and veins (the first drug to do so) and apparently improves response when added to other drugs, but whether it will further reduce mortality has yet to be seen.

All the research clarifying the effects of various drugs hasn't reached many doctors, however. At the 1993 scientific meeting of the American Heart Association, it was reported that calcium channel blockers are prescribed in one third of cases of CHF, despite the fact that these drugs have been shown to worsen symptoms and increase the risk of serious episodes. Despite evidence of their value, on the other hand, beta blockers are used only 5 percent of the time.

CAN DRUG TREATMENT PREVENT CHF?

Several studies are, at this writing, still in progress to determine whether early medication can prevent CHF. In one, people who have a reduced ejection fraction (a test that shows the heart isn't pumping normally) but as yet no signs of CHF, are being given the ACE inhibitor enalapril, and compared with a placebo group to see whether symptoms appear. In another, two thousand people will be started on an ACE inhibitor or placebo shortly after a heart attack (which frequently precedes CHF), and followed for some years.

Positive findings from these and similar studies could have a significant impact on rates of—and deaths from—CHF.

Prevention is on many minds these days—as it should be. Noting that coronary heart disease is the most common cause of CHF, an editorial in *The American Journal of Cardiology* (March 1, 1993) suggested the second heart attack could be best forestalled by preventing the first. "I suspect that more congestive heart failure will be prevented by lipid-lowering medicines earlier than will be helped by the more conventional anticongestive heart failure medicines later," the editor wrote.

CAN EXERCISE HELP CHF?

Fatigue and shortness of breath limit the ability of people with CHF to be active, and this has a serious impact on quality of life. According to an article in the *British Heart Journal* (1992, no. 67), CHF apparently affects the muscles themselves, making them less responsive and less able to metabolize oxygen.

For many years, it was thought that exercise training could impair heart function further and make symptoms worse. But more recently, a number of studies have shown that exercise, if planned properly, could benefit even people with severe CHF, with limited risk.

In one controlled crossover study that compared an exercise program to activity restriction, eleven people with moderate to severe heart failure (caused by coronary heart disease) significantly increased the length of time they could remain active, as well as their peak oxygen consumption (a measurement of aerobic condition), over an eight-week training period. Their heart rate slowed (another sign of improved fitness), and their general symptoms improved significantly, too.

"The authors conclude that simple home-based training is a feasible and effective way to improve fitness, exercise tolerance, and symptoms in patients with moderate to severe heart failure, secondary to ischemic heart disease," the researchers wrote (*Chest*, May 1992).

They pointed out, however, that exercise could be dangerous for some

people with heart failure (such as those with certain heart rhythm disturbances) and urged that its use "be determined on an individual basis and
used with caution."

Especially if heart failure is severe, exercise must be tailored carefully
to the individual. Most people can exercise safely at home, without supervision, but it may be important to monitor heart rate for safety's sake.

Although some researchers think that a regular exercise schedule can
reverse some of the biochemical changes that make CHF progressively
worse, and may even prolong life, this hasn't yet been shown.

WHEN SHOULD HEART TRANSPLANT BE CONSIDERED?

Improvements in recent decades have made heart transplant a far safer and
more effective procedure that can be done in centers across the country.
It is reserved, however, for the 10 to 15 percent of people whose severe
CHF is unresponsive to medical treatment, and who face death without
the surgery.

Although some suggest that earlier transplantation would spare other
organs the cumulative damage of impaired circulation, the scarcity of hearts
for transplant will probably keep this a last-chance option for the foresee-
able future.

◆ CORONARY HEART DISEASE
(Diagnosis and Treatment)

A half century ago, there wasn't much to be done once you had coronary heart disease. You'd probably be given nitroglycerin to ease your angina (the chest pain that occurs when too little blood gets to the heart). If you had a heart attack and survived, you'd be advised to retire, take it easy, and, in effect, wait for the inevitable.

Things couldn't be more different today. There's a whole arsenal of drugs to keep the heart functioning as normally as possible. Surgery to replace vessels blocked by atherosclerosis has become commonplace, and ingenious procedures to open up affected vessels without major surgery are increasingly popular. Most exciting of all, there's the evidence diet and exercise can actually reverse the process of heart disease.

As so often happens in medicine, however, practice runs far ahead of research—and sometimes in a different direction. To choose between options in a confusing, life-or-death field, you have to know the facts.

DO I HAVE HEART DISEASE?

Whether chest pains are intense or relatively mild, the idea that they herald heart disease is always terrifying. But a surprising percentage of the time, the source of the pain isn't your heart at all. Many people have added needless anxiety and pointless medication to their pain because the true cause wasn't diagnosed. In a nationwide survey of six hundred thousand angiograms—dye-assisted X ray to investigate chest pain—the coronary arteries were normal in as many as 30 percent of cases.

About half the time, according to a study in *Annals of Internal Medicine* (January 1, 1989), these people have gastroesophageal reflux—the back-flow of stomach juices into the esophagus, which ordinarily causes heartburn (see Heartburn).

Prosaic as it sounds, acid reflux (possibly along with the esophageal spasm it triggers) can cause pain that's an easy match for angina in severity. (Angina is the chest pain caused by constricted coronary arteries.) It can be brought on by exercise, just like angina, or by emotional distress. And it can't be distinguished without appropriate tests.

What's more, just because you have one condition doesn't mean you can't have the other. A study reported in *Annals of Internal Medicine* (1992, 117:824–30) described thirty-four people with documented heart disease who continued having chest pain despite surgery or aggressive medication. In twenty cases, some of this pain was found to be caused by gastroesophageal reflux; thirteen improved substantially after eight weeks of treatment to suppress acid production in the stomach.

Another cause of chest pain that can be hard to distinguish from angina—or even heart attack—is panic disorder (see Anxiety). According to an article in *American Family Physician* (September 1992), more than one third of people who have chest pain and whose coronary arteries are normal on arteriography suffer from this disorder.

Other heart disease mimics include drugs (either licit, like the migraine drug ergotamine, or illicit, like cocaine and amphetamines) and certain kinds of osteoarthritis of the upper spine.

AM I GETTING OPTIMAL MEDICATION?

Medication and surgery are the usual options for heart disease severe enough to cause pain. The most common prescriptions include nitrates that open up coronary arteries, allowing more blood to reach the heart; and beta-blockers and calcium channel blockers, both of which reduce the heart's need for oxygen. If used properly (usually in some kind of combination), they relieve symptoms effectively and make normal life possible for many people.

But drugs are not used properly—or, in any case, optimally—much of the time, according to Dr. Thomas B. Graboys, the cardiologist who directs the Harvard-affiliated Lown Cardiovascular Center in Brookline, Massachusetts. Many of the hundreds of people referred to his clinic for treatment-resistant angina simply haven't had the right kind of medication—or, in some cases, any medication.

"When we bring these people into the hospital and put them on the right medication, the so-called refractory unstable angina goes away," Dr. Graboys said in an interview.

WHAT DOES A SURGICAL PROCEDURE OFFER ME THAT MEDICATION DOESN'T?

Coronary bypass surgery, in which healthy blood vessels are grafted into the heart's circulation to bypass obstructed coronary arteries, has become a widespread treatment for heart disease: 368,000 bypass operations were performed in 1989, up from 137,000 a decade earlier. It's major surgery that requires a substantial hospital stay and lengthy recuperation. And it's not cheap: at forty thousand dollars each, it adds significantly to the nation's health-care bill.

There's an alternative procedure to open up the coronaries that's less invasive, less traumatic, and less expensive than bypass: angioplasty. In angioplasty, a catheter is threaded into the affected artery and a tiny balloon is expanded to squeeze and break up the fatty deposits that are blocking the arteries. The rise of angioplasty has been even more spectacular: in 1980, 5,000 were done; in 1989, that number had risen to 258,796.

Both of these procedures do what drug therapy tries to do, and they customarily do it well: they relieve the symptoms of heart disease, notably angina. But neither *cures* heart disease any more than medications do. The disease process continues; arteries that were not operated on are unimproved. If coronary spasm is responsible for angina, the operation may have little effect on that condition. Sooner or later, the same arteries may become blocked again—what doctors call *restenosis.*

After angioplasty, restenosis often occurs sooner than later. It has been reported that 40 percent of treated arteries are constricted again in six months. And according to a 1992 article in the *Journal of the American College of Cardiology,* restenosis is probably inevitable in everyone who has angioplasty. An editorial accompanying that study called restenosis "probably . . . a fundamental healing or scarring process that is a limitation inherent to the procedure itself."

Although angioplasty is safer than bypass surgery—the mortality rate, 3 percent, is conspicuously low for this field of endeavor—it's not risk free. Angioplasty can trigger a heart attack or may require emergency bypass surgery. It has also become clear, as more women undergo angioplasty, that women's mortality rate is higher than men's: 5 percent.

Whether the risk, the hospitalization, and the expense are worth it probably comes down to the question: will having bypass surgery or angioplasty prolong life or prevent a heart attack?

A person with demonstrated narrowing of coronary vessels may be told he or she is "sitting on a time bomb," risking death without the surgery. It certainly makes sense. But in fact, repeated studies have confirmed that for most people, surgical procedures have no such advantage over medication. "There are no data to prove that the patient will live longer or is less likely to have a heart attack by having the procedure, as opposed to just continuing drug therapy," Dr. Graboys says of angioplasty.

Even people who have had a heart attack, recovered with the help of clot-dissolving drugs, and are now symptom-free but still have an artery blockage won't necessarily benefit from angioplasty. A large, randomized study in *The New England Journal of Medicine* (March 11, 1993) found that they did *better* just taking medication.

Angioplasty or bypass can indeed prolong life and prevent heart attack under some circumstances—in particular, when the left main coronary artery is blocked, or when severe symptoms of heart disease persist despite medication. Ask your doctor to demonstrate whether this applies in your case.

HOW CAN I GET A SECOND OPINION?

As Dr. Graboys wrote in a paper in the *Journal of the American Medical Association* (November 11, 1992), doctors are doing angioplasty and surgery far more readily than before: "Evident over the past decade is the ever-lowering threshold for carrying out bypass as well as angioplasty. Initially, these interventions were justified for severe or intractable angina pectoris. At present, even symptomless patients are not exempt."

In an atmosphere of rampant medical enthusiasm, a second opinion can offer at least some protection. To minimize the likelihood that the second opinion will simply rubber-stamp the first, don't go to another cardiac surgeon. A cardiologist who *doesn't* do angioplasty may be a good choice.

HOW MIGHT TESTING RESULT IN BETTER TREATMENT?

Always a good question; in the area of heart disease it's essential. Cardiology has become a technology festival in recent years, and expensive, often invasive, tests have proliferated. They all can tell the doctor something about the state of your heart and circulation, but not all of this information has practical value in all cases. Just because the doctor is there, you're there, and your health insurance is there doesn't mean that everything possible should be done.

It's more than just a question of trouble and expense. An unnecessary test all too easily leads to an unnecessary operation. This is a particular risk with angiography, in which dye is injected, through a catheter, to make the coronary arteries visible on X ray. When the test reveals a blockage in the artery, this quickly becomes characterized as a "time bomb," with angioplasty the logical next step.

It's easier to keep the cautions of the preceding few pages in mind before the doctor tells you what bad shape your coronary arteries are in. Dr. Graboys says that many angiograms aren't in fact indicated, and avoiding them is the best way to keep out of the operating room. He urges getting a second opinion *before* you undergo angiography.

HOW CAN I ADOPT A HEALTHIER LIFESTYLE?

Many people seem to think that once they've developed heart disease, it's too late for a healthy diet, exercise, and stress reduction to do any good. Their doctors apparently share that belief. According to an article in the *Journal of the American College of Cardiology* (April 1992), just 17 percent of people who undergo angioplasty or bypass have been counseled seriously on reducing risk factors, by lifestyle change or cholesterol-lowering drugs.

But in fact, people who already have heart disease have more to gain from preventive measures than anyone else. The reduction in heart attacks and death from cardiovascular disease (by reducing cholesterol, for example) is far more substantial in high-risk people than in the healthy. Interventions to change stress-prone "Type A" behavior have lowered the rates of second heart attacks (see Coronary Heart Disease—Prevention).

Noting that a study in the same issue showed that the risk of death after heart attack was five times higher for people who are depressed, an editorial in the *Journal of the American Medical Association* (October 20, 1993) urged further research to explore psychological interventions to lower the heart disease toll.

IS IT POSSIBLE TO REVERSE HEART DISEASE?

In contrast to bypass surgery and angioplasty, lifestyle changes actually influence the heart disease process. A number of studies have shown that a low-fat diet and regular physical exercise can slow or halt the progression of heart disease. In one study, people who had angina were put on a program of aerobic exercise and low-fat diet for a year. Artery blockage progressed in nine participants, remained unchanged in eighteen, and actually regressed in thirteen; significantly better results than in a control group (*Circulation,* July 1992).

Even more hopeful are reports that a rigorous program of lifestyle change can reverse heart disease. In the Lifestyle Heart Trial, forty-eight people with documented heart disease were randomly assigned either to a group that got the usual care or to an aggressive experimental program to reduce heart risk factors.

Those in the latter group gave up smoking, ate a very low-fat (10 percent of calories) vegetarian diet, exercised regularly (three hours per week, usually brisk walking) and practiced a relaxation technique for an hour a day.

The program was demanding, but the results, as reported in *The Lancet* (1990, no. 336), were striking. After one year, coronary artery obstruction had regressed in 82 percent of the experimental group. Equally important, their symptoms markedly improved: frequency of angina attacks dropped by 91 percent. Often, improvement in symptoms was noticeable within weeks.

It's important to note that this program, designed by Dean Ornish, M.D., attacks heart disease on three fronts: diet, stress, and exercise. A key element is strong support, with regular group sessions, that may play an important role in helping participants stay with it.

Critics object that while Dr. Ornish's results are indeed impressive, it's hopeless to expect most people to do the same, insofar as the majority of Americans seem to have great difficulty in just cutting fat intake down to 30 percent. In interviews, Dr. Ornish has conjectured that big changes are, paradoxically, often easier to stay with than small ones, and that the prompt relief of symptoms—which you don't see when you cut fats modestly—is a better motivator than all the data in the world.

Similar programs are beginning elsewhere, many directed by doctors trained in the Ornish program. Health insurance companies are reimbursing them. If this approach interests you more than heart surgery, ask your doctor where you can get the support you'll need. And take a look at Dr. Ornish's book, *Dr. Dean Ornish's Program for Reversing Heart Disease* (New York: Random House, 1990).

◆ CORONARY HEART DISEASE
(Prevention)

Heart disease is still the number-one killer in America, but it has been steadily losing its punch. In 1991, the mortality rate was 146 per 100,000 people, nearly 20 percent lower than 1985 and half the rate of 1963.

At least some of the improvement can be attributed to success in publicizing and modifying the risk factors that make coronary heart disease (far and away the most widespread kind of heart disease) more likely.

If you don't know what these risk factors are (cigarette smoking, high cholesterol, hypertension, lack of exercise, overweight, stress, diabetes), it can only be because you haven't been paying attention to public service ads, public health campaigns, and television specials.

Although you can't do much about your inherited risk of heart disease (it's greatest if a parent died of it prematurely) or your gender (men with heart disease greatly outnumber women until quite late in life), there's a lot about your lifestyle that you can change to improve your chances of escaping this killer.

Some ways to reduce your risk of heart disease are explored in other chapters (see High Cholesterol; High Blood Pressure—Hypertension; and Diabetes).

HOW MUCH EXERCISE DO I NEED?

Exercise has long been recognized as a weapon against heart disease—as important, some say, as quitting smoking. According to a meta-analysis of forty-three studies, active people are just half as likely to get heart disease as the sedentary (*Annual Review of Public Health,* 1987, no. 8).

Aerobic exercise (like running, biking, or swimming) that brings your heart rate up and keeps it there continually for twenty minutes or more is the classical prescription for heart health. But a considerable body of evidence indicates that exercise needn't be continuous, strenuous, or very long for considerable benefit.

The Multiple Risk Factor Intervention Trial (MRFIT), which followed over twelve thousand men for seven years, found that those who were moderately active had less than two thirds as many episodes of heart disease, and just over two thirds as many deaths as the least active third of the group. "Moderately active," in this study, didn't necessarily mean organized exercise. It also included things like gardening, walking, climbing stairs, yard work, and dancing (*Journal of the American Medical Association,* November 6, 1987).

Just how exercise moderates heart risk isn't clear. It appears to reduce low-density lipoprotein (LDL) and increase high-density lipoprotein (HDL) cholesterol, to increase the heart's pumping capacity, and to reduce the levels of stimulatory chemicals like adrenaline that put wear and tear on the heart.

The important thing isn't going to a health club or training to run a marathon, but staying active regularly, in whatever way fits your taste and lifestyle. Walking about half an hour a day is a popular and valuable approach. Your doctor may have some helpful suggestions about the amount and kind of exercise that's right for you.

HOW CAN I REDUCE STRESS?

The role of stress in heart disease can be as dramatic as emotional upset triggering a massive and fatal coronary, or subtle as a stress-prone personality trait that accelerates the decades-long process of arterial narrowing.

For years, attention has been focused on "Type A" personality and behavior—the short-tempered syndrome of hurrying, worrying, and driving hard that, research in the 1970s showed, was typical of many heart attack victims.

More recently, researchers have honed in on one part of the picture as the toxic core that's largely responsible for Type A damage: what they call "hostility." This is a combination of attitude (a mistrustful cynicism of people and their motives); emotion (anger and anxiety); and behavior (expressions of temper and irritability). Repeated studies have found a strong association between hostility and heart disease.

It's not hard to understand why. People with a mistrustful, cynical attitude live in a threatening world, and their bodies respond appropriately, staying in a state of arousal that raises blood pressure, speeds the heart, and generates stress hormones that raise cholesterol and promote its deposition on the artery wall.

Hostile attitudes and behavior aren't likely to attract lots of friends, and a vast body of research links isolation to increased risk of illness, including heart disease. A large study reported in the *American Journal of Epidemiology* (1988, no. 128), for example, found that men with the least social contact had nearly two and a half times the risk of death from heart disease as those with the most.

A connection between acute stress and heart attack has been known at least since the time of ancient Rome, which recorded the deaths of two emperors in the grip of emotional turmoil. More recently, a study of nearly a thousand men who had already had heart attacks, reported at a 1991 scientific meeting of the American Heart Association, found that those who scored high in measures of ''emotional arousability'' were more than twice as likely to die suddenly.

In highly arousable people, the researchers conjectured, strong emotion triggers an outpouring of stress hormones like adrenaline that can fatally disrupt the heart rhythm.

Changing attitudes and reactions to protect your heart isn't easy, but it can be done. Programs to reduce hostility and Type A behavior have been shown in one study to lower the risk of second heart attacks by nearly half. In particular, cognitive-behavioral therapy, which teaches you to identify negative thoughts that turn ordinary experiences and interactions into heart-threatening stress and substitute healthier thought patterns, seems to be helpful.

Self-help approaches can be useful, too. One of the effects of exercise is to reduce levels of stress hormones that trigger emotional arousal, and regular practice of meditation or other relaxation techniques apparently calms your body's response to demanding situations. The whole range of stress-reducing strategies, from getting a pet to getting religion, can work for some people.

CAN ASPIRIN OR VITAMINS LOWER MY RISK?

The Physicians' Health Study, which has been following twenty-two thousand male doctors for years, was the first to find that a very low dose of aspirin (the equivalent of one standard pill every other day) can reduce the risk of heart attack. More recently, the Nurses' Health Study confirmed the same effect in women. Most likely, aspirin's anticlotting properties keep thromboses from forming and blocking arteries.

Further analysis of the original set of data, however, showed that the benefits were limited to men of age fifty and older (*The New England Journal of Medicine,* July 20, 1989). Aspirin at that dose should have no adverse effects (unless you're allergic to it or have gastrointestinal problems), but no one really knows the consequences of taking it for decades. Some experts recommend the aspirin approach only for people with other risk factors.

Findings from the same study also suggested that beta-carotene, the precursor of vitamin A, might also reduce heart attack risk. Among the 333 doctors who had already had heart attacks, those who took 50 milligrams of beta-carotene daily had half as many heart attacks, strokes, sudden cardiac deaths, and heart surgeries as those who didn't. Whether the same protection might be seen in people who don't yet have heart disease is yet to be investigated.

Beta-carotene is an antioxidant, and it appears to fight heart disease by preventing the conversion of LDL-cholesterol into a more toxic form. Other studies have found that vitamin E, vitamin C, and a diet rich in fruits and vegetables (which contains all three antioxidants) can reduce heart disease rates, too.

CAN ALCOHOL WARD OFF HEART DISEASE?

Interest in the power of alcohol to lower heart attack risk largely began with research publicizing the "French paradox"—the finding that the French, despite their predilection for cheese, pâté, and heavy sauces, had less heart disease than others, including Americans. The Gallic taste for wine was given the credit, and before you could say *Vive la différence!*— the liquor industry had built a major marketing campaign.

The FTC hyped them down, but the advantage of alcohol seems more than a fluke. Research supporting the idea includes a 1992 study of 130,000 adults reported in *Annals of Internal Medicine,* which found heart disease deaths 30 percent lower among those who had one or two drinks daily, compared to teetotalers.

The "French paradox" report and some others suggested that wine had special cardioprotective virtues, but most researchers doubt that. One study pointed out that wine drinkers differ from those who prefer beer or bourbon in education, diet, and lifestyle—which could readily account for differences (*American Journal of Cardiology,* February 15, 1993). The alcohol in two shots of liquor (one and a half ounces each), two glasses of wine (four ounces each), or two bottles of beer (twelve ounces each) emerged as the responsible component.

The research is quite consistent, and a good reason to keep on taking wine with your dinner, if that's your custom. Whether you should overcome an aversion to alcohol for your heart's sake is another matter. Even modest drinking can raise blood pressure and increase the chance of stroke, and people with heart rhythm disturbances may run additional risks. Alcohol consumption also may contribute to obesity, which is a cardiac risk factor in its own right.

When you start having more than two drinks a day, in any case, the health risks quickly overtake the benefits, and heavy drinking can inflict heavy damage on your heart and other organs. If you've had trouble with alcohol or other drugs, or there's a family history of alcoholism, you may be wise to take up jogging instead.

◆ DEPRESSION

An estimated one person in five—twice as many women as men—will suffer an episode of major depression during their lifetime, and more will be less profoundly depressed, but more persistently, for years. And the picture is getting bleaker. According to an article in the *Journal of the American Medical Association* (April 21, 1989), depression rates have increased among people born after World War II, and the average age at which the disorder strikes is growing younger.

Depression is not to be taken lightly; it can be life-threatening. An estimated 15 percent of people suffering from major depression kill themselves. And according to a study of 11,242 people with significant depressive symptoms, the condition caused as much or more disability than chronic medical conditions that are often taken more seriously, such as heart disease, diabetes, arthritis, and high blood pressure (*Journal of the American Medical Association,* August 18, 1989).

Although existing treatments can help an estimated 80 percent of people with depression, relatively few receive their benefit: two thirds of depressed people never seek help, and just half of those who do are accurately diagnosed and adequately treated.

COULD DEPRESSION BE CAUSING MY PHYSICAL SYMPTOMS?

Most depressed people see their regular family doctor or internist first, and all too often, these physicians handle the situation poorly. According to the 1993 *Clinical Practice Guidelines for Depression in Primary Care,* published by the Agency for Health Care Policy and Research, only one third to one half of depressions are detected by primary care practitioners.

A study sponsored by the RAND Corporation found that doctors in HMOs did particularly badly: they diagnosed only 46 percent of the depressions they saw, compared with 51 percent by solo practitioners. Mental health professionals picked up depression 78 to 87 percent of the time (*Journal of the American Medical Association,* April 21, 1989).

While we customarily think of depression in terms of mood, its symptoms often appear physical: fatigue, insomnia, loss of appetite, sexual dysfunction, and such assorted aches and pains as headache, backache, and persistent upset stomach. These may bring you to the doctor, but if you're reluctant to talk about your feelings, and the doctor isn't alert enough to inquire, the depression can pass unnoticed and untreated.

HAS MEDICAL ILLNESS BEEN RULED OUT AS A CAUSE OF MY DEPRESSION?

On the other hand, depressive symptoms can be biologically caused by any number of diseases and drug reactions. According to the Agency for Health Care Policy and Research (AHCPR) guidelines, such symptoms are seen in 12 to 16 percent of people with medical conditions. Among the illnesses most likely to cause depression are under- or overactive thyroid, diabetes, autoimmune disorders, heart disease, vitamin or mineral deficiencies, and some malignancies.

For this reason, a complete history, followed up with whatever physical exam and lab tests are indicated, should be part of the evaluation for depression.

Depression is among the side effects reported with many medications, such as antihypertensives, hormones (including oral contraceptives), steroids, tranquilizers, and ulcer drugs cimetidine and ranitidine. You may react to a drug that most people take without difficulty, so make sure the doctor knows all the medications you're taking.

Substance abuse frequently causes depression. Studies have found that 10 to 30 percent of alcoholics, for example, are depressed at the time they are evaluated. The depressive symptoms sometimes disappear, but not always, after the abused substance is discontinued.

SHOULD I SEE A SPECIALIST?

Depression often goes unrecognized by the family doctor, studies show, and too often inappropriate drugs, such as tranquilizers, are prescribed. But this doesn't mean that all primary care doctors should be avoided in favor of a specialist. A 1995 RAND study found that primary care physicians can treat depression with success equal to that of a psychiatrist or a psychotherapist, as long as the appropriate treatment is delivered (*Journal of the American Medical Association,* January 4, 1995). According to the RAND analysis of published studies on depression, the combination of antidepressant drugs and counseling, though initially more expensive, is not only the most effective way to treat depression but also cost saving in the long run.

The 1993 practice guidelines from the Agency for Health Care Policy Research, however, note that some depressions merit a referral to, or at least consultation with, a mental health specialist such as a psychiatrist or psychologist. This is true for psychotic depression and for manic depressive illness (in which the same person also experiences episodes of abnormal energy, euphoria, and poor judgment). A suicidal person should see a mental health specialist.

Family physicians and internists can prescribe antidepressant medication, but they (with very few exceptions) aren't qualified to do real psychotherapy or give specialized treatments like light therapy or electroconvulsant therapy. For that matter, a person who fails to improve on two different antidepressant drugs should see a specialist.

Even with these qualifications, not everyone agrees with the role advocated for primary care physicians. An article in the January 1994 *American Psychologist*—a publication of the American Psychological Association (APA)—urged that the AHCPR guidelines be withdrawn and revised to eliminate what the authors called a bias in favor of drugs and against psychotherapy. If depression is diagnosed or suspected, the APA proposed, a primary care physician should consult with a mental health professional.

Others have suggested that the emphasis on primary care treatment of depression will lead to overuse of medication (because that's the treatment family doctors and internists are qualified to provide), or to incompetent attempts at psychotherapy. The research supporting the effectiveness of depression treatment, they point out, was done almost entirely in mental health settings, not doctors' offices.

WHAT TREATMENT MAY BE BEST FOR ME?

The standard treatments for depression are antidepressant drugs, psychotherapy, or a combination of both. For most depressions, drugs and certain kinds of psychotherapy are comparably effective.

In a randomized trial involving 239 depressed people, two kinds of psychotherapy worked nearly as well as antidepressants, eliminating serious symptoms in 50 to 60 percent of people. Among the people with more severe depressions, medication was somewhat more effective than psychotherapy. All three treatments were significantly more effective than placebo (*Archives of General Psychiatry,* November 1989).

The psychotherapies tested were short term and rather new: cognitive therapy, which aims to change thought patterns; and interpersonal therapy, which tries to improve interactions with other people.

The AHCPR guidelines suggest that medication should be the "first line treatment" when depression is severe or if it includes psychotic symptoms like delusions or hallucinations, because "there is strong evidence for the efficacy of medication and little or none for the efficacy of psychotherapy alone." Similarly, they say that a person with melancholic depression (where physical symptoms like sleeplessness, appetite loss, and fatigue predominate) will do better with drugs.

Your own feelings are often the deciding factor. If you don't like taking medications or fear their side effects (more on this later), or if you just prefer what therapy has to offer, the choice is yours. On the other hand, you may believe that drugs seem the appropriate approach, or simply don't want to enter therapy.

If you do decide to go on antidepressants, you should consider whether some concurrent psychotherapy to deal with the problems that may have made you vulnerable to depression might also be helpful to you.

WHAT KINDS OF PSYCHOTHERAPY ARE OFFERED?

Beside cognitive and interpersonal therapy, there are many other kinds of psychotherapy used to treat depression, none of which have as much research support. In a number of trials, behavior therapy was effective for 55 percent of people with depression, and brief dynamic therapy for 35 percent. A randomized controlled trial found that behavioral marital therapy was superior to no therapy. Isolated studies also support the effectiveness of such diverse approaches as dance therapy and logotherapy (using self-help books).

HOW DO I DECIDE WHICH ANTIDEPRESSANT TO USE?

Randomized controlled trials have found most antidepressants comparably effective; each one generally works in about half of cases of depression. But individuals differ: one person may not respond to Tofranil but do well on Prozac, while someone else may react in the opposite way. Certain kinds of depression (where the person sleeps too much, rather than too little, for example) are said to respond better to particular drugs. All antidepressants have side effects, and the choice often comes down to the one that will cause least distress.

Their relative lack of side effects is largely responsible for the great popularity of Prozac and similar drugs (Zoloft and Paxil) that have come along in recent years. They are less likely to cause the sedation, dry mouth, constipation, weight gain, and other side effects that often accompany the older tricyclics (such as Tofranil, Elavil, and Sinequan), or require the strict diet control of the other major group, monoamine oxidase inhibitors (MAOI).

This isn't to say that Prozac, etc., are without adverse effects. Anxiety, insomnia, stomach upset, headache, and sexual dysfunction occur in significant numbers of people who use these drugs. And since they are relatively new, there is less research supporting their safety and effectiveness (two randomized controlled trials of Zoloft, compared to over a hundred of Tofranil), and little data on the consequences of extended use. In addition, because the older antidepressants are available in generic form, they are considerably less expensive.

ARE ANTIDEPRESSANTS DANGEROUS?

Most antidepressant side effects are unpleasant rather than dangerous, but there are some important cautions. The tricyclics can cause heart rhythm disturbances, which may make them dangerous for people with certain heart conditions and may require follow-up tests like electrocardiogram (this is especially important for children and adolescents). Anyone taking an MAOI must strictly avoid certain foods, like aged cheeses and red wine, or risk triggering a sudden, dangerous elevation of blood pressure.

The great popularity of Prozac in the late 1980s was followed by frightening reports of bizarre behavioral changes, including suicidal and homicidal behavior. Talk shows, magazine articles, and court cases resulted, but extensive clinical studies haven't provided evidence that Prozac, rather than the disease it was treating, was responsible. An FDA panel concluded that Prozac was no more likely to cause suicide or the rest than other antidepressants, but some members expressed alarm at the careless way the drug was apparently being used by some doctors.

Again, individual reactions to drugs differ, and extreme idiosyncratic adverse effects may occur in isolated cases. This makes it essential to maintain good, open communication with your doctor about how you're feeling. Keeping a close watch on your reactions to drugs is another good argument to see a psychotherapist regularly while you're depressed.

DO ANTIDEPRESSANTS REALLY WORK?

There have been some conspicuous dissents from the almost universal acceptance of antidepressants. One researcher, psychologist Roger P. Greenberg, Ph.D., of the State University of New York, Syracuse, believes that the vast majority of clinical trials are flawed in methodology; in particular, because antidepressants cause distinct side effects, studies comparing them to placebo aren't really "double-blind." "Obviously, if patients actually know they are getting a placebo rather than the real drug, they'll bias the outcome of the study," Dr. Greenberg said in an interview.

His meta-analysis of twenty-two antidepressant studies, published in the *Journal of Consulting and Clinical Psychology* (October 1992), found that the effectiveness of the drug was modest at best, and that in the better-designed trials, there was no advantage over placebo. The few studies that used a placebo that duplicated antidepressant side effects, for more effective blinding, showed "very little to no antidepressant effects beyond the placebo," and the role of drug therapy in depression should be much more limited, he believes.

HOW DO I KNOW THAT TREATMENT ISN'T WORKING?

Neither antidepressants nor psychotherapy are instant cures. Most people feel somewhat better in a few weeks, and the AHCPR guidelines suggest that someone who has responded minimally or not at all after six weeks may need a different medication, the addition of drugs (if psychotherapy was the first treatment), or psychotherapy (if drugs were the first treatment).

If treatment is successful, symptoms should be gone altogether after twelve weeks, and a number of randomized, controlled studies indicate that six to nine months of continued treatment will minimize the risk of relapse.

HOW CAN RECURRENCE BE PREVENTED?

Depression is often a recurrent disorder: 50 percent of people who have one episode of depression will go on to have another; if you've had two episodes, you have a 70 percent chance of recurrence; if three or more, a 90 percent chance.

Maintenance treatment with the antidepressant that relieved the depression appears to prevent a substantial number of recurrences. In one study, 22.6 percent of people had recurrences during three years that they continued to take imipramine, compared with 78.2 percent who were given placebo (*Archives of General Psychiatry,* 1990, no. 47, pp. 1093–99). A continued reduction in recurrence risk was seen in the same group of people when maintenance was extended for two more years (*Archives of General Psychiatry,* 1992, no. 49, pp. 769–73).

Continued psychotherapy may be beneficial in reducing the risk for relapse or recurrence, but the evidence isn't strong, according to the AHCRP report. The 1990 *Archives of General Psychiatry,* for example, found that continued interpersonal therapy delayed, but didn't prevent, depression from returning.

The decision on whether to continue maintenance medication or therapy should take into account the risk of recurrence—specifically, how many episodes you've already had, how severe they were, your family history and how early your illness began.

Resources

Call the AHCPR hotline, (800) 358-9295, and request the clinical practice guidelines on depression.

◆ DIABETES

Diabetes (full name: diabetes mellitus) is a major—and growing—health problem in the United States. There are an estimated fourteen million diabetics today, and it is projected that rates will increase: from 7 percent of the population in the early 1990s to about 10 percent by the end of the century.

Diabetes is a disease of sugar metabolism, the essential source of energy for virtually all the cells of the body. The process depends on insulin, a hormone secreted by certain cells in the pancreas. The vast majority of diabetics have what's called Type II or Non-Insulin Dependent Diabetes Mellitus (NIDDM), in which the pancreas secretes too little insulin, and/or the body's cells are unusually resistant to absorbing it. About 10 percent have Type I or insulin-dependent diabetes, in which the pancreas secretes no insulin at all.

It's uncertain what causes the two types of diabetes. Heredity clearly plays a predisposing role, and environmental factors such as diet, weight, and certain infections may be important, too. But possible consequences of diabetes are clear—and severe.

People with diabetes have a much higher rate of circulatory disorders than the general population. Blood vessels leading to the heart (coronary), the brain (carotid), and eyes are affected. Consequently, diabetes substantially increases the risk of stroke and kidney disease, and is the leading cause of blindness in the United States. Its impact on nerve function and blood flow may lead to amputation. It raises the likelihood of coronary heart disease—by 70 percent in men and 200 percent in women—and is a principal cause of impotence in older men. (Some believe that the higher rate in women is deceptive because this is a disease of older age and women tend to live longer than men. Also, the demands of childbearing may strain insulin reserves, predisposing women to diabetes later in life.) Recent studies have documented with increasing clarity, however, that effective care can substantially reduce the risk of some complications.

Type I diabetes is a dramatic disease and hard to miss. It is estimated, however, that only half of the people with Type II diabetes have been diagnosed: in the others, even if they have no symptoms, elevated blood sugar may be silently doing its damage.

HOW CAN I REDUCE MY RISK OF DIABETES?

To reduce your risk of Type II diabetes, which is usually diagnosed in middle age, do not allow yourself to become overweight. Obesity is a known risk factor. Although the greater weight-to-height ratio among people who develop diabetes probably reflects, to some extent, the effects of the disease, weight loss is highly recommended as a way of reducing risk. Fat tissue is somewhat insulin-resistant; people who are overweight need more insulin, which in turn strains the pancreas to accommodate the increased need.

Another risk factor that has received increasing attention during the last decade is exercise. In a five-year study of 21,271 male American physicians, ages forty to eighty-four, who exercised (vigorously enough to sweat) at least once a week were just two-thirds as likely to develop diabetes as those who were more sedentary. And the more active the men were, the lower their risk. Those who worked out five times or more weekly had just over half the risk of the sedentary group (*Journal of the American Medical Association,* July 1, 1992).

"These data suggest that, in the general U.S. population, in which more than 60 percent of adults do not exercise regularly, at least 25 percent of the incidence of NIDDM may be attributable to sedentary lifestyle," the authors wrote.

Many have suggested that various nutritional factors (refined sugar and fiber among them) could raise or lower the risk of diabetes, but none of these theories has been scientifically supported. One interesting study reported in a U.S. Department of Agriculture publication (*Food and Nutrition,* July–September 1990) suggested that getting the recommended dietary allowance of the mineral chromium could improve the body's ability to metabolize sugar, making Type II diabetes less likely. Wheat germ, brewer's yeast, and calves liver are good sources of chromium.

Your genetic endowment clearly affects the risk of getting both Type I and Type II diabetes: it's notably higher if you have a first-degree relative (parent or sibling) with Type II diabetes, for example.

Not everyone who is genetically susceptible will develop diabetes, however. There is substantial evidence that environmental factors can trigger Type I diabetes in those who are vulnerable. Among the suspects are certain viral infections: Type I diabetes appears to be an autoimmune disease, and the infection may lead the body to produce antibodies that then attack insulin-producing cells in the pancreas.

Not enough is known about possible environmental triggers to put into action to prevent Type I diabetes.

SHOULD I BE TESTED FOR DIABETES?

You ought to be aware of the classic symptoms of diabetes, which include excessive and unusual thirst, frequent urination, weight gain or loss, extreme tiredness, or vaginal itching. If you have any of these symptoms, seek medical attention to find out if diabetes is to blame.

Be aware, however, that Type II diabetes often has few or no symptoms, even while it progresses toward serious complications. It isn't considered economically feasible to screen everyone for diabetes, but people who are at increased risk probably should be tested regularly. This includes anyone who has diabetes in the family, is markedly overweight, or suffers from recurrent infections.

Many women become diabetic during pregnancy (gestational diabetes). Even if your blood sugar returns to normal afterward, as it often does, you should be considered at increased risk of diabetes, and tested accordingly. The same goes for anyone with a history of temporary glucose intolerance. According to an article in *Patient Care* (September 15, 1988), women who have given birth to large infants (over nine pounds) or had difficult pregnancies should also be screened.

Screening is a relatively simple matter: a single blood sample is drawn after you've fasted overnight, and the sugar level is tested. Further tests may sometimes be needed to establish the diagnosis.

IF I HAVE DIABETES, HOW CAN I MANAGE MY CONDITION?

It's extremely important for someone with Type I diabetes to find a specialist, either an endocrinologist or a diabetologist, who will work closely with you. Insulin-dependent diabetes is a very individualized condition: what works for one person may not work for another. You must be as knowledgeable as your doctor, and your doctor must be willing to *listen* as well as to instruct.

HOW CAN I KEEP COMPLICATIONS TO A MINIMUM?

A large study, reported in 1993, showed that very close control of diabetes could reduce the rate of complications dramatically.

It had long been thought that keeping blood sugar as close to normal as possible—by insulin injections, other drugs, and diet—was the ticket to sparing diabetics the dire health complications that often come after years of living with the disease. The Diabetes Control and Complications Trial confirmed it.

The study compared over fourteen hundred people with Type I diabetes for ten years; one group received the usual counseling, medical treatment, diet, and insulin schedule—one or two doses daily. This approach keeps blood sugar generally normal, but allows rather wide fluctuations.

The other group was put on a "tight-control" program that involved either three to five insulin injections daily or an implanted insulin pump; they tested their own blood sugar as often as seven times a day and kept in touch with nurses, dieticians, and doctors at least once a week.

The "tight-control" group suffered less than one half the serious complications of the "routine-care" group, such as damage to the retina of the eye, the kidney, and the nerves. In some cases, mild degrees of kidney damage that had already taken place could be reversed.

The participants in the Diabetes Control and Complications Trial all had Type I diabetes, but the investigators think it highly likely that those with Type II, who are subject to the same complications, will benefit from the same strategy.

The tight-control method has its drawbacks. All diabetics who use insulin sometimes suffer hypoglycemia; but tight control triples the risk of episodes severe enough to cause loss of consciousness. The method attempts to keep blood sugar levels within a normal range, thus a decrease would be experienced as more drastic. Many people in this Diabetes Control and Complications Trial found the tight-control program to be stressful; the dropout rate in this trial was high.

The method demands a lot from people with diabetics, and from the health-care system: its annual cost, for that matter, is double the average for diabetic care. But the cost, both human and economic, of diabetes complications is far greater.

The effectiveness of tight control in reducing the risk of heart disease and stroke isn't clear, and these are the biggest causes of death among diabetes. So it's especially important for you to follow the risk-reducing lifestyle that's recommended for all Americans: adjust your diet to keep weight and cholesterol down; exercise regularly; and give up cigarettes, in particular, because smoking contributes to cardiovascular disease.

WILL I NEED INSULIN?

Type I diabetes, in which the pancreas has totally lost the ability to secrete insulin, requires insulin injections as a primary therapy. Type II, despite its name (non-insulin dependent), may require injections as well.

The first treatment for Type II diabetes is usually diet and exercise. Increasing your physical activity apparently makes cells more sensitive to insulin, so even if your body's supply has dwindled, your blood sugar may drop toward normal. With a carefully controlled diet, if you bring your weight down, you may need no further treatment.

When diet and exercise aren't enough, oral medications called sulfonylureas are generally the next step: they increase the rate at which the pancreas secretes insulin, and the rate at which the cells of the body use it. Newer sulfonylureas have fewer side effects than the original medications.

Doctors today may start drug therapy earlier than they did in the past. It appears that elevated blood sugar itself tends to damage the insulin-secreting cells of the pancreas, in a kind of vicious cycle, so a quicker switch to medication may, at least in theory, slow the progression of the disease. If you're taking these drugs, it's important to be tested periodically. If stress or physical activity levels have changed, you may be able to take less. Studies have shown that both physical and emotional stress can cause blood glucose levels to rise.

Insulin is usually reserved for people whose blood sugar remains too high despite diet, exercise, and oral drugs.

WHAT SHOULD I KNOW ABOUT THE DRUG COMMONLY PRESCRIBED FOR TYPE II DIABETES?

Diabinese, the oral drug presribed to control mild to severe Type II diabetes, should not be taken by anyone over age sixty. The drug has a long duration of action. In an older person, Diabinese stays in the body longer, which can cause severe and prolonged hypoglycemia. It is one of twenty medications singled out by a panel of experts that should never be given to people over sixty in any dose and for any length of time (*Journal of the American Medical Association,* July 27, 1994). Most Type II diabetes can be controlled by diet.

WHAT'S THE BEST DIET FOR ME?

The prevailing thinking about diets for diabetics has changed in recent years. The American Diabetic Association now calls for an individualized diet based on a person's food preferences, lifestyle, and medication. The best amount of carbohydrates, for example, may differ from person to person: some studies have found that raising carbohydrates higher lowers fasting glucose and insulin needs, but for some people, apparently, the effect is opposite. The recommended amount of protein may be limited if you have kidney problems.

Most experts feel that complex carbohydrates—starches, usually including some fiber—are best. The effectiveness of fiber per se in reducing blood sugar is unclear. Two articles in one issue of the *British Medical Journal* (1990, no. 300, pp. 1334–1336) came down on opposite sides of the question. The editor commented that, while the evidence that high intakes of certain kinds of fiber can improve diabetic control "seems indisputable," the real question is how many people are willing to change their diet sufficiently.

Whatever its exact constituents, a carefully designed, consistent diet is a keystone of diabetic treatment. For your own best health, you will want to seek out the help of a good dietician or nutritionist experienced in working with diabetics.

WILL I NEED MEDICAL CARE FROM SPECIALISTS?

Given the complexity of good diabetic management and the wide range of possible complications, many experts advocate a team approach. Since self-care is such a vital part of diabetes management, and most doctors have limited time to speak with the people who come to see them, they often have a nurse or other staff person specially trained as an educator. You may also consult with an exercise therapist, and you should see a dietician.

Your doctor will probably keep an eye out for signs of complications, but you may also be well advised to see certain specialists regularly. Foot problems are extremely common in diabetes, the result of the disease's effect on the vascular system; if left untreated, they can lead to serious infections, even amputation. A well-trained podiatrist can help you learn optimal foot care, prescribe shoes that will minimize problems, and treat them quickly and effectively when they come up.

Regular eye examinations are a must. Retinal damage may lead to blindness, but prompt treatment, perhaps using laser, can cut the risk of significant vision loss by half. A specially trained ophthalmologist can diagnose and treat these potentially devastating conditions.

WHAT MUST I KNOW FOR SELF-CARE?

It's absolutely essential for you to be aware of the early signs and symptoms of diabetic complications, so you can get prompt medical attention when needed. If you take insulin, you must know the signs that your blood sugar is dropping to hazardous levels. In addition, you should be fully informed of your diet and exercise needs, and how changes in these can affect your need for insulin or other medications.

Since home glucose monitoring is a central part of tight control, you should understand it fully. In just about any chronic disease, people do best if they become active partners in their care. In diabetes, it's mandatory.

♦ DIVERTICULOSIS AND DIVERTICULITIS

Many things can go wrong in the complex digestive highway that carries food, and then waste matter, through the body. Toward the end of the road is the colon, or large intestine, and it's here that tiny pouches (diverticula) can bulge out through weaknesses in the wall. This is what's called diverticulosis.

Like so many other illnesses, diverticulosis is primarily a condition of advancing age and a diet of refined foods; about one third of people will have it by age fifty and two thirds by eighty. The average age of a person visiting the doctor for diverticulosis is sixty-two, according to one study.

Diverticulosis may be "one of the most common diseases seen in western civilization," as a paper in *Medical Clinics of North America* (September 1993) put it, but to a great extent, it's a disease without symptoms. An estimated 80 to 90 percent of persons with diverticulosis suffer no pain or serious disruptions in bowel habits, and for the most part remain unaware that there's anything wrong with their large intestine.

For the others, diverticulosis can be painful, disabling, even life-threatening. The most common complication, *diverticulitis,* develops when the pouches become inflamed or infected. The infection is believed to be due to feces getting caught in the pouches on the way through the colon.

Diverticulosis can be prevented by eating a high-fiber diet. The hard stool produced by a person on a low-fiber (refined foods) diet requires high pressure in the intestine in order to push it along. This high pressure causes the pouches to develop along the outer surfaces of the colon wall; whereas a high-fiber diet produces softer, more bulky stool which passes through the colon more easily, with less pressure.

Diverticulosis was rare before this century and is still rare in many parts of the world. The key, many researchers have concluded, is diet. The switch to refined grain products and sugar in the modern Western diet has drastically reduced the amount of fiber, and thus the bulk, that the colon should have in order to take the strain out of its contractions. The theory is supported by migration studies. In Japan, where the diet has more fiber, diverticulosis is uncommon; the rate rises to American levels, however, for ethnic Japanese who are born in Hawaii and eat the American way (*Surgical Clinics of North America,* October 1993).

IF I HAVE NO SYMPTOMS, WHAT'S TO BE DONE?

Sometimes, diverticulosis is discovered when the large intestine is examined by endoscope (a long, thin, hollow instrument) or X ray, routinely or for another condition. Less than one quarter of people with diverticulosis found in this manner are likely to ever experience symptoms, according to a review article in the *British Medical Journal* (May 1992).

On the other hand, diverticulosis may cause some chronic or periodic digestive distress resembling that of irritable bowel syndrome—pain in the lower or central abdomen, gas, bloating, and constipation—but it doesn't become infected or inflamed, or cause more acute problems.

There's no treatment for asymptomatic diverticulosis, and little that needs to be done for the uncomplicated condition. You're well advised, however, to follow a high-fiber diet (a good idea for just about anyone).

IS IT TOO LATE TO PREVENT DIVERTICULOSIS?

No. A high-fiber diet can prevent *diverticulitis* from occurring in people who already have *diverticulosis*. According to the 1993 Surgical Clinics of North America paper, several studies have indicated that getting onto a high-fiber diet will reduce the frequency of recurrent symptoms to 10 percent. By passing the stool along more easily, a high-fiber diet can help keep existing pouches free of stool obstructions that can lead to infection. A high-fiber diet should include plenty of fruits and vegetables, whole-grain breads, and wheat-bran cereals. Changing to this type of diet can help symptoms of diverticulosis subside in as little as two weeks. Don't forget to drink lots of water (six to eight glasses a day) when you increase your fiber intake.

WHEN DO I NEED TREATMENT?

If you have diverticulitis, you probably won't need much encouragement to seek medical attention. Pain usually comes on abruptly; it is most often in the left lower area of the abdomen (because diverticula are commonly in the far end of the intestine), but can be anywhere in the abdomen. In Asians, it's more common for diverticulitis and its accompanying pain to occur on the right side. Fever and an increased number of white blood cells are caused by the infection.

DO I NEED TO BE HOSPITALIZED?

If your attack of diverticulitis is relatively mild (most are), you will probably do fine on several days of antibiotics at home, with a liquid diet to allow your digestive system to rest and recover.

A more serious episode may require a hospital stay, so that antibiotics, fluids, and perhaps nutrients can be given intravenously, and to allow close observation. Prolonged or repeated inflammation of the bowel wall could eventually obstruct normal bowel action. The inflamed part of the bowel may be brought in contact with other abdominal organs, and a passage between them, or fistula, may be created. This most commonly happens to the bladder and leads to repeated urinary tract infections and distressing symptoms.

The most dangerous complication is peritonitis. A breakthrough in the colon wall allows infectious and fecal matter to enter the abdominal cavity. Mortality in this situation can be as high as 35 percent.

An attack that doesn't get substantially better in a day or two may involve an abscess or other complication and may require more intensive treatment, perhaps surgery. A colostomy, the surgical removal of part or all of the colon, is performed in the more severe cases in order to remove the source of infection. It should be reserved for people with diverticulitis that has not responded to less drastic treatments.

If your immune system is impaired by disease or drug therapy (such as corticosteroids), the risks from diverticulitis are heightened considerably. Peritonitis is more likely to develop, and surgery at this time carries higher risks of complications and death. Some studies have shown that people who take nonsteroidal anti-inflammatory drugs (NSAIDs) are also significantly more prone to serious complications, possibly because the symptoms of diverticulitis are masked by the NSAIDs until the condition progresses. Be careful with NSAIDs, because they are known to aggravate or cause other gastrointestinal complaints, such as bleeding ulcers and dyspepsia.

IF I HAVE ONE ATTACK OF DIVERTICULITIS, WILL I HAVE OTHERS?

About 70 percent of people treated medically for one episode of diverticulitis will have no more. Of the others, 90 percent will have recurrences within the next five years, according to a follow-up study of 455 people. Even if you don't have another attack, you may experience low-grade, chronic bowel symptoms.

Before having elective surgery, make sure your doctor has fully established that diverticulitis is in fact responsible for your symptoms. Even if you have *diverticulosis,* if the bowel is not inflamed, the problem may be due to something else, like irritable bowel syndrome. According to the 1993 *Surgical Clinics of North America* article, one researcher found there was no evidence of inflammation in one third of colons subjected to diverticulitis surgery.

HOW SAFE AND EFFECTIVE IS THE SURGERY?

The colostomy is considerably safer when done electively, after the bowel has been prepared thoroughly, than when done as an emergency operation in the midst of a severe attack. It's also simpler, as the emergency procedure must sometimes be done in stages, with the diseased colon section removed, and a temporary colostomy created so the organ can recover before the ends are reconnected.

The risk of death with such surgery depends largely on the severity of the disease, the circumstances under which the surgery is done, and the health of the person to whom it is done. Safety has improved over the years. A study reported in the German journal *Zentralblatt fur Chirurgie* (1993, no. 118) found that the mortality rate dropped from 24 percent for a series of operations done during the 1970–80 period, to 7 percent in the next decade.

Even after surgery, diverticulitis can recur in parts of the bowel that were left behind. Several studies have found recurrence rates varying from 7 to 15 percent, even after the procedure was apparently successful.

♦ EATING DISORDERS (Anorexia and Bulimia)

It's hard to be sensible about food; a sizable proportion of Americans are overweight, and diet books, plans, and programs are perennial money-makers, leading some people to characterize the eating disorders anorexia and bulimia simply as exaggerations of common concerns about weight.

But they're not. Anorexia (drastic restriction of food intake that leads to dangerous emaciation) and bulimia (binges of eating and purging to keep weight normal) are psychiatric disorders, serious emotional illnesses that can be fatal. They aren't willful self-indulgence, failures of character, or shameful idiosyncracies, anymore than depression or panic disorder. They need—and often respond to—treatment.

Both disorders are far more common in women, but also occur in men. Bulimia is the more common of the two disorders; an estimated 4 to 20 percent (depending on how strictly the condition is defined) of women will have suffered from bulimia by the time they reach college age. Anorexia affects about one in a hundred women.

AM I AT RISK?

According to an article in *The Lancet* (June 26, 1993), anorexia is currently believed to be "multifactorial": the result of psychological, biological, social, and family influences working together. Studies have shown that identical twins are more likely to share the disease than fraternal twins, suggesting that some aspect of the disorder is inherited.

Both psychology and biology are apparently at work in bulimia as well, according to a paper in *The New England Journal of Medicine* (September 15, 1988). A study reported in the same issue suggested a defect in a bio-chemical appetite control mechanism in bulimia. As you eat, your small intestine normally secretes a chemical, cholecystokinin (CKK), that builds up and signals the brain that you're full. In bulimics, the response is blunted: they may eat prodigiously without feeling satisfied. Other studies have pointed to abnormal levels of serotonin, a neurochemical involved in mood and eating behavior.

Our society, with its "you can't be too thin" premium on slim, youthful appearance, has been indicted as a cause of eating disorders, in women particularly. The power of its influence, however, is uncertain. Anorexia, after all, was first identified in England a hundred and fifty years ago—a very different culture with very different esthetic standards. *The Lancet* article suggests that "some variant of anorexia nervosa may be traced back to medieval times."

Certainly, reports of anorexia and bulimia have greatly increased in recent decades, but the extent to which this represents a true increase or simply heightened awareness is unclear. A study of reported cases of anorexia in Rochester, Minnesota (*Mayo Clinic Proceedings,* May 1988), found that the incidence of the disorder remained stable from 1935 through 1979.

Both anorexia and bulimia are predominantly diseases of white, middle-class young women, and they typically appear during adolescence. But they are seen in people of all races and socioeconomic classes and have been known to develop as early as age five and as late as age sixty. Often, the disorder appears during a time of profound change, such as leaving home to start college, or unusual emotional stress.

CAN MEN GET THESE DISORDERS?

An estimated 5 to 10 percent of eating disorders occur in men; that adds up to several hundred thousand in the United States. Although people with anorexia and bulimia are rarely eager to seek help, the problem of shame and denial is compounded in men, who as a group are unlikely to visit doctors for emotional problems, particularly for what's generally thought of as a "women's disease."

Eating disorders appear to be more common in gay than straight men, but athletes may also be prone to binging/purging cycles, particularly in sports with rigid weight requirements, like wrestling.

ARE EATING DISORDERS REALLY THAT DANGEROUS?

The impact of what amounts to prolonged starvation in anorexia wreaks havoc all over the body. Heart, kidneys, bone marrow, brain, and nervous system all can be seriously affected. Hormone levels drop, and menstruation usually ceases. Disruption of the normal balance of minerals can lead to fatal heart arrhythmias; serious infections can follow a decline in immune function. Muscles waste away and bones thin, leading to stress fractures. Besides the physical buffeting, the emotional anguish of anorexia causes some to attempt suicide.

An estimated one anoretic in thirty will die of the disorder within ten years of diagnosis. Not a cheery statistic, but it represents a substantial improvement over past mortality rates, according to a 1989 article in the *British Medical Journal*.

Because bulimics usually keep their weight close to normal, they are spared the starvation damage of anorexics. The condition is far from benign, however. Repeated binging and purging (typically, by self-induced vomiting or with laxatives) disrupts the normal mineral balance, much as severe diarrhea would, and can cause heart arrhythmias or seizures. Frequent vomiting may damage the digestive system severely, and the stomach acid will erode tooth enamel.

Although anorexia and bulimia are distinct disorders, it is possible to have both. It appears that a substantial number of anorectics also have the binge/purge behavior pattern, and that the proportion increases the longer they are sick. Needless to say, binging and purging compounds the physical damage of anorexia.

DOES TREATMENT DO ANY GOOD?

Eating disorders, particularly anorexia, usually require extensive treatment, and the outcome is guardedly hopeful. Most people can be successfully helped through the acute phase of anorexia, but fewer than half are considered recovered four years later, and eventually, as many as one quarter are chronically disabled, physically and/or psychiatrically, by their persistent condition.

Some programs have much better success, however. A study that appeared in the *American Journal of Diseases of Children* (November 1989) followed forty-nine adolescent girls who had been hospitalized for anorexia. An average of six and a half years later, fewer than 15 percent had persistent problems with the eating disorder. Their education and employment hadn't been adversely affected by their illness.

The best treatment for anorexia appears to be a multifaceted approach, which combines psychotherapy, nutritional counseling, and family therapy. People with anorexia typically have severe self-esteem difficulties; they may have a legacy of childhood trauma to contend with, and are trapped in self-defeating habits of thought and behavior. Psychotherapy may be helpful in addressing all of these issues. A support group led by a trained professional can also be beneficial to many anorectics. Although hospitalization isn't always necessary, it's frequently the only way to start changing the anorectic self-destructive way of living.

Bulimia is less likely to require hospitalization, insofar as it is rarely so directly life-threatening. Various kinds of psychotherapy, both individual and in groups, apparently relieves symptoms reasonably well in the short term. But bulimia tends to come in cycles, and relapses are common, according to an editorial in *The New England Journal of Medicine* (September 15, 1988).

For either disorder, early diagnosis and treatment improves the outlook. The longer an eating disorder continues, the worse the prospect for lasting recovery, and the greater the physical damage that has already been inflicted.

CAN DRUGS HELP?

No drug has been approved specifically for eating disorders, but some medications are used, generally in conjunction with psychotherapy.

Antidepressants have been shown to be somewhat successful in treating bulimia. Bulimics often report feeling depressed and anxious before binges, and better afterward. Research has suggested a biochemical explanation, linking symptoms of bulimia to low levels of serotonin, a neurotransmitter that regulates mood and appetite. The new generation of antidepressants (Prozac, Zoloft, and Paxil) are targeted to increase serotonin specifically, and some studies suggest they can effectively reduce bulimic symptoms.

Similar drugs are sometimes given to anorectics, but their malnourished state makes side effects more pronounced and problematic.

Resources

American Anorexia/Bulimia Association
293 Central Park West, Suite 1R
New York, NY 10024
(212) 501-8351 M-F 9 A.M.–5 P.M. eastern time

Information—by phone or mail
Referrals (nationally)
Support groups (nationally)
Newsletter

National Association of Anorexia Nervosa and Associated Disorders (ANAD)
Hotline: (708) 831-3438 M-F 9 A.M.–5 P.M. central time

Referral and Information Service
Maintains a national list of eating disorder specialists
National network of support groups
Free information packets

✦ ENDOMETRIOSIS

Endometriosis is a common gynecological condition, but just how common is impossible to say. One estimate puts the prevalence at 2.5 to 7.5 percent of American women of ages fifteen to fifty-four. While it may cause severe pain and impair fertility, the disorder is often discovered in the course of a laparoscopic examination for other reasons. During this minor surgical procedure, the surgeon can view the ovaries, fallopian tubes, and uterus, via a long telescopelike device, which is inserted through a small incision in the navel. Reported cases of endometriosis have risen dramatically in recent years, but to an extent, this probably reflects increasing use of laparoscopy, rather than increased incidence of the disease.

Exactly what causes endometriosis—implantation of cells from the lining of the uterus elsewhere in the abdominal cavity—is unclear, but one widely held hypothesis links it to the backup of menstrual blood into the fallopian tubes. The menstruation connection would also help explain the increase in the number of cases, according to an article in the *British Medical Journal* (January 16, 1993): "Women now experience over 450 menstruations during their reproductive lifetime rather than the 30 to 50 that would be expected without contraception and with long periods of lactation."

The average age at which endometriosis is discovered is the late twenties, but it is relatively common in adolescents (found in 47 to 65 percent of women under twenty who have chronic pelvic pain or pain during intercourse) and probably peaks in the early forties. Some of the cells from the lining of the uterus migrate to other organs, attaching themselves to the surface of the uterus, the tubes, bladder, and bowel, where they continue to thrive under the stimulation of ovarian hormones. Because the symptoms of endometriosis are dependent on these hormones, menopause generally puts an end to the problem (except when hormone replacement is given).

IS ENDOMETRIOSIS THE CAUSE OF MY PAIN?

The relief of severe abdominal pain is the most appropriate reason to treat endometriosis. But just because you have pain and a laparoscopic examination shows that you have endometriosis doesn't mean the second is responsible for the first.

Pain around the time of menstruation is the most typical pattern in endometriosis; it may also be triggered by sexual intercourse or defecation. Abdominal tenderness on physical examination, or the presence of a physical mass strengthens the probability that endometriosis is to blame for pelvic pain.

All too often, however, the pain of endometriosis isn't relieved because the diagnosis isn't made. At the Third World Congress on Endometriosis, held in Brussels in 1992, a retrospective study of American women with the disorder reported that 27 percent had symptoms for six years or longer before they were diagnosed. "The delays were caused by doctors failing to recognize the importance of symptoms and claiming that women were overreacting," according to an account in *The Lancet* (June 20, 1992).

If your doctor isn't taking your symptoms seriously, find another.

WHAT TREATMENT IS RECOMMENDED FOR ENDOMETRIOSIS?

There are several approaches, and each has its side effects and limitations. Danazol (brand name: Danocrine), a testosterone derivative, has long been the preferred treatment. It reduces the amount of circulating female hormones, which stops menstruation, shrinks the endometrial deposits, and improves symptoms. According to the 1992 *Lancet* paper, 60 to 100 percent of women taking danazol report fewer symptoms, and laparoscopic examination shows a reduction in endometrial deposits in 51 to 94 percent of cases.

The side effects of danazol can be distressing, however: weight gain, acne, and increased appetite are most common; voice changes and hirsutism are rarer, but mean that the treatment must be discontinued. A rise in cholesterol is also seen. These side effects aren't always reversible.

Progestin (a female hormone that suppresses ovulation) works about as well as danazol, but with such side effects as abnormal uterine bleeding, breast tenderness, nausea, and depression.

The newest approach is gonadotropin-releasing hormone (GnRH), which inhibits production of estrogen by the ovaries, producing a "medical menopause." This is comparable to danazol in symptom relief and disease regression, and its side effects are like those of menopause, the most serious being a significant reduction in bone mass (which usually returns to normal six to nine months after the drug is stopped). The side effects of GnRH drugs are apparently less distressing than those of danazol. In trials involving both drugs, the women who were assigned to danazol were more likely to drop out than those assigned to GnRH.

Whatever drug is chosen, adverse effects generally limit it to short-term use. After the drug is discontinued, symptoms may stay away for a time, but they often return eventually. Five years later, symptoms recurred in half of women who had been treated with drugs or with conservative surgery.

Conservative surgery, that is, the destruction or removal of endometriotic deposits or the release of adhesions (internal scar tissue), has relieved pain in 70 to 100 percent of women in uncontrolled trials, but longer-term follow-up has found that deposits reappear in 28 percent of women after eighteen months; adhesions form again in 40 to 50 percent; and pain recurs in 34 percent over a five-year period.

WILL TREATING ENDOMETRIOSIS RESTORE MY FERTILITY?

Endometriosis is often treated in women who have difficulty conceiving, but here the decision to treat with any of the above-mentioned approaches is on shakier ground. "None of the published randomized trials have shown that medical [drug] treatment improves fertility," and there are no randomized studies of the effectiveness of endometriosis surgery, according to the 1993 *British Medical Journal* article.

One study, cited in a review article in *The New England Journal of Medicine* (June 17, 1993), found surgery to be no more effective than drug therapy for women with mild or moderate endometriosis, but significantly better in restoring fertility when the disease was severe.

Among the effects of endometriosis are pelvic adhesions and other distortions of reproductive tract anatomy, which can interfere with the mechanics of conception. In this situation, surgery specifically undertaken to restore the pelvis to a more normal condition may improve fertility, according to a review article in *The Lancet* (November 21, 1992). Unfortunately, surgery itself can cause adhesions.

I HAVE NO SYMPTOMS. WHAT HAPPENS IF I DO NOTHING?

To quote the title of the 1993 *British Medical Journal* article, "Endometriosis should not be treated just because it's there." Three controlled studies of medical treatment found that in the placebo group—the control group that had no therapy at all—endometriosis got worse about half the time. In the other half, it stayed the same, got better, or disappeared altogether. It was impossible to identify the women in whom the disease would progress.

What's more, treatment with drugs like danazol can be given only for limited periods of time, and there is evidence that it does no more than suppress the disease; the endometriosis often returns after treatment ends.

COULD MY BIRTH-CONTROL METHOD WORSEN THE CONDITION?

Some research has suggested that oral contraceptives protect against endometriosis because they prevent ovulation and stop menstruation. Unfortunately, the protection only lasts as long as the pills are taken. In a study following 17,032 women who had come to a family planning clinic for up to twenty-three years, those who were taking oral contraceptives had about 40 percent of the risk of endometriosis of the others, but two to four years after they stopped taking the pill, they had nearly twice as much disease.

There was no association between the length of time that women had been on the pill and their risk of endometriosis. Oral contraceptives apparently neither cure nor cause the disease. "We suggest that endometriosis is suppressed during current and recent pill use but that the disease subsequently emerges after the pill is stopped," the authors wrote (*British Medical Journal,* January 16, 1993).

A similar pattern emerged in women who used IUDs: they had less than half the risk of endometriosis while using the device, but nearly one and a half times as great the risk four to six years later. In this case, the authors speculate, bleeding and pelvic pain actually due to endometriosis are assumed to be caused by the IUD. The symptoms improve when the IUD is removed, and it may be years before continued problems lead to a workup and diagnosis of endometriosis.

In the study, use of a diaphragm had no effect on endometriosis rates.

One thing to keep in mind no matter what contraceptive you choose: since endometriosis may worsen with time and impair fertility, pregnancy shouldn't be delayed for too long.

IS HYSTERECTOMY EVER A CONSIDERATION?

Given all the drawbacks of this major surgery (see Hysterectomy), the approach should be considered a last resort for women whose pain is extreme and resistant to other treatment. The fact that an increasing proportion of hysterectomies (now 20 percent) are done for endometriosis suggests that the procedure is overused. Although widely viewed as the definitive treatment for severe endometriosis, the total hysterectomy (ovaries included) has never been subjected to a controlled clinical trial to determine efficacy in treating endometriosis.

According to *The New England Journal of Medicine* 1993 review of uncontrolled studies, surgical removal of the uterus, the ovaries, and endometriosis deposits leaves 10 percent of women still in pain. Leaving the ovaries in place increases the risk of recurrent symptoms (to as much as one third in women with advanced disease).

Resources

The Endometriosis Alliance of Greater New York, Inc.
P.O. Box 326 Cooper Station
New York, NY 10276-0326
(212) 533-ENDO (3636)

A self-help organization with crisis call counseling that will refer women in the Greater New York area to support groups. The alliance will answer questions on the phone (if you call and leave your name and phone number, the organization will call you back collect) and send information to women living outside of New York.

Endometriosis Association
8585 N. 76th Place
Milwaukee, Wisconsin 53223
(800) 992-ENDO (3636)

International self-help organization with local chapters throughout the United States.
Support groups.
Information clearinghouse.
Newsletter.
Call and leave name and address on the answering machine to receive a free information packet.

✦ ENLARGEMENT OF THE PROSTATE

Most organs shrink as we get older. The prostate, which produces a fluid vital for male fertility, grows. This walnut-shaped gland surrounds the urethra—the tube that carries urine from the bladder to the penis—so its enlargement can interfere with normal urination. About 75 percent of men over fifty have some symptoms of prostate enlargement: difficulty in starting or maintaining urination, increased frequency (that often interferes with sleep), or the sudden urge to urinate.

The excess prostate tissue is neither malignant nor premalignant, which is why the condition is technically called *benign* prostatic enlargement (BPH). But the symptoms can range from annoying to life-disrupting. If the blockage progresses, it may abruptly close off the urethra and make it impossible to urinate altogether, an acute crisis that requires catheterization. Retention of urine in the bladder can lead to infection, and increased pressure may cause permanent damage to the bladder or kidneys.

SHOULD I BE TREATED FOR BPH?

Prostate enlargement in itself doesn't necessarily require treatment. "Just because someone has BPH, that doesn't mean anything," says Mark Solloway, M.D. "What is important is the severity of the symptoms and their inconvenience." If your urinary difficulties are mild enough for you to tolerate, in other words, perhaps you should do just that—tolerate them.

What's more, there are steps you can take on your own to make BPH easier to live with. For one, eliminate caffeine, which is a potent diuretic (in addition to coffee and tea, cola drinks, and chocolate, contain appreciable amounts). Restrict your fluid intake. In particular, avoid caffeine, alcohol, and liquids at night, to minimize sleep disturbance.

The side effects of certain drugs can make urination difficult, aggravating the symptoms of BPH. Among these are antihistamines (included in most over-the-counter cold remedies), tranquilizers, and certain antidepressants. Discuss whatever drugs you're taking with your doctor; it may be possible to switch to alternatives that will work as well without the drawbacks.

IF I WANT TREATMENT, WHAT'S BEST?

Treatment options have broadened substantially in recent years. The original surgery, in which the abdomen or the perineum was opened and the prostate removed, has largely been replaced by transurethral resection of the prostate (TURP), a less invasive procedure. There are other, more experimental methods which use microwave or the pressure of an inflated balloon to destroy or compress excess tissue. There are drugs to shrink the prostate. And there's the conservative approach called "watchful waiting."

Which is best? A clinical trial is currently in progress comparing surgery, drug therapy, the balloon method, and watchful waiting. The fact of such a trial means that, as far as medical science is concerned, there's no clear evidence—yet—that any one of these options is better than the others. Results from the study are expected to provide more definite answers.

Some treatment options that are not included in the trial may also be worth considering, such as the microwave method, and TUIP (transurethral incision of the prostate).

WHAT IS "WATCHFUL WAITING"?

Rarely does BPH require immediate surgery or drug therapy. If you don't have repeated infections, urinary retention, or signs of bladder or kidney damage, you may choose to wait and see if symptoms worsen or improve.

If left alone, some BPH does get better, perhaps because bladder muscles strengthen to compensate for the obstruction, or men learn to live with their symptoms and use self-help measures (cutting back on caffeine or bedtime fluid intake). Over one quarter of men with moderate symptoms report that their symptoms have improved to "mild" after a year of watchful waiting (they worsened to "severe" in 16 percent of cases, and another 9 percent of the men decided to have surgery). Severe symptoms improved in nearly half of men who took this approach for a year, and 17 percent had surgery.

It's important to understand that "watchful waiting" doesn't mean doing nothing. It should be an *active* approach, with regular return visits to the doctor to report on symptoms, plus tests to monitor kidney function to make sure no damage is taking place.

The risks of watchful waiting are relatively small. In a Veterans Administration study, 7 percent of men developed acute urinary retention during five years of watchful waiting. No severe urinary tract infections were reported in similar studies. It may be, however, that if surgery is deferred and then becomes necessary, risks of complications are greater because you're now older or in poorer health.

IS TURP THE BEST SURGERY?

Whether transurethral resection of the prostate (TURP) is the best surgery is unknown; clearly it is the most common treatment. A thin tube is threaded up the penis and urethra; guided by fiberoptics, the surgeon scrapes away the part of the prostate that is constricting urine flow.

TURP can be done under spinal block, and is less invasive than old-fashioned "open surgery," which meant general anesthesia, an incision in the abdomen, and removal of the entire prostate. Recovery is quicker (most men are out of the hospital in several days), and complications are fewer. In particular, impotence and incontinence, which were major drawbacks to prostatectomy, are less likely.

But they do happen. About one man in twenty becomes impotent after TURP (it's unclear whether this is a physical or psychological reaction), and a small number (4 percent in one prospective study) suffer some incontinence, which is usually mild. Most men, however, experience retrograde ejaculation. Because the bladder neck no longer closes completely as a result of the surgery, sperm is ejaculated into the bladder during intercourse, rather than out the penis. This may be disconcerting (the next time you urinate, it will be foamy), but not harmful. It does cause infertility, however.

When TURP was first developed, its safety was a major selling point. The chance of dying during or in the weeks after surgery is, in fact, less than one in a hundred. Studies that followed men for longer, however, found mortality rates of 4 to 9 percent in the three to twelve months after surgery. And men who have TURP were more likely to die of various causes, including heart attack, during the next eight years, than men who had open surgery.

Although TURP usually relieves symptoms effectively in the short run, for some men the improvement doesn't last. The procedure can scar the urethra, causing constriction that produces the same symptoms, or prostate tissue may grow back. As many as 10 percent of men who have TURP must repeat the procedure within five years.

There are some men—those whose prostates are extremely enlarged—who are not candidates for TURP.

WHAT ABOUT PROSCAR?

The approval by the Food and Drug Administration (FDA) of a pill to reduce prostate enlargement without surgery made big headlines a few years ago. Proscar (the generic name is finesteride) blocks the enzyme that converts testosterone, the male hormone, into dihydrotestosterone, a derivative that stimulates prostate growth.

More than a hundred thousand men, it is estimated, now take Proscar for BPH. At about two dollars a day—presumably for life—it's not, in the long run, a cheap treatment. How well does it work?

The study, published in *The New England Journal of Medicine* that led to Proscar's approval by the FDA, found that the drug shrank the prostate by an average of 20 percent, and reduced the level of hormones that increase prostate size by 60 percent.

Yet the clinical results—the improvement in symptoms and urine flow—were "not impressive," to quote Paul H. Lange, M.D., the urologist from the University of Washington who wrote an editorial in the same *Journal* issue that carried the report. "Such minimal gains do not begin to compare with those achieved by transurethral resection of the prostate," he wrote.

The response to Proscar, as to most drugs, differs from one person to the next. If you like the nonsurgery approach, you might want to see how well it works for you. You'll have to wait, however; it takes as long as six months for results to show.

And, as with any medication, there are side effects: 3 to 5 percent of men in the studies experienced reduced sexual desire, smaller ejaculations, or impotence. Because it is a new drug, the risks and benefits of long-term Proscar treatment are not known.

One last concern: Proscar may distort the results of prostatic specific antigen (PSA) testing, which is used to detect prostate cancer (see Prostate Cancer).

ARE THERE ANY OTHER DRUGS FOR BPH?

Another type of medication that appears to improve symptoms of prostate enlargement is the alpha-blocker. These drugs, long used for high blood pressure, relieve urethral constriction by relaxing smooth muscle in the prostate.

The most interesting of these drugs, Hytrin (terazosin), has the advantage of long action—you need to take only one pill a day. In a four-week study of 237 men, symptoms and urinary flow improved significantly more on Hytrin than with a placebo. The effect appears more robust than with Proscar, but the drugs have not been directly compared (such a study is now under way). In any case, therapy with Hytrin is considerably less expensive.

Hytrin has a greater variety of side effects than Proscar, most involving the cardiovascular system. Dizziness, headache, weakness, tiredness, and impotence have been reported in one third of men taking Hytrin for BPH. In a study that compared Hytrin to placebo, however, only postural hypotension (blood pressure drops when you stand up, causing dizziness) was significantly more common with the drug.

ARE THERE ALTERNATIVES?

Several other ways to relieve BPH symptoms have been developed, but there are less data and experience with them. Some are options only for men with relatively modest prostate enlargement.

In one such treatment, balloon dilation of the prostate, a tube, like the one used for TURP, is threaded up the urethra, and a balloon is expanded to widen the passage. Studies are inconsistent. Some show symptom improvement in 40 to 70 percent of men who have the treatment, while others have found no advantage over placebo. Long-term results have been disappointing. The study with the longest follow-up found lasting improvement in less than one third of men.

Another new approach is microwave therapy, in which a urethral tube delivers microwave radiation that rapidly heats and destroys excess prostate tissue. A study of forty men reported in the *British Medical Journal* (May 15, 1993) found that symptoms were reduced by nearly two thirds in men who had the treatment, significantly more than those who had a sham procedure. The men were followed for only three months, however.

Microwave therapy is still considered experimental, so you can receive it only by participating in a clinical trial that is under way in several medical centers. Ask your urologist for a referral.

Transurethral incision of the prostate (TUIP) works much like TURP, but instead of removing parts of the gland, the surgeon inflicts a number of slits in it to relieve pressure on the urethra. Like balloon dilation, it's an option only for men whose prostates are just moderately enlarged. The procedure appears to offer as much symptom relief as TURP, with less risk of complications. But whether results hold up in the long run is not yet clear.

Resources

For a free copy of the pamphlet "Treating Your Enlarged Prostate," call the Agency for Health Care Policy Research at (800) 358-9295.

◆ EPILEPSY

An epileptic seizure can be a dramatic thing: involuntary sounds, collapse, loss of consciousness, convulsive movements. But actually, there are many kinds of seizures, most of them quite subtle and limited. An arm or leg may twitch uncontrollably, a person may see things or hear voices, or a child may lose touch with her surroundings and stare absently into space.

In centuries past, epilepsy seemed frightening and mysterious, and was often ascribed to some sort of possession—by a god, according to the ancient Greeks, or a demon, in the Renaissance. Although epileptics aren't burned at the stake these days, many still suffer from the ignorance, fear, and superstition of others.

What all kinds of epileptic seizures have in common is disorganized, uncontrolled brain activity. Neurons—brain cells—normally communicate by passing electrical impulses from one to another. In epilepsy, a group of neurons fire at once, far more rapidly than normal. If the activity is localized, the result is a "partial" seizure; if it spreads throughout the brain, a convulsive grand mal or petit mal (absence) seizure occurs. The latter, which occurs primarily in children, is so subtle that its manifestations include a blank stare, eyelid fluttering, and fine mouth and hand movements.

WHAT CAUSES EPILEPSY?

This chronic neurological disorder—the most common, afflicting about two million Americans—can result from any number of things that damage cells in the brain. Disruption of oxygen to the baby just before or during birth, or head injury later in life are frequently responsible. Infection, toxicity, tumor, or stroke may cause the damage.

An inherited predisposition is apparently involved in up to 50 percent of cases, but here, too, it may take some kind of accident or injury to bring it out. While 75 percent of epilepsy first occurs in childhood, the disorder may appear at any time.

Epilepsy can be prevented—or the risk reduced, anyway—by taking precautions against head injury (wear a helmet when biking and playing sports like football), and having immunizations against childhood infections that cause high fevers.

IF I HAVE A SEIZURE, DOES IT MEAN I HAVE EPILEPSY?

By definition, epilepsy is a chronic condition—seizures recur over time, and a first such episode may also be the last. A British study of 564 people who had had one seizure found recurrences in about two thirds within a year, and in 78 percent, within three years.

The risk of recurrence was higher when the seizure was associated with a congenital neurological abnormality (100 percent in the next twelve months), and lower when it followed a head injury or stroke (40 percent). People under sixteen and over fifty-nine were more likely to have recurrences than those in between, and partial seizures were more likely to recur than the big generalized ones (*The Lancet,* November 24, 1990).

While just two seizures may be enough to fit the diagnosis of epilepsy, this doesn't always mean a chronic disease. "In many individuals the total number of seizures experienced is small," the authors of the study said.

CAN FEVER CONVULSIONS CAUSE EPILEPSY?

Convulsions caused by high fever (febrile convulsions) are not uncommon in infancy and early childhood, and some fear that they reveal or may even cause the brain damage that leads to epilepsy. Not that long ago, some doctors advocated giving prophylactic anticonvulsant medication to some children, at least, who had had febrile convulsions.

It's become quite clear, however, that the vast majority of febrile convulsions are neither ominous nor harmful. In a group of nearly fifteen thousand children in England, 2.7 percent had had at least one such episode by the age of ten. After excluding those who were known to have neurological abnormalities before their attack, only 2.4 percent of the children who had a fever convulsion went on to develop epilepsy (*British Medical Journal,* November 30, 1991).

Some types of convulsions, however, apparently should be taken more seriously than others, because they are associated with a significantly higher risk of later epilepsy (over 6 percent). They are convulsions that lasted more than fifteen minutes, convulsions that recurred during the same illness, and focal convulsions, which are partial seizures with motor or sensory effects that reflect the affected part of the brain. Very possibly, fever convulsions take these forms in children who have an inherited predisposition to epilepsy or a neurological abnormality that later leads to the disease.

HOW DO YOU KNOW IT'S EPILEPSY?

It's not always easy to tell. Seizures can have other causes, and they're sometimes hard to distinguish from epilepsy. An estimated 20 percent of people referred to one specialized center for "resistant" epilepsy who didn't respond to treatment actually had some unrelated disorder.

Other neurological conditions, including migraine, may produce episodes that resemble partial seizures, as can certain kinds of heart disease or severe hypoglycemia. Attacks may be emotional in origin. Acute anxiety can cause similar symptoms, and brief spells of fainting may be an unconscious "cutoff" device to escape from painful memories or situations. The vast majority of these, it's important to remember, are no more intentional or conscious than epilepsy itself.

The best way to diagnose epilepsy is an electroencephalogram (EEG) taken during the attack, which shows abnormal brain waves (ideally, with a videotape to record concurrent behavior). Such studies can be done in a clinic, where various means are used to trigger a seizure, or with a portable unit that a person wears during the day.

Other high-tech aids, like computerized tomography (CT) and magnetic resonance imaging (MRI), may be indicated if it seems possible that a cyst or excess fluid in the brain is responsible for epilepsy, or to identify the abnormal part of the brain more precisely in considering surgery.

CAN THE RATIONALE, BENEFITS, AND ADVERSE EFFECTS OF MEDICATION BE DISCUSSED HONESTLY AND OPENLY?

Medication to prevent seizures by modifying biochemical and electrical activity in the brain is the standard approach. Among the most commonly used anticonvulsant drugs are carbamazepine, phenytoin, valproic acid, phenobarbital, and Valium-like compounds. The choice will depend on factors like the type of seizures you have, and your susceptibility to various side effects.

Whenever possible, most doctors prefer using a single anticonvulsant, but combinations may be effective when no one drug works well enough at a tolerable dose. It may take some trial-and-error patience to find the drug or drugs that work for you, but drug therapy eventually controls seizures in about three quarters of cases.

A review article in *The New England Journal of Medicine* (June 18, 1992) suggests that one third to one half of people with epilepsy don't take medications as prescribed, and that this is a significant cause of uncontrolled seizures. Unpleasant side effects like dizziness, insomnia, and nausea often make this understandable, but it's still unwise. If you're unhappy with how your medication affects you, discuss it with your doctor. There are almost always alternatives. (If you don't feel comfortable bringing it up, find a doctor with whom you will feel comfortable.)

Above all, don't abruptly stop taking anticonvulsants. Sudden withdrawal can cause repeated, lengthy, and potentially dangerous seizures.

HOW CAN SIDE EFFECTS BE KEPT TO A MINIMUM?

Adverse reactions occur in about one fifth of people using a single anticonvulsant, and double that when two are used. Although they can have a serious impact on your quality of life (sedation is common), these effects are rarely dangerous and may improve when the dose is adjusted. But serious toxicity (such as a drop in white blood cells or a change in liver function) does occur with some of these drugs, and you may need regular blood tests to ensure safety.

Anticonvulsants can interact with other medications, including some antibiotics, ulcer, and cardiac drugs, reducing the potency of one or the other. Certain ones, such as carbamazepine, can make oral contraceptives less effective. You may need to take a stronger oral contraceptive, or use a different method of contraception.

Women are advised to continue taking antiepileptic drugs during pregnancy. An epileptic attack can pose a great threat to the developing fetus by temporarily cutting off the blood supply and causing brain damage. However, antiepileptic drugs increase the risk of birth defects—to two to three times the rate in the population at large. Among the most common defects are cleft lip palate, congenital heart disease, spina bifida, and mental retardation. Single-drug therapy appears to be considerably safer than combinations of drugs. Only one drug, trimethadione (brand name: Tridione), is considered dangerous enough to recommend terminating pregnancy during its use. Women using other antiepileptic drugs are encouraged to continue their pregnancies. "More than 90 percent of such pregnancies are uneventful and will result in a healthy baby," according to an article in *The Lancet* (June 1, 1991). However, women with epilepsy should consult with their doctor before trying to become pregnant.

WILL I HAVE TO TAKE ANTICONVULSANTS FOR THE REST OF MY LIFE?

Epilepsy eventually remits in a fair number of people. According to a review article, twenty years after the diagnosis, about half of those with epilepsy have been seizure-free without anticonvulsants for at least five years.

Anticonvulsants may be discontinued after seizures have been controlled for several years. But there is the risk of recurrence; new seizures will occur in up to 60 percent of adults and 25 percent of children. Tapering the drugs gradually, over a period of months, seems associated with reduced chance of relapse.

People with seizures that first appeared during childhood were easily controlled with drugs, and were not very frequent at any time have the best chance of lasting remission when drugs are withdrawn. The longer seizures have been controlled with drugs, the less likely a relapse will occur when they are withdrawn. Relapses of some kinds of seizures are more likely than others.

When a relapse does occur, resuming medication almost invariably brings seizures back under control. Even without renewed medication, in fact, a single relapse may be an isolated event. About half of relapses occur while the anticonvulsant dose is being reduced, suggesting that the seizure is actually the result of withdrawal. Some studies found fewer relapses if the withdrawal period was extended (*Clinical Pharmacy,* October 1990).

WHAT ACTIONS SHOULD BE TAKEN IF A SEIZURE OCCURS?

Frightening as they may be, seizures almost always run their course and cause no damage to mind or body. There is nothing you can do to stop a seizure once it has begun, but there are steps you can take to prevent injury from occurring. The most important step is to ensure that breathing is unobstructed. Contrary to previous views, it is not necessary to put anything, such as a leather belt, in the person's mouth to protect him or her from biting the tongue. In fact, rather than preventing tongue injury, this action might push the tongue to the back of the throat and block the airway. Vomiting also poses a threat to unobstructed breathing; if the person having a seizure vomits, try to clear the mouth and nose (using something other than your fingers, for you might get bitten). It is a good idea to loosen clothing around the neck. A person having a seizure is also at risk of self-injury from violent jerking motions. It is not necessary to restrain all movement, but the person can be protected by cushioning the blows with pillows, towels, or extra clothing.

For people with a history of epilepsy, it is probably unnecessary to call 911 when a seizure occurs, although a doctor should be consulted immediately afterward. Prolonged or rapidly repeated seizures, however, require prompt and effective treatment. This condition, *status epilepticus,* affects between fifty and sixty thousand people each year, and is fatal for 3 percent of children and 10 percent of adults who develop it, according to a report by the Epilepsy Foundation of America (*Journal of the American Medical Association,* August 18, 1993).

The longer the episode continues, the poorer the outcome; urgent drug treatment to relieve *status epilepticus* should be begun whenever a seizure has lasted more than ten minutes, the authors of the Epilepsy Foundation of America report recommend.

Any seizure may be dangerous if it occurs at the wrong time: when driving a car, for example. The risk of accidents may be less than previously estimated, however. A study of 30,420 people with and without epilepsy and diabetes found that epilepsy and diabetes raised the risk of traffic accidents, but only slightly (*The New England Journal of Medicine*, January 3, 1991).

WHEN IS SURGERY RECOMMENDED?

Surgery can reduce or eliminate seizures by removing the brain cells whose uncontrolled electrical activity initiates them. Such procedures can only be done if the brain area is small and doesn't control vital functions like speech or hearing. The risk of death is under 5 percent.

According to a 1990 Consensus Report of the National Institutes of Health, surgery should only be considered an alternative when all attempts at medication have failed—that is, for about 10 to 20 percent of people with epilepsy. A very thorough evaluation is essential to guide the surgery safely and effectively.

Resources

Assistance and counseling, service referrals, and free information packets are offered by:

Epilepsy Foundation of America
4351 Garden City Drive
Landover, MD 20785
(800) 332-1000 or (301) 459-3700

The *Epilepsy Foundation Library* will research epilepsy and related topics and mail out information. The library is open to the public.

Same address as above
(800) 332-4050

Service referrals, literature, support groups, legal advocacy, and newsletter are available through:

Epilepsy Institute
257 Park Avenue South
New York, NY 10010
(212) 677-8550

◆ FIBROMYALGIA

Widespread musculoskeletal pain, persistent fatigue, and nonrefreshing sleep feel bad enough in a passing illness, such as the flu. When these symptoms are chronic, as they are in fibromyalgia, they can be devastating. Until fairly recently, the defining criteria for this condition were vague, and many doctors treated it as a "diagnosis of exclusion"—it was what they figured you had if they couldn't find anything else.

But now it's well accepted that fibromyalgia is a genuine disorder that is more common than rheumatoid arthritis. It afflicts more than 10 percent of people who come to general medical clinics, and 15 to 20 percent of those who visit rheumatology clinics. The pain is often accompanied by tenderness and stiffness in the muscles and tendons, which may be so severe that normal movement is impaired. People with fibromyalgia often have other disorders, such as irritable bowel syndrome, headaches, and premenstrual syndrome.

The cause of fibromyalgia is unknown. Some researchers suspect that the pain comes from microscopic muscle tears, to which some people are genetically susceptible. Possibly, an imbalance of neurotransmitters—messenger chemicals in the brain—and an excess of substance P, which carries pain messages, is at the root of the disorder.

Although the overall incidence isn't known, among sufferers who seek medical treatment, at least, it's far more common in women than men. About 90 percent of fibromyalgia is diagnosed in women. Typically, it comes on during the childbearing years, although onset may also be in childhood or later life.

Misdiagnosis is still a serious problem. Experts believe that fibromyalgia is overlooked more often than it is detected, and sometimes long, fruitless treatment, including surgery, results.

HOW CAN I TELL IF I HAVE FIBROMYALGIA?

Typically, a person with fibromyalgia has generalized muscle pain, persistent fatigue, and difficulty sleeping. But unlike screening for arthritis (with which it is readily confused), X rays, joint examinations, and laboratory tests are normal.

This doesn't mean, however, that there's no test for fibromyalgia. According to a report of the multicenter criteria committee of the American College of Rheumatology, diagnosing the disorder depends on finding "tender points" in specific areas of the body, which hurt when pressed (*Arthritis and Rheumatism,* 1990, no. 3).

There are eighteen of these points, distributed around the upper back, neck, and chest, near the buttocks and at the elbows and knees. By the American College of Rheumatology criteria, eleven must be tender to pressure that would not seem painful elsewhere in the body to justify the diagnosis.

WHY IS DIAGNOSIS SO DIFFICULT?

Sometimes, the pattern of symptoms is confusing. If pain is concentrated in one part of your body, both you and your doctor may overlook less severe, more generalized, achiness. People have had unnecessary surgery to relieve neck, back, or wrist pain that actually is the tip of the fibromyalgia iceberg.

In particular, fibromyalgia is easily confused with other diseases that cause fatigue and generalized pain, and for which diagnostic tests are not totally reliable. One such illness is Lyme disease, which can cause a kind of arthritis. In one study, seventy-seven of seven hundred people seeking treatment at a Lyme disease center actually had fibromyalgia.

Fibromyalgia often occurs along with other disorders; an estimated 10 percent of people who visit rheumatologists for fibromyalgia also have diseases like arthritis.

IS FIBROMYALGIA PSYCHOSOMATIC?

Many doctors used to believe so (one misnomer for the condition was "psychogenic rheumatism"), but no longer. One study found that people with this disorder are no more likely to be depressed or anxious, or to have any emotional disorder than those with arthritis (*American Journal of Psychiatry,* 1991, no. 148). Like any chronically painful condition, of course, fibromyalgia is liable to *produce* emotional distress.

HOW CAN I DEAL WITH STRESS?

Clearly, stress plays a role in fibromyalgia. Like arthritis, it's a disorder that flares up and dies down, and stress may trigger exacerbations. It certainly makes pain more difficult to bear. Techniques of stress control, such as muscle relaxation, meditation, or counseling to help deal with the pain and life disruptions of the condition can be extremely helpful.

What's more, severe stress—emotional or physical—appears connected to the onset of fibromyalgia about half the time. It's not unusual for symptoms to appear first soon after the death of a loved one, a divorce, or an automobile accident. After a physical trauma, pain may initially be focused on the injured part of the body, but may spread generally within several months.

Infection is another bodily stress that has been linked to fibromyalgia. One study found, for example, that symptoms appeared not long after certain viral infections (*Arthritis and Rheumatism,* 1991, no. 34). In another, 22 of 287 people treated for Lyme disease also had fibromyalgia, which apparently had been triggered by that infection (*Annals of Internal Medicine,* August 15, 1992).

Probably none of these stresses actually *cause* fibromyalgia, but they bring it out in people who are genetically susceptible.

IS FIBROMYALGIA PROGRESSIVE?

Painful as it may be, fibromyalgia doesn't damage joints or muscles the way a disease like arthritis does. Symptoms may get worse for several years, especially if the diagnosis was early in the course of the illness. But fibromyalgia won't kill you or cripple you. It's extremely important to be aware of this.

The impact of fibromyalgia shouldn't be dismissed as trivial, however.

Job change and unemployment are more common as a result of this disorder than arthritis, although good management can make a real difference.

IS THERE A CURE?

No medication, physical therapy, or psychotherapy is known that will get at the root of the disorder and relieve symptoms permanently. But treatment can make a real difference in how well you can live with fibromyalgia's symptoms.

Probably the most important treatment is one you administer yourself: exercise. Inactivity deconditions muscles, which increases pain and fatigue, leading into a vicious cycle, but proper exercise can improve symptoms. Low-impact aerobic activity, such as biking, brisk walking, or (ideally) swimming is considered best.

If you're exhausted, in pain, and in poor condition from your disease, it may take a major effort to become active. Start slowly—as little as five minutes of nonstraining exercise per day—building up to a half hour three or four times weekly. Stretching beforehand can make exercise easier and safer. Some advocate the gentle stretch-and-relax benefits of yoga.

SHOULD I HAVE PHYSICAL THERAPY?

As with arthritis, a physical therapist can be a most helpful trainer in getting into exercise safely and effectively, particularly if your symptoms are severe or you have become deconditioned from inactivity. He or she (or your doctor) can also teach you principles of body mechanics—how to stand, sit, walk, and work—to minimize strain and keep going longer without fatigue.

Hands-on physical therapy has a role, too, but it is a limited one. Heat, electrical stimulation, and massage can ease pain, as can the "spray-and-stretch" technique in which the therapy anesthetizes a painful region with ethyl chloride, and then stretches it by hand. But these strategies are best used just for a week or two for flare-ups, until regular exercise becomes possible again. Being in control of your illness, remember, is the goal.

A Swiss study reported that electroacupuncture helped control the pain of fibromyalgia (*British Medical Journal,* November 21, 1992). This is a modern version of traditional Chinese acupuncture in which needles stimulated by electrical current are inserted into certain parts of the body.

WHAT DRUGS DO YOU PRESCRIBE?

There is no medication that treats the actual disease of fibromyalgia, although painkillers, such as standard doses of acetaminophen (Tylenol), are recommended. Nonsteroidal anti-inflammatories (NSAIDs), like ibuprofen and naproxen, are often prescribed, but they are ineffective in treating fibromyalgia, which is not an inflammatory disorder. Low doses of the tricyclic antidepressant amitriptyline (some brand names: Elavil, Amitril) have been proven effective in reducing the pain of fibromyalgia, as has alprazolam (Xanax), a mild tranquilizer (*Journal of Musculoskeletal Pain*, 1994, no. 1).

The other reason for drugs is to address the sleep problems that seem a central part of fibromyalgia. Be careful with Xanax; this drug is highly addictive.

WHY IS SLEEP SO IMPORTANT?

Any condition that causes pain may rob you of sleep. In the case of fibromyalgia, the situation is apparently more complex. Nonrestorative sleep (you may get enough hours, but you don't feel rested) is almost universal with this disease, and many think sleep disturbance is at the core of the disorder.

In fibromyalgia, there's apparently a deficiency of stage four sleep, the deep slumber that your body needs for rest and renewal. In fact, the symptoms of fibromyalgia can be experimentally induced in healthy persons by repeatedly waking them when they enter this phase of the sleep cycle. Some researchers speculate that stress or other illnesses may trigger fibromyalgia by interfering with deep sleep.

Improving sleep is an important strategy for relieving symptoms. Allow time for a good eight hours of sleep, and follow lifestyle practices that promote it: keep a regular schedule, don't take midday naps, and avoid caffeine, alcohol, and tobacco at night.

If your sleeping remains poor, medication may be prescribed, at least for the short term. Small doses of tricyclic antidepressants, taken at bed-time, apparently promote vital stage four sleep, as does cyclobenzaprine, a muscle relaxant. Sedatives and benzodiazepines (a family of mild tran-quilizers which includes Valium) may disrupt the kind of sleep you need most.

◆ GALLSTONES

The gallbladder stores bile en route from the liver to the intestine (where it aids in digestion). The organ can also be the source of severe pain, and has become the center of a lucrative—and controversial—surgical industry.

When components of bile (most often cholesterol, but sometimes calcium and bilirubin) become too concentrated to remain dissolved, they begin to solidify, forming gallstones. Intense pain occurs when a stone blocks the outlet of the gallbladder. It generally lasts for several hours and is likely to recur within several months.

On the other hand, gallstones may be "silent," causing no pain or other symptoms, and are discovered accidentally in the course of routine examination. About 10 to 15 percent of American adults—more than twenty million people—have gallstones (twice as many women as men, and more older than younger people). Most never know they have them.

MUST SYMPTOMLESS GALLSTONES BE TREATED?

Most experts agree that if your gallstones were discovered incidentally, by ultrasound for example, and cause no symptoms, there's no reason to do anything about them. One study that followed 123 people with symptomless gallstones found that just 18 percent developed any symptoms at all over the next twenty years.

In its guidelines for the treatment of gallstones (*Annals of Internal Medicine*, October 1, 1993), the American College of Physicians recommends "expectant management" (i.e., watching and waiting) for patients with symptomless stones, regardless of age or sex. "The effort and minor risks of surgical and nonsurgical intervention still outweigh their corresponding benefits," the report says.

The one justification for prophylactic gallbladder removal is cancer prevention. But the risk of gallbladder cancer for people with gallstones is actually quite low: one per one thousand people per year.

According to the American College of Physicians and a consensus statement by the National Institutes of Health (*Journal of the American Medical
Association,* February 24, 1993), prophylactic removal should be an option
in the rare situations when cancer risk is unusually high—when the gallbladder is calcified, for example, or when the person belongs to an ethnic
group at increased risk, like the Pima Indians. Certain anatomical abnormalities and exceptionally large stones (over 3 centimeters in diameter)
may also raise cancer risk.

IF MY GALLSTONES CAUSE PAIN, DO I NEED SURGERY?

The most obvious and permanent solution to gallbladder pain is to remove
the offending organ, because otherwise the problem is likely to recur and
may progress (25 percent in ten to twenty years) to complications requiring
urgent surgery.

Some 30 percent of people who have had one gallbladder attack, however, never have another, even after ten years or longer. You may choose
to wait and see if the pain recurs before deciding what to do.

Of course, you want to be sure that your pain is the result of gallstones.
Many symptoms popularly associated with the gallbladder—intolerance to
fatty foods, bloating, belching, flatulence—actually have nothing to do with
that organ (even if ultrasound shows you have gallstones).

Classic gallbladder pain is usually severe and in the upper right side of
the abdomen. It doesn't respond to the usual digestive remedies, often
peaks around midnight, and goes away by itself after several hours. Chronic
pain is unlikely to be related to gallstones.

When stones lead to acute inflammation of the gallbladder, severe
abdominal pain is usually accompanied by nausea, vomiting, and fever.
Because of the risk of gangrene and gallbladder perforation (rupture), and
a 30 percent chance of a repeat episode within the next three months,
removal of the gallbladder is strongly advised in this situation.

WHAT KIND OF SURGERY IS BEST FOR ME?

Before 1989, there was just one procedure for cholecystectomy (gallbladder removal) in the United States: ''open surgery.'' This operation requires

a six-inch abdominal incision, up to seven days in the hospital, and three to six weeks of convalescence.

Then laparoscopic cholecystectomy arrived from France. Its advantages over open surgery were clear. Instead of a big incision, several small ones are made. Then the gallbladder is removed through a long, hollow fiber-optic device fitted with a television camera, which allows the surgeons to view their magnified work field on a video screen. Because it involves a tiny incision rather than abdominal surgery, convalescence is much quicker—you're out of the hospital in a day or two—and postoperative pain is much less.

The new procedure was a major hit. With some help from aggressive marketing by equipment manufacturers and hospitals, by 1992, 80 percent of gallbladder removals were done laparoscopically. "Seldom has a new surgical procedure gained acceptance so quickly," according to an article in the *Journal of the American Medical Association* (September 22/29, 1993).

Was acceptance *too* quick? Statistics compiled by the New York State Department of Health revealed that the rate of injuries to the bile duct, bladder, intestine, liver, aorta, and other structures has increased markedly since laparoscopic cholecystectomy came upon the scene.

In a six-month period, there were thirty-five bile duct injuries during cholecystectomy, compared with just one in all of 1988, the last year that all gallbladder removals were done by open surgery. In eighteen months, there were six deaths with the new procedure. Although a head-to-head comparison has never been made, it seems very possible that complications, including death, are more likely with laparoscopic than open cholecystectomy.

CAN LAPAROSCOPIC CHOLECYSTECTOMY BE SAFER?

One possible explanation for these unattractive statistics is that, in their haste to get in on a good thing, many surgeons have picked up their laparoscopy tools with inadequate training. "The surgeons would train in this technique rather minimally, often at a weekend conference at a resort hotel," according to Peter Slocum, director of public affairs for the New York State Department of Health. "Then they operate on a couple of pigs, and then they do it on their patients."

Although quick study is something of a surgical tradition ("See one, do one, teach one," goes an adage), critics point out that the principle seems questionable for laparoscopic surgery, which with its tiny tools, precise demands, and limited visibility requires an unusual amount of skill.

The price of inexperience ("a steep learning curve," in professional parlance) was suggested by a study released by the Southern Surgeons Club (*The New England Journal of Medicine,* April 18, 1991). Their analysis showed a 2.2 percent bile duct injury rate on the first thirteen patients operated on by newly trained surgical teams, which dropped to 0.1 percent in later patients.

Some of these figures have begun to sink in, it seems. The New York State Department of Health has issued hospital guidelines to make sure surgeons performing laparoscopic cholecystectomy are adequately trained. And innovations to enhance safety are under study. A national survey to assess quality of care, coauthored by Mohan C. Airan, M.D., professor of surgery at Chicago Medical School, found that the complication rate drops sharply when two experienced surgeons perform the procedure together.

The TV system of the laparoscope provides "a binocular view of the gallbladder rather than a three-dimensional view, and the tactile feel of the hands inside the abdomen is also lost," Dr. Airan explained. "But when two surgeons are looking at the monitor, each is looking at a different portion of the screen and consulting with the other as they go along."

In six hundred laparoscopic procedures, Dr. Airan said, he and his partner have not had a single bile duct injury.

If you decide to have laparoscopic cholecystectomy, you can enhance your safety by making sure the surgeon has undergone rigorous training and proven his or her competence. (The New York State Department of Health, for example, requires the surgeon to have done ten procedures under direct supervision by an experienced laparoscopist and been monitored for the first three months on his or her own.) Better still, get two competent surgeons to do it.

WHAT DOCTOR SHOULD I SEE FOR GALLBLADDER PAIN?

Dr. Airan, himself a surgeon, advises against seeking the first evaluation for possible gallbladder pain from a member of his specialty. A primary care physician (internist, gastroenterologist, general practitioner, or family practitioner) can best give you (or refer you for) a workup that will determine whether gallstones are indeed involved, and help you decide what to do next.

Keep in mind that, even though laparoscopic surgery has a short hospital stay and a rapid convalescence, it's not to be taken lightly or done more readily than open surgery. Soon after the new procedure took hold, gallbladder removals in the United States made a quantum leap, from a half million to six hundred thousand per year.

In one study (*Journal of the American Medical Association,* September 22/29, 1993), the rate of cholecystectomies done in an HMO rose from 1.35 per 1,000 enrollees (in 1988) to 2.15 (in 1992). It's unlikely that an explosion of gallstones was responsible.

ARE THERE ALTERNATIVES TO SURGERY?

Gallstones can be dissolved with bile acids, taken by mouth over a six-month to two-year period, or by direct contact solvents introduced into the gallbladder with a catheter. Gallstones can be shattered by ultrasonic waves (extracorporeal sound-wave lithotripsy), usually with the help of oral bile acids. This last procedure hasn't been approved by the FDA.

Bile acids and lithotripsy are noninvasive and painless (although lithotripsy is followed by at least one episode of pain in one third of those who have it done), and direct contact solvent therapy is far less extensive than surgery. But these approaches are applicable only for stones of limited size and certain composition, and recurrence rates are estimated at 10 percent per year for five years.

Several years ago, the manufacturers of oral bile acid tablets (Actigall) actively promoted the use of their product for symptomless stones, claiming it would forestall the danger of progression to pain and emergency surgery. The FDA made them stop. The fact is, if gallstones are causing no trouble, there's no more excuse to use solvent therapy or lithotripsy than to do surgery.

✦ GENITAL HERPES

In the early 1980s, genital herpes was discovered. The sexually transmitted disease, which had actually been around (largely ignored) for centuries, suddenly seemed to be spreading wildly. Proclaimed "the new scarlet letter" by *Time* magazine (complete with a glowing *H* on the cover), herpes had millions of Americans thinking fearfully about their dating habits.

Today, far stronger reasons to worry—AIDS and hepatitis, to name two—have made it easier to think rationally about herpes. Caused by a virus, herpes simplex, related to those that cause chickenpox, shingles, and infectious mononucleosis, genital herpes is virtually identical to a cold sore, but in a more emotionally charged area.

It is almost always a benign disorder, and for the vast majority of those infected, occasionally troublesome, if at all. Like similar viral diseases, however, it isn't curable; once you have it, it may recur, and you can transmit it to others.

What has become obvious in the last decade is that far more people have been exposed to the virus than had been believed. According to an epidemiological survey in *The New England Journal of Medicine* (July 6, 1989), one adult in five, ages thirty to forty-four, has the antibodies that indicate infection. The rates are higher among women than men, and among blacks than whites.

CAN I HAVE HERPES WITHOUT KNOWING IT?

The classic symptoms of genital herpes, when you are first infected, are a blistering, sometimes painful, sore in the genital area, often accompanied by mild flulike symptoms including fever. Recurrent lesions, which are almost always less severe, appear occasionally, frequently, or not at all. The majority of people infected with the disease have "silent herpes," investigators now believe. The first episode was mild enough to escape notice, and there were no (or very mild) recurrences.

A study of 779 women at a sexually transmitted disease clinic in Seattle found that nearly half had positive blood tests, indicating they had been infected with herpes. But only 22 percent of the infected women had symptoms of infection at the time they were examined, and another 16 percent reported a history of herpes symptoms. Nearly two thirds, in other words, had no clinical signs or history that would show they were infected.

CAN I TRANSMIT HERPES WITHOUT SYMPTOMS?

It used to be thought that herpes was contagious only while there was an actual sore, or in the few days preceding (often heralded by early symptoms of itching or burning). Recent years, however, have led to a more distressing conclusion: a substantial number (estimates range from 17 to 50 percent) of people with herpes can shed virus—and therefore transmit the disease—at least some of the time when they are without symptoms.

According to a study of 306 women reported in *Annals of Internal Medicine* (March 15, 1992), symptomless viral shedding is more common in the first three months after the disease is acquired. An unknown proportion of people with "silent herpes" shed the virus and can transmit the disease. It appears that symptomless transmission, in fact, is the principal way that herpes is spread.

WILL A CONDOM PROTECT ME AGAINST HERPES?

Herpes is transmitted by direct, skin-to-skin contact with a sore, or with the area that is shedding the virus. If a condom is covering that spot, it offers protection. If the spot is elsewhere in the genital area, it doesn't. The bottom line: wearing a condom (or having your partner wear one) provides limited protection.

WHEN IS ACYCLOVIR PRESCRIBED?

Acyclovir (Zovirax) is the only drug approved by the FDA for the treatment of herpes. It's an antiviral—it interferes with the synthesis of DNA, and thus with the virus's ability to replicate—and while it has been shown to reduce the frequency of recurrence, it won't eradicate the organism that causes herpes.

The effectiveness of this therapy is well established. Oral acyclovir is a standard treatment for the original infection: it shortens the duration of pain, healing time (from fourteen days to eight days), and viral shedding. Intravenous acyclovir works a bit better, but it requires hospitalization and is usually reserved for people with immune disorders who are at risk of severe complications.

For recurrences, acyclovir can be applied topically, in a cream. It reduces viral shedding, but does little for symptoms. Oral medication, taken within a day of an episode's onset, shortens viral shedding and healing time (from seven days to six), but has little if any effect on symptoms (*The New England Journal of Medicine,* September 10, 1992).

Increasingly, daily doses of acyclovir have been used to prevent recurrences, particularly in people who have them frequently. In one randomized, placebo-controlled multicenter study of people who previously had six or more recurrences yearly, the average number of episodes dropped from twelve per year at the start of the study to one in the third year; nearly two thirds had no episodes during that final year; and one quarter of the participants had no recurrences at all during the entire study (*Journal of the American Medical Association,* February 13, 1991).

Even when recurrences are suppressed by acyclovir, asymptomatic shedding of the virus—and transmission—can still occur.

IS ACYCLOVIR SAFE? HOW LONG CAN I TAKE IT?

Acyclovir is what's called a "prodrug"—it is an inactive compound that is activated inside the body. Cells infected with the herpesvirus convert acyclovir into the active drug, but other cells don't. This should make the compound relatively nontoxic.

Adverse effects are generally mild: nausea, diarrhea, headache, rash, weakness, dizziness, and abdominal pain have been reported. In the 1991 *Journal of the American Medical Association* study, they were not common (4.8 percent had nausea in the first year; 2.4 percent diarrhea); the other side effects were less frequent and became less so as the study progressed. Abnormalities in blood count, kidney function, and liver function tests were rare, and no more common in the third year than the first.

In an extension of the study, acyclovir therapy remained safe and effective for five years: recurrences dropped to an average of .8 per year in the final year, and adverse effects remained mild and few (*Archives of Dermatology,* July 1993).

Apparently, the herpesvirus in otherwise healthy people rarely becomes resistant to acyclovir, according to *The New England Journal of Medicine* 1992 review. This has been a problem, however, among people with immune problems (such as AIDS) who are treated with heavy intravenous doses of the drug.

IF I BECOME PREGNANT, HOW CAN I PROTECT MY BABY?

The herpes simplex virus is transmitted to her baby by an infected mother, either during pregnancy or at delivery, in an estimated one in seventy-five hundred to thirty thousand births; 40 percent of these babies die or sustain neurological damage.

Until the mid-1980s, the practice was to do weekly cultures of women with a history of herpes infection, to see if virus was being shed. Since then, however, this expensive procedure has been largely abandoned. The current recommendation is to perform a cesarean section only if the mother has a lesion at the time of delivery. (A 1992 survey, however, found that 38 percent of a random sample of American obstetricians still did screening cultures.)

An analysis of past studies reported in the *Journal of the American Medical Association* (July 7, 1993) concluded that little was to be gained by doing a cesarean in the case of women with recurrent herpes lesions at the time of delivery; the reduction in infant mortality was more than offset by the surgical risk to the mother. The authors recommended cesarean delivery only for women who were having a first episode of herpes at the time of birth.

An editorial in the same issue of the *Journal,* however, called some of the data in the analysis questionable, and advised cesarean for any woman with a lesion, new or recurrent, at delivery.

Oral acyclovir, given to reduce the likelihood of a recurrence late in pregnancy, has been found safe in small trials. But, as the editorial authors point out, most babies with herpes are born to mothers with "silent herpes," who have no history of infection. The most effective way to protect infants would be to culture *all* women in labor, to see if they are shedding the herpesvirus. But no fast, accurate, and economically practical method for doing this now exists. The standard practice is to give acyclovir injections to infants who show signs of herpes.

HOW CAN I DEAL WITH THE PAIN AND DISTRESS OF HERPES?

Although genital herpes is almost invariably a minor ailment from a physical point of view, the same can't be said about its emotional impact. Particularly when recurrences are frequent, people infected with herpes may suffer shame, guilt, and anxiety that can come with any sexually transmitted disease. Confusion about how and when to inform potential sexual partners can lead to social withdrawal.

Psychotherapy and support groups have helped many people take herpes in stride, and learn to live with it. Your doctor, or the resource listed below, may help you to find the appropriate therapy.

Therapy or counseling may also reduce the actual frequency of recurrences. Various studies have strongly suggested a role for stress in triggering episodes, and learning to reduce stress may be helpful.

Resources

Herpes Resource Center
c/o American Social Health Association
P.O. Box 13827
Research Triangle Park, NC 27709
(919) 361-8488

◆ GLAUCOMA

Glaucoma is the third largest cause of blindness in the United States. An estimated 15 million Americans have the condition; 1.6 million suffer visual impairment; and 150,000 become blind as a consequence, according to the Baltimore Eye Survey. The risk rises with age; it is rare before age forty, while 2 to 3 percent of the elderly have open-angle glaucoma. This is the most common type of glaucoma, characterized by increasing intraocular pressure leading to a gradual loss of vision.

A fluid called aqueous humor normally circulates through the part of the eye around the lens. In chronic open-angle glaucoma, the fluid doesn't drain properly, causing pressure to build up within the eye and, in the worse-case scenario, damage to the optic nerve. The field of vision shrinks, beginning at the periphery, at an average rate of 1 to 3 percent per year.

Glaucoma can be treated with medication and with surgery. But first it must be detected, and this is complicated by the fact that symptoms of the disorder do not usually appear until substantial nerve damage has taken place. Visual acuity is not affected until fairly late in the disease. Symptoms like headache, blurred vision, pain and halos around light are, contrary to popular belief, not related to the condition.

HOW ACCURATE IS THE TEST FOR GLAUCOMA?

If you've had a standard eye exam, it probably included tonometry, a test of pressure within the eye, which is a way of screening for glaucoma. Tonometry measures intraocular pressure by testing the eye's resistance to a slight amount of force applied by a metal device. High intraocular pressure would indicate a buildup of fluid within the eye, which may be a sign of glaucoma.

The connection between increased pressure (also known as intraocular hypertension) and glaucoma is not simple, however. Some people have abnormally high intraocular pressure, and do not develop glaucoma, while others (25 to 50 percent with the disease) suffer damage although their pressure remains within normal limits. It is more accurate to say that intraocular hypertension is a *risk factor* for glaucoma.

What's more, the pressure tester used in most mass screening is not the most accurate available, which requires the use of eyedrops, a skillful operator, and more time than is usually allotted.

Other tests for glaucoma are ophthalmoscopy and visual field testing. In the first, a hand-held instrument makes it possible to examine the optic disc for abnormalities; the second tests your ability to see flashes of light at the edge of your field of vision.

These tests are more accurate than tonometry, because they are intended to spot the actual physical and visual changes that are caused by the disease process. But even they aren't entirely free from false positives: the optic disc may be abnormal or visual field limited for reasons other than glaucoma.

IF MY EYEBALL PRESSURE IS RAISED, SHOULD I BE TREATED FOR GLAUCOMA?

Not necessarily. In view of the variable connection between pressure and glaucoma, "intraocular pressure above the normal range . . . is no longer part of the definition of the disease," according to a review article in *The New England Journal of Medicine* (April 15, 1993).

For reasons that are not understood, some eyes apparently can tolerate "abnormal" pressure without damage, while others deteriorate at pressures considered normal.

To diagnose glaucoma, it's considered wisest to weigh the evidence from the various examinations of eye structure and function and to rule out other possible causes of abnormalities. Other risk factors may be taken into account: the rate of the disease appears to be higher in people with high blood pressure, diabetes, or (the connection is less certain here) myopia.

It seems likely that the tendency toward glaucoma runs in families. A defective gene (on chromosome 1) was identified in one family where twenty-two of thirty-seven members in five generations suffered from a severe form of the disease. There are probably other genes involved in other variants of glaucoma (*Journal of the American Medical Association*, June 2, 1993).

Race clearly affects the risk of glaucoma. By a conservative estimate, the incidence of glaucoma is four times higher among African Americans than among whites. One survey found that over 11 percent of African Americans over age eighty had evidence of nerve damage from glaucoma. The disease is apparently undertreated in this population, leading to blindness rates as much as eight times higher than in whites (*The New England Journal of Medicine*, November 14, 1991).

CAN GLAUCOMA BE TREATED EFFECTIVELY?

The various medical and surgical treatments for glaucoma all have a common goal: to reduce intraocular pressure. Although this has been the standard approach since the nineteenth century, the ability of treatment to actually halt optic nerve damage and vision loss has never been conclusively proven.

One expert summarized the situation this way: "The available data from clinical studies suggest that there is a significant reduction in the rate of initial injury when eyedrops are used to lower pressure. The protective effect is not absolute, however, and not all trials show a significant effect" (*The New England Journal of Medicine*, April 15, 1993).

There are apparently individual differences: some people with suspected glaucoma may go untreated for years without loss of vision; others (10 percent, by one estimate) lose their sight despite treatment. Still, pressure-lowering treatment is the best bet to protect vision when glaucoma is diagnosed or is strongly suspected.

The most common treatment is beta-adrenergic blockers eyedrops (Timoptic, Blocadren, Timolide) taken daily, which reduce the formation of fluid in the eye. Other popular options are epinephrine, which reduces inflow and improves outflow of fluid, and pilocarpine eyedrops, which increase the aqueous outflow.

Although these are topical medications—placed directly in the eye, where they are needed—all are absorbed by the body and can have systemic side effects. Like similar drugs used to treat high blood pressure, the beta-blockers can cause breathing difficulties, irregular heart rhythm, depression, weakness or fatigue, or sexual dysfunction. Epinephrine may produce headache, tremor, increased blood pressure, or heart rhythm disturbances.

It's important to discuss side effects with your physician, particularly if you have other medical problems or are taking other drugs.

A new approach—with an old drug—may improve glaucoma treatment. Ethacrynic acid, a diuretic, appears to improve fluid drainage from the eye by cleaning out the "sludge" that blocks the exit structure called the trabecular meshwork. A single yearly dose may be sufficient. If clinical trials are successful, the treatment may be available in 1995.

WHEN IS SURGERY INDICATED?

Surgery to create a permanent canal that helps drain fluid from the eye is generally used when drugs fail to reduce pressure adequately. Typically, pressure control remains effective in 75 percent of people, five years after the surgery. Innovations to improve the rate, such as drugs to keep the canal open, are currently being tested. The risk of permanent vision loss after surgery may be as high as 5 percent.

Another alternative, midway between eyedrops and surgery, is laser. The application of laser to the trabecular meshwork doesn't destroy tissue, apparently, but stimulates the release of chemicals that hasten outflow of fluid. The treatment is generally successful, but pressure rises again in up to half of treated eyes within five years, and repeated laser treatment is not always helpful.

CAN I DO ANYTHING TO HELP MYSELF?

Although controlled studies are lacking, lifestyle changes apparently assist medical intervention to lower eye pressure. Because hypertension causes increased fluid pressure in the eye, it is important to maintain normal blood pressure through diet, exercise, and cessation of smoking. Diabetes is also associated with glaucoma; efforts to control this condition, such as maintaining normal weight, are important.

◆ HAY FEVER

Hay fever is doubly misnamed: it has nothing to do with hay and it doesn't cause fever. *Seasonal allergic rhinitis* is the accurate term for this periodic condition of inflammation, congestion, and sneezing that affects an estimated twenty-two million Americans.

Like other allergies, hay fever is an immune reaction to normally harmless substances, in this case, pollen from trees, grasses, and/or weeds, particularly ragweed. You suffer symptoms when the pollen to which you're sensitive is in the air, depending on the season: tree pollen in spring; grasses in early summer; ragweed in late summer and fall.

Allergies to other substances can cause the same symptoms: molds (specifically, the airborne spores by which they reproduce), dust, and pets are common culprits. This can be seasonal (like pollen, mold is most abundant during the warm months), or year-round.

The tendency to allergic rhinitis runs in families: if one of your parents has it, your chance of getting it is 30 percent greater than average; if both parents have it, the risk is higher. People with hay fever also are prone to other allergic disorders, such as eczema, food allergy, and asthma.

HOW CAN I AVOID THINGS THAT GIVE ME HAY FEVER?

The first treatment for allergic rhinitis is simple and logical: stay away from the things to which you're allergic. If this is successful enough, you may need no medication.

But avoidance isn't always easy. In the case of pollen allergy, it's nearly impossible, because these tiny particles spread far and wide and even invade the air indoors. You can reduce the intensity of your symptoms, however, by using strategies to minimize your exposure. Stay indoors in the late mornings and afternoons of dry, sunny, breezy days, when pollen is most abundant. Schedule outdoor exercise for early morning or evening.

Air conditioning can limit the amount of pollen that enters your home, and an electronic air cleaner may further reduce the concentration of these tiny particles. Pollen can hitchhike on clothing and skin, so shower before bed, if you've spent time outdoors, and leave the day's clothing outside your bedroom.

Molds proliferate outdoors, from spring to late fall, and all year round in warm climates, as well as in damp indoor areas. If you're allergic to them, a dehumidifier may reduce your exposure in your house.

Dust is almost ubiquitous; what causes the allergic reaction is actually the waste products of dust mites, near-microscopic organisms that live in the dust. The "dust" you see floating in a beam of sunlight is actually dead mites and mite excrement.

Reducing dust in your bedroom can improve symptoms. Among the strategies recommended by the National Institutes of Health for dust-allergic people are to encase mattresses and box springs in a plastic dust-proof cover and to use Dacron pillows and washable blankets. Avoid wool or feather-stuffed comforters, and leave the floor uncarpeted. Keep as little as you can in the room. If possible, store clothes and shoes elsewhere; otherwise, put clothes in zippered plastic bags and shoes in boxes.

The room should be cleaned every day and aired thoroughly once a week, then kept closed except when occupied. Leave windows bare, or put up lightweight curtains and wash them every week. Keep pets out of the bedroom.

CAN CHANGING MY DIET HELP MY HAY FEVER?

Some people feel that milk products worsen hay fever symptoms, by increasing the production of mucus. The validity of this theory hasn't been documented, but if you feel reducing or eliminating dairy may help you, there's no harm in trying.

Certain foods may, however, make a difference. If you're allergic to pollen, you are likely to react allergically to chemically similar proteins in certain foods, making sneezing worse, or producing itching or digestive symptoms. Wheat is in the same family as grasses, and melons carry proteins that resemble those of ragweed. If you're allergic to birch pollen, you may react badly to apples, during the pollen season.

WILL OTC DRUGS HELP ME?

After avoidance, the simplest treatment of allergic rhinitis is taking over-the-counter drugs to relieve the symptoms. Antihistamines block the action of a chemical, histamine, that induces mucus production, sneezing, and itching; decongestants constrict blood vessels to reduce swelling in nasal tissues.

Both types of drugs work, often quite well, but at a cost. According to a review article in *The New England Journal of Medicine* (September 19, 1991), the most important side effect of antihistamines is sedation, which is reported by 20 to 35 percent of people using one common compound. Other adverse reactions include dry mouth, constipation, blurred vision, and accelerated heart rate. Children may become hyperexcited rather than drowsy.

Decongestants often cause insomnia and irritability. Use them carefully, if at all, if you have high blood pressure, heart disease, epilepsy, or hyperthyroidism; if you're on other medication, check with a doctor first. Decongestants, particularly nose drops and nasal sprays, shouldn't be used for more than a few days at a time. Your body adjusts to them quickly, and before long, you'll be more congested than before.

ARE PRESCRIPTION DRUGS ANY BETTER IN CONTROLLING SYMPTOMS?

No, but they may have fewer side effects. Several antihistamines—Seldane, Hismanal, and Claritin—have been developed that have less sedation than the older products. They are considerably more expensive and available only by prescription.

For people with severe nasal congestion due to allergy, doctors often prescribe nasal sprays that cause fewer side effects than antihistamines and decongestants. Cromolyn, a common ingredient in sprays which apparently blocks a step in the inflammatory process behind the sneezing, runny nose, and congestion, "has the fewest adverse effects of any antiallergic medication," according to *The New England Journal of Medicine* review article. When it works, it's about as effective as an antihistamine. But it doesn't work for everyone.

Corticosteroids are the strongest drugs for allergic rhinitis. Taken orally, they have potentially serious side effects and are rarely used for this purpose, but nasal steroids work just about as well and generally cause little trouble. Because the steroid is applied directly to the nose, absorption is minimal and side effects are local. About 10 percent of people who use it have some nasal irritation, burning, or sneezing, and occasionally, perforation of the wall between the nostrils develops with long-term use. But in clinical trials, there were no systemic side effects.

Currently, antihistamines and decongestants are usually the first line of attack, if simply avoiding the offending substances doesn't make symptoms better, but cromolyn nasal spray is at least as safe and sometimes works well. Most doctors reserve steroid nasal sprays for situations when antihistamines and other preparations don't work, but some may prescribe them first, in light of their few side effects and effectiveness.

WHAT ABOUT THOSE HOMEOPATHIC REMEDIES SOLD OVER THE COUNTER?

Homeopathic medicine was shown to be more effective than a placebo in treating 144 people with hay fever, according to a study conducted in Glasgow, Scotland (*The Lancet,* October 18, 1986). Several other well-designed studies have published similar results (*British Medical Journal,* February 9, 1991). Homeopathic medicine, though practiced by M.D.'s, approaches the treatment of illness in a manner that is entirely different from conventional medicine. Instead of drying up the mucus membranes, for example, a remedy will be chosen for the opposite effect. The idea is to mimic the body's own defense system which is flushing out the offending substance.

Homeopathic remedies are much-diluted substances given in the form of tiny pills or tinctures. According to the principles of homeopathy, the smaller the dose, the more powerful the effect.

DO I NEED TO KNOW WHAT I'M ALLERGIC TO?

It's often pretty obvious what's causing your misery, and there's no point in putting yourself through testing. If symptoms peak in the fall, you can assume that ragweed allergy is to blame. But people who are allergic to one thing are often allergic to others, and these can have a synergistic effect: a cat allergy may ordinarily cause no more than mild stuffiness, but it "primes" your nasal membranes so your reaction to pollen will be much more intense than it would be otherwise.

The main reason to undergo testing is to pinpoint your allergies so you can plan strategies to reduce exposure. Be aware, however, that allergy tests have not been subjected to careful study to prove safety and effectiveness.

The skin-prick test is most widely used: drops of various allergens are introduced just beneath the skin; an inflammatory reaction identifies those to which you're allergic. Injecting the allergen a bit deeper (intradermal testing) is more sensitive, but "carries a small but definite risk of a systemic reaction," according to a position paper of the American College of Physicians (*Annals of Internal Medicine*, February 15, 1989).

The RAST (radioallergosorbent test) is a lab test that measures the specific antibodies involved in allergy. It requires drawing a single sample of blood, rather than repeated pinpricks, but it is more expensive than skin testing. The American College of Physicians paper notes that RAST is somewhat less sensitive than skin testing.

Allergy testing, particularly lab tests like RAST, is most accurate when directed by your particular symptoms (rather than a "scatter shot" approach) and their history.

WHAT IS THE ROLE OF ALLERGY SHOTS?

Immunotherapy can be effective for people with *severe* hay fever that has been unresponsive to less risky treatment. Allergy shots can be quite effective—more than antihistamines or cromolyn. They appear to be as effective as steroids, though no well-designed comparative studies have proven this definitively.

In a series of injections, you are given increasing doses of the substance to which you are allergic, gradually building up your body's tolerance. A dose that is too high can trigger a massive, life-threatening allergic reaction. There have been forty-six immunotherapy deaths in a forty-year period in this country. Clearly, this treatment should be reserved for resistant cases and should be administered under careful conditions. The serious reactions usually occur within minutes of the injection, and they can be reversed with an immediate injection of adrenaline. A two-hour wait in the doctor's office after each injection is recommended. More than 90 percent of people improve after immunotherapy, if they've been properly diagnosed and treated, *The New England Journal of Medicine* review article says. The treatment reduces or eliminates the allergic response to the specific substances to which you're being desensitized, but not others, which makes accurate testing essential. Allergy shots involve a lot of time, trouble, and expense: injections are at first weekly, then every two to four weeks, all year round.

In the United Kingdom, wariness about immunotherapy has led to considerable restrictions in its use. A report of the British Society for Allergy and Clinical Immunology recently recommended that the treatment only be given by experienced physicians in a clinic where emergency resuscitation equipment is available. People with asthma, the paper noted, are particularly vulnerable to adverse effects of immunotherapy (*British Medical Journal,* October 9, 1993).

IF I AM A CANDIDATE FOR ALLERGY SHOTS, HOW LONG WILL I NEED THEM?

Symptoms generally improve for a year or two, and most doctors continue immunotherapy for two or three years longer. What happens when the shots are discontinued is hard to say. Studies have been few, poorly controlled, and inconsistent: some show that symptoms usually stay away for years; others that they return quickly.

In general, the lack of sound data makes it difficult to choose whether or not to undergo immunotherapy. "Controlled studies directed toward the rational use of immunotherapy are virtually nonexistent," *The New England Journal of Medicine* review article said.

CAN HAY FEVER TURN INTO SOMETHING WORSE?

The connection between hay fever and asthma is uncertain. An estimated twenty-two million people have hay fever and ten million have asthma, and many are the same people. Some doctors believe that hay fever in childhood, particularly if poorly treated, increases the likelihood of asthma in a person who is genetically susceptible to the breathing disorder, but this hasn't been proven.

There is good evidence, however, that early exposure to house-dust mites and cats (both often potent allergens) may increase the risk of asthma, and it makes sense to keep children away from pollen, to which they're allergic, too.

Very clearly, the congestion of hay fever can promote or exacerbate other problems like sinusitis. (Sinusitis is a bacterial infection with yellow-green, often foul-smelling, nasal discharge.) In children, fluid in the ear that can interfere with hearing (and learning) is often linked to allergy.

◆ HEADACHE

Everyone gets a headache from time to time, but forty-five million Americans have them chronically. Tension headaches are most common, and migraine next. A particularly troublesome variety is the "mixed headache," in which sufferers have episodes of migraine superimposed on chronic muscle tension headache.

A tension-type headache is typically a dull, aching pressure on both sides of the head, and often includes tightness in the neck and shoulders. It may be gone in an hour or may linger for days. Some people have them daily.

Migraines generally strike one side of the head or face (but not always the same side), with pain most often described as "intense," "throbbing," or "pounding." The headache is frequently accompanied by nausea and vomiting, and sensitivity to light and noise.

In 10 percent of people who suffer from migraines, the attack is preceded by an "aura"—he or she sees flashing lights and dancing lines, feels numbness or tingling, or experiences other signs of disturbed neurological function. (It has been suggested that the painter Vincent van Gogh's migraine auras inspired his famous painting *Starry Night*.)

The pain of cluster headache, which is also usually concentrated on one side, is said to be even worse than migraines. Cluster headaches can last up to four hours, and come in bouts of four to twelve weeks, followed by lengthy pain-free periods. Migraines are more common in women, cluster headaches in men.

WHAT'S CAUSING MY HEADACHE?

There are twelve recognized types (and sixty subtypes) of headache. In addition to being disorders in their own right, headaches can be symptoms of a wide spectrum of illnesses—sinusitis, infection, constipation, and high blood pressure, to name a few. Chronic or frequent headaches are also common expressions of emotional disturbance, particularly anxiety and depression.

Headache can be a side effect of many diverse medications, including heart drugs and antidepressants, and some you might least suspect, like OTC decongestants taken for sinusitis. Ironically, headaches can be caused by taking too many headache medications (see next-to-last question).

Lifestyle factors can be involved—in particular, caffeine intake. Drinking too much coffee or cola can give you a headache, but so can *missing* your morning cup of java. Caffeine is actually an addictive drug, and the headache that coffee drives away (caffeine is an ingredient in some pain remedies) is probably a withdrawal symptom. Cut out caffeine entirely for a week to see if that cures your chronic headaches.

WHAT KIND OF HEADACHE REQUIRES A THOROUGH EVALUATION?

Rarely, headache signals a serious health problem that merits prompt medical attention. A severe headache that comes on suddenly, a headache much worse than any you've had before, or a general increase in intensity, duration, and frequency of headaches should be evaluated thoroughly. Also, if your headaches are accompanied by numbness, weakness, or other signs of neurological dysfunction, you should find out whether these symptoms are due to migraine or something more serious.

Computerized tomography (CT) scan and magnetic resonance imaging (MRI) are widely used nowadays to examine the head for tumors and anatomical abnormalities, when symptoms suggest the possibility that these are responsible for headaches. They aren't used routinely, however, when the pattern of symptoms points clearly to migraine or tension-type headache.

You should seek a medical evaluation if a persistent headache comes after a head injury, or any time the pain is severe enough to interfere with your normal life.

HOW CAN I CHANGE MY LIFESTYLE TO REDUCE HEADACHES?

Stress is clearly a factor in persistent, severe headaches, not only for the tension type, but for migraines as well. Making a commitment to fit leisure time into a crowded schedule, and other stress-reducing strategies have been reported to reduce migraine frequency. Scientific evidence for the effectiveness of biofeedback and hypnotherapy is limited, according to an article in the *British Medical Journal* (July 15, 1989), but many people feel they benefit from them.

Some people with migraine have a paradoxical pattern: their headaches come on not during the period of high stress, but when it's over. "Weekend headaches" are a reported phenomenon.

Migraine appears sensitive to a number of lifestyle factors. Many people find that missing a meal will precipitate an attack, as will lack of sleep— or too much. Keeping to a regular routine can be helpful. But individuals differ: some find their attacks are triggered by certain smells, by cigarette smoke, or by excessive noise.

CAN CHANGING MY DIET REDUCE MY HEADACHES?

It's well established that certain foods are often among the triggers of migraine headaches. Caffeine, chocolate, cheeses, nuts, processed meats that contain nitrites, monosodium glutamate (MSG), and alcohol (especially red wine) are the most common. But some people also respond poorly to such diverse foods as citrus fruits, lima beans, sourdough bread, and bananas. Individuals differ markedly, so it's best to keep a food/headache diary to see what dietary changes are helpful for you.

Some headache specialists feel that the majority of persistent headaches, even the "tension-type" and those attributed to sinusitis, are actually variants of migraine, caused by the same process: dilation of blood vessels in the head. They suggest trying the same strategies that work for migraine: eliminating foods that may bring on an attack, and making an effort to maintain a regular schedule of eating, sleeping, and exercising.

SHOULD I TAKE ASPIRIN TO PREVENT HEADACHES?

A couple of aspirin may not do much for a major migraine, but one large study suggests that just one aspirin every other day may prevent them. The Physicians' Health Study, which followed 22,071 male physicians, found that those who took this low dose of aspirin had significantly fewer migraines than those who took placebo: 6 percent had a migraine during a five-year period, compared with 24 percent who took placebo (*Journal of the American Medical Association,* October 3, 1990).

While noting some of the gaps in the study (it didn't report frequency or severity of the headaches, for example), an editorial in the same *Journal* issue counseled physicians "to incorporate into your practice low-dose aspirin prophylaxis for men with significant and presumably migrainous attacks that occur at least weekly."

WHAT DRUGS ARE PRESCRIBED?

OTC analgesics and anti-inflammatory drugs are effective against many headaches, but they may not help a severe migraine or cluster headaches. Ergotamine tartrate is a standard treatment for migraine, but it is effective in only half of people, according to a review article in *The New England Journal of Medicine* (November 11, 1993). A related drug, dihydroergotamine, is more effective in aborting attacks, but it must be injected.

When migraines are frequent (more than two or three a month) and severe, despite diet and lifestyle changes, and they don't respond well to treatment, many doctors prescribe prophylactic therapy. A number of drugs, taken regularly, have been shown to prevent migraine attacks. According to *The New England Journal of Medicine* review, beta-blockers (antihypertensive and antianginal drugs) "should be considered the treatment of choice . . . especially in patients whose attacks of migraine are related to stress." About one third of people don't respond to them, however. Other prophylactic drugs are certain antidepressants (amitriptyline); methysergide; and nonsteroidal anti-inflammatory drugs (NAISDs, e.g., ibuprofen). Calcium channel blockers (primarily used for heart disease and high blood pressure) were more widely prescribed several years ago than they are now. "Their effect has been unimpressive," the *Journal* article says.

They appear to improve headache frequency, but not severity; it may take months before they make a perceptible difference; and, ironically, they can cause severe headaches of their own.

Some of the same drugs may help block cluster headaches. And some doctors say these drugs can reduce symptoms in people with persistent headaches of virtually any description.

SHOULD SUMATRIPTAN BE PRESCRIBED?

The big news in migraine treatment is sumatriptan, which is usually injected (you learn to do it yourself) when the headache begins. This drug affects the receptors of a certain nervous-system chemical (serotonin) that apparently plays a role in the blood vessel changes that bring on migraine. Sumatriptan, which was recently approved by the FDA, relieves both the headache and the nausea of migraine better than placebo. Some researchers feel it is quicker and more effective than other medications given for an acute attack.

In one study involving people with severe migraine from ten headache and neurology clinics, sumatriptan relieved pain in up to 80 percent of people within one hour, compared with 24 percent with placebo. Nausea and light-sensitivity also improved (*Archives of Neurology*, December 1992).

The drug also seems effective for cluster headaches, which often resist other treatments. In one study, thirty-nine people with cluster headaches were randomly assigned to receive either sumatriptan or a placebo injection; neither they nor their doctors knew who was actually receiving the sumatriptan. The headache severity diminished within fifteen minutes of sumatriptan injection in 74 percent of the attacks, compared with 26 percent with placebo; with the drug, 46 percent of the people were pain-free by this time (compared with 10 percent with placebo) (*The New England Journal of Medicine*, August 1, 1991).

Sumatriptan isn't without adverse effects, however. Although most are mild and short-lived, 3 to 5 percent of people who use the drug experience chest discomfort, including pain. Sumatriptan apparently constricts coronary arteries, although not dramatically. The drug shouldn't be given to people with coronary heart disease or high blood pressure, *The New England Journal of Medicine* 1993 review suggests; and if you're in a group that may have unrecognized heart disease (men over forty, women past menopause, smokers at any age), the first dose should be given under medical supervision.

Another drawback is the tendency of headaches to recur. Sumatriptan is a quick but short-acting medication: headache recurs in 38 to 46 percent of people within twenty-four hours. A second injection may work again, but the FDA approval cautions against more than two injections in twenty-four hours.

Although some doctors now regard sumatriptan as the treatment of choice for acute migraine episodes, it hasn't been evaluated as a preventive drug, and shouldn't be used that way.

CAN HEADACHE DRUGS MAKE THINGS WORSE?

A substantial number of chronic headaches are actually worsened by overuse of painkilling medication, even ordinary aspirin and acetaminophen. These "analgesic rebound headaches" are most likely to occur when such painkillers are combined with caffeine, as in such OTC preparations as Excedrin and widely used prescription drugs, like Fiorinal. Overuse of ergotamine is another frequent offender.

The headaches won't go away until you escape the vicious cycle. Many doctors suggest tapering off slowly, to prevent disabling headaches during the withdrawal period, but others have gotten good results with abrupt discontinuation (supported by NSAID and amitriptyline to lessen the symptoms) (*The Lancet,* June 15, 1991).

Withdrawal, even if the analgesic involved is an over-the-counter drug, is a serious business that you shouldn't attempt alone. If you've been taking a barbiturate or opiate painkiller, withdrawal must be managed carefully to avoid seizures.

To keep from getting onto the analgesic rebound merry-go-round, Alan M. Rapoport, M.D., assistant clinical professor of neurology at Yale University School of Medicine, suggests limiting your use of painkillers to three days a week. Try nondrug alternatives, such as biofeedback, relaxation, massage, and exercise whenever possible.

And if you continue to have disabling headaches, consider the prophylactic measures described above: they don't cause rebound problems.

HOW ARE MENSTRUAL MIGRAINES TREATED?

A link between migraines and female hormones probably accounts for the fact that they're twice as common among women, and that one third of women say their migraines began along with menstruation.

For many, migraines are timed to the menstrual cycle: they only occur or are worse at the beginning of a period, midway through, or at the time of ovulation. It may help to use migraine prevention strategies (watch your diet, alcohol consumption, sleep, and other trigger factors) at these times, or even to go on prophylactic medication for this period each month. NSAIDs are especially effective for the pain of menstrual migraine.

Hormone preparations, including oral contraceptives, can also trigger migraines; work with your doctor to find out if these are involved and, where possible, make appropriate changes.

Resources

National Headache Foundation
5252 North Western Avenue
Chicago, IL 60625
(800) 843-2256 or (312) 878-7715

◆ HEARTBURN (Gastroesophageal Reflux)

The discomfort of heartburn is at least an occasional trouble for millions of people. In a Gallup poll, 44 percent of Americans reported symptoms: typically, a burning sensation behind the breastbone, often rising up to the back of the throat, at least once a month; and 18 percent of these took some kind of medication for it twice weekly or more.

The ads for antacid pills like Tums, Gelusil, and Maalox call heartburn "acid indigestion," but actually, the problem is more complicated than that. In the vast majority of cases, heartburn is a symptom of gastroesophageal reflux (GER): stomach fluids containing acid and digestive enzymes back up past the valvelike sphincter that separates the stomach from the esophagus, causing pain.

Occasional reflux is normal. According to an article in *Hospital Practice* (January 15, 1992), it happens to almost everyone, usually after meals, exposing the esophagus to stomach juices no more than 5 percent of the time during the day. The juices are quickly cleared by swallowing before they can do harm or cause more than momentary discomfort.

In some people, however, reflux is more frequent and distressing, not necessarily because they have excess stomach acid, but because the sphincter is too loose, the stomach empties more slowly than usual, or the lining of the esophagus is more sensitive to damage. In these cases, heartburn can continue despite OTC drugs, may interfere with sleep, and may cause physical damage to the esophagus lining.

DO I NEED TESTS TO DETERMINE WHAT'S WRONG?

Only a small proportion of people with heartburn ever consult their doctors about it, according to an article in the *World Journal of Surgery* (1992, no. 16), and fewer still undergo any kind of systematic testing. When symptoms follow the typical pattern—discomfort within a half hour after eating, or brought on by exercise or lying down—and are uncomplicated by weight loss, blood loss, or difficulty swallowing, most doctors will

186

assume that GER is to blame, and will treat it accordingly.

But sometimes, particularly if these symptoms are present, tests are required to see if something more serious, such as peptic ulcer or cancer, may be wrong. Pain caused by GER also may be sharp and severe enough to be mistaken for heart disease. According to a review article in the *British Journal of Clinical Practice* (Winter 1991), up to one third of people hospitalized with suspected heart pain actually have an esophageal problem like GER.

Heartburn may not be the chief complaint for some people with GER. It has been found to be an aggravating factor in asthma, hoarseness, coughing, and sore throat.

Particularly if symptoms are severe or include difficulty swallowing, and don't respond to the usual measures (see below), testing may be advisable to determine if the esophagus is visibly damaged. This condition, esophagitis, occurs in about two thirds of people with GER. Such testing will also show if the passage is narrowed or obstructed by a tumor.

An upper-gastrointestinal series, an X-ray examination of the esophagus, is the simplest test. It involves swallowing liquid barium sulfate to block the X rays, thus allowing the esophagus to show up on the X ray. But endoscopy (a flexible tube allows the doctor to look directly at the esophagus) is more sensitive. Like the upper-gastrointestinal series of X rays, this test does not involve anesthesia or an overnight stay in the hospital, though you are likely to receive pain medication and a sedative through an intravenous line in your arm.

GER that occurs even when these tests are normal may be documented by twenty-four-hour pH monitoring, in which a tiny electrode is placed above the esophageal sphincter to record the amount of acid backing up, and to determine how closely this is associated with symptoms. Because it is expensive and tedious, this test is usually saved for situations when other tests are negative and symptoms persist.

CAN I FEEL BETTER WITHOUT DRUGS?

Often, heartburn can be effectively reduced or prevented by some simple diet and lifestyle adjustments. Weight loss often helps. Smaller, more frequent meals reduce the volume of stomach contents, so there's less pressure to reflux.

Certain foods promote heartburn, but contrary to popular belief, spicy dishes aren't always the culprit. Fats, chocolate, coffee, and alcohol relax the esophageal sphincter. Avoid them if you find they're linked to heartburn. Cigarette smoking can have the same effect. Some people find that citrus fruits and tomatoes or their juices cause symptoms.

Many people are particularly troubled by heartburn at night. It's a good idea not to eat for two hours before bedtime. In addition, you may gain relief by sleeping with your head elevated by about six inches, either by lifting the head of the bed with blocks, or by raising your head and shoulders with a wedge-shaped pillow. This will more quickly return refluxed gastric juices to the stomach.

Some medications may worsen heartburn by loosening the esophageal sphincter. Valium (diazepam) not infrequently has this effect, as do some antidepressants, heart drugs, asthma drugs, and hormone preparations that contain progesterone. You may be able to switch medications to get the therapeutic benefits you need without the digestive distress.

DO ANTACIDS HELP?

OTC drugs that neutralize stomach acid are, for most people, the first line of defense against heartburn. There's nothing wrong with them (if you heed the limitations on the label), and many people feel they help. In fact, however, controlled studies haven't shown that antacids prevent symptoms any more effectively than placebo, according to the 1992 *Hospital Practice* article.

Some preparations combine antacids with alginic acid, a compound that foams when in contact with stomach acid. In theory, the foam will rise into the esophagus instead of the gastric juices. But controlled studies find no advantage over simple antacids.

Some people find that just drinking water or milk will dispel symptoms.

ARE PRESCRIPTION DRUGS ANY BETTER?

More powerful treatment is indicated when the above approaches fail to relieve symptoms, and is important when tests show esophagitis. If untreated and chronic, esophagitis can lead to complications like stricture (permanent narrowing of the stomach opening), which often makes swallowing difficult. Permanent changes in the lining of the esophagus raise the risk of cancer.

The same stomach acid-reducing drugs often used for peptic ulcer, such as cimetidine (Tagamet) and ranitidine (Zantac) are the standard prescription drugs for GER. They reduce stomach acid secretion and have been shown to be significantly better than placebo both in relieving symptoms and in healing mild to moderate esophageal inflammation, according to a paper in the *American Journal of Medicine* (May 27, 1992).

When esophagitis is severe, a double or triple dose of Tagamet or Zantac is sometimes more effective. This is expensive, however (perhaps two to three hundred dollars per month), and carries greater risk of side effects. For example, nervous agitation and confusion are possible side effects when these drugs are taken by people over the age of sixty.

Drugs to tighten the esophageal sphincter and hasten stomach emptying (such as metoclopramide) are also used, particularly for severe GER, but findings on its effectiveness are "mixed" according to the *American Journal of Medicine* article.

A new addition to the drug arsenal is omeprazole, which blocks stomach acid secretion more completely than the standard prescription drugs for GER. It is significantly more effective than other drugs in healing esophagitis, particularly when severe. Because of questions about its safety (laboratory studies have found that the drug can cause tumors in rats), omeprazole shouldn't be prescribed for more than three months.

Whatever drug is used, relapse is a problem after the drug is discontinued. Even with the most potent treatments, omeprazole and high-dose H2 blockers, esophagitis returns in 80 percent of patients within six months after they stop taking the drug.

WHEN WOULD SURGERY BE INDICATED?

If used appropriately, surgery to correct anatomical defects in the esophageal sphincter can improve severe GER more effectively than medical treatment, according to a study reported in *The New England Journal of Medicine* (March 19, 1992). In a randomized group of 207 people with significant complications of GER, those who had surgery had better healing of esophagitis, and were more satisfied with their treatment than the medication group.

In view of the fact that medication for severe GER must be taken pretty much indefinitely and must be accompanied by regular testing, surgery appears to be less expensive in the long run, suggests an editorial in the same issue of *The New England Journal of Medicine.*

But surgery isn't for everyone. For one thing, tests must definitively establish that a defective sphincter is actually to blame—which, according to an article in *World Review of Surgery* (1992, no. 16), is the case in 50 to 60 percent of people with GER disease. If other abnormalities (of the stomach, for example) are responsible for the problem, antireflux surgery won't help.

In addition, surgery often produces some unpleasant effects. According to another article in the same issue of *World Review of Surgery,* bloating, difficulty swallowing, or other persistent digestive problems occur in 30 percent of cases.

The relative advantages of surgical, and possibly lifelong, medical treatment of severe GER may depend on such factors as age and the presence of complications or chronic illness. The choice is often up to you, so make sure you're thoroughly informed on the risks and benefits of both approaches.

According to *The New England Journal of Medicine* study, the experience of the surgeon can make a significant difference in the effectiveness of the surgery. Question your surgeon carefully about his or her experience in performing the type of operation you are considering.

◆ HEMORRHOIDS

If you don't know what hemorrhoids are, you must not own a TV. According to Ralph Nader's Public Citizen Health Research Group, Americans spend over a hundred million dollars on over-the-counter hemorrhoid remedies each year, and they are promoted heavily. In fact, most people have hemorrhoids, and an estimated one in three persons (one in two over age fifty) have symptoms that cause greater or less distress.

Quite simply, hemorrhoids are varicose veins in the area of the anus—veins, that is, that have become enlarged. They may hurt, bleed, or cause no symptoms at all. Internal hemorrhoids, under the mucus membrane of the rectum, may bleed or protrude. External hemorrhoids, under the skin of the anus, can be extremely painful.

A predisposition to hemorrhoids (like varicose veins of the legs) appears to be inherited. The traditional low-fiber American diet contributes to their development, probably by promoting constipation. Contrary to popular belief, prolonged sitting, standing, and heavy lifting don't cause hemorrhoids, although those things may aggravate symptoms.

DO I NEED TO SEE A DOCTOR?

Hemorrhoids are not dangerous, nor are they a warning sign of more serious illness. If you have persistent pain or any bleeding, however, you need to have it checked out, to make sure hemorrhoids are actually to blame. Anal fissure (an infected crack in the anal lining), abscess, or spasm can be responsible for the pain, and these may require treatment.

Bleeding from hemorrhoids is typically bright red; it may appear just on the toilet paper after a bowel movement, or drip into the toilet bowl. Dark red blood, particularly mixed into the bowel movement itself, suggests bleeding further up in the large intestine, perhaps caused by a tumor. But because it is impossible to know for sure, bleeding should never be ignored.

Despite the ads for hemorrhoid remedies, anal itching is almost always caused by something else: most commonly, skin disease or allergy.

CAN I TREAT HEMORRHOIDS MYSELF?

Once you've established that hemorrhoids are indeed the cause of your discomfort, self-treatment may be all you need. A diet high in fiber (best supplied in whole-grain products, vegetables, and fruits), along with adequate intake of water (six to eight glasses daily), will prevent the constipation and straining that inflames hemorrhoids and makes them worse.

Take pressure off hemorrhoids by not spending excessive time or straining on the toilet.

Sitz baths can ease hemorrhoids by reducing the swelling. Sit for fifteen minutes, two or three times a day, in very warm (but not uncomfortably hot) water. There are devices that fit over the toilet to make this easier.

Hemorrhoids may make it difficult to clean properly after bowel movements, and traces of stool and body secretions can lead to itching, irritation, and infection. Clean the anal area with mild soap and water, at least once a day. Pat, don't rub the area dry, to minimize irritation.

DO OTC REMEDIES HELP?

Not much. And you can get at least as much relief as they provide at far less expense. Preparation H, claimed by its manufacturer to shrink hemorrhoidal tissues, accounts for more than half of the entire national outlay on such products, but its active ingredients are "unconvincing in their effectiveness," according to the Public Citizen Health Research Group. Nor are Anusol, Hemorrin, and the like any better.

The shark liver oil in Preparation H is a lubricant that can afford limited protection to sensitive anal tissues. But it's no more effective than petroleum jelly or zinc oxide, which are vastly cheaper.

Some products contain topical anesthetics, like benzocaine. These relieve discomfort temporarily, but they don't do anything for the underlying disorder. And those who use them can develop an allergy to all related compounds, including novocaine.

WHAT IF SELF-HELP DOESN'T WORK?

Going further is up to you. Internal hemorrhoids don't hurt because the inner rectum has no pain-carrying nerves. They can protrude, however, and become irritated or create a hygiene problem. And they can bleed: not only is this distressing, if ignored long enough, it can cause anemia.

Acutely painful hemorrhoids are the external ones that develop clots. The clot—and the pain—invariably disappear eventually, but it may take weeks or months. A quicker solution is having the clot removed, which can be done under local anesthesia in a doctor's office.

There are a number of office procedures available to destroy internal hemorrhoids. The most popular is rubber-band ligation. Using a special instrument, the surgeon detaches the vein from the rectal wall and slips a tiny rubber band around it. With its blood supply cut off, the hemorrhoidal tissue shrivels and dies. The procedure is painless and needs no anesthesia. Life-threatening infections can develop within several days after this procedure, but they are extremely rare: fewer than one in ten thousand.

Alternative methods use infrared light to coagulate the hemorrhoid or lasers, freezing, or electricity to injure the hemorrhoid so it will atrophy. With sclerotherapy, the same result is achieved by injecting a chemical to scar the hemorrhoid tissue.

All of these methods work, but not permanently; hemorrhoids commonly return several years later. In a study that appeared in the *American Journal of Gastroenterology,* data from five trials involving 863 patients were analyzed. When rubber-band ligation, sclerotherapy, and infrared coagulation were compared, similar numbers of patients remained symptomless one year after treatment. Those who had rubber-band ligation required least additional treatment for returning symptoms, but they also had significantly more post-procedure discomfort. Infrared coagulation caused fewest and mildest complications.

SHOULD I HAVE SURGERY?

Surgical removal of the hemorrhoid and adjacent skin, the most drastic treatment, has declined dramatically in popularity in recent decades and is now reserved for the most bothersome hemorrhoids that keep on coming back after more conservative measures such as rubber-band ligation.

The recurrence rate after hemorrhoidectomy is low (1 to 2 percent), but the procedure must be done in the hospital under anesthesia, although an overnight stay is no longer required, and the aftermath may be quite painful. You'll probably have to miss some days of work. Surgery is not something to rush into before alternatives are thoroughly explored. Get a second opinion.

✦ HEPATITIS

Hepatitis—inflammation of the liver—is extremely common throughout the world, particularly in Asia and developing areas. The name actually describes a broad spectrum of diseases, with causes as diverse as infection and drug reaction, and severity ranging from an asymptomatic condition, detected only by blood tests, to severe illness that causes liver destruction and death.

Five different viruses have been identified as causes of infectious hepatitis. Hepatitis B is the most common, with three hundred million people across the world carrying a chronic infection that, even without symptoms, may be transmitted to others by blood transfusion, sexual activity, or close personal contact. The disease itself is often mild, but can lead to a lifelong chronic infection state that may have dire consequences, including cirrhosis or liver cancer.

Hepatitis A is transmitted by contaminated food and water or from person to person, like typhoid or cholera. It is common in developing nations, far less so in the United States and other developed countries, but still a persistent cause of disease in some inner-city areas. Raw shellfish can be a source of infection.

The existence of another virus was deduced in the mid-1970s, among blood transfusion recipients who developed hepatitis but also tested negative for hepatitis B. It's now recognized that three different viruses can cause "non-A, non-B hepatitis"; the one responsible for 84 percent of cases has been designated "hepatitis C."

Hepatitis can also be caused by excessive alcohol consumption, which causes liver damage, or as a side effect of certain drugs, such as antibiotics. Like most viral diseases, hepatitis is resistant to effective treatment. Fortunately, most cases will—in time—go away on their own.

WHAT ARE MY RISKS OF CONTRACTING
HEPATITIS A WHILE TRAVELING?

According to an article in *The Lancet* (May 16, 1992), 40 to 50 percent of hepatitis A in industrialized countries is linked to international travel. One Italian study found that the risk varied markedly with destination: a person voyaging to southern Italy had over two and a half times the chance of contracting the disease as someone who stayed home; travelers to Eastern Europe had nearly six times the risk; and those to Africa, Asia, and Latin America, twenty-five times the risk. Hepatitis A infection is more likely among backpackers and under primitive living conditions.

HOW CAN I PROTECT MYSELF FROM HEPATITIS A?

The usual precautions against contamination should be observed by anyone visiting an area where sanitation is doubtful and the chance of contracting hepatitis or other food and water-borne diseases is significant. Beyond that, an injection of immune globulin (a blood product rich in antibodies against hepatitis A) has long been advised for travelers abroad. It only provides protection for several months, however.

Recently, a vaccine against hepatitis A has been licensed. Made from the killed virus, it builds up far higher blood levels of antibodies, lasts far longer, and appears to protect about 97 percent of people treated. (Because the vaccine was developed only recently, how long it remains effective is unknown.)

HOW CAN I PROTECT MYSELF AGAINST
HEPATITIS B?

Intravenous drug use is now the principal way that hepatitis B is transmitted in this country. It's also a sexually transmitted disease. You can get it even from someone who is a carrier but has no symptoms (another reason to use a condom and limit your number of sexual partners). Health-care workers, family members of infected persons, people who receive multiple blood transfusions or hemodialysis, drug addicts who share needles, and people confined to institutions and jails are also at increased risk. Rarely, outbreaks occur because of contaminated water. The disease can be transmitted via contact with any bodily fluid of an infected person.

A vaccine for hepatitis B has been available for over a decade and is recommended for people at high risk. It has been added (by the American Academy of Pediatricians) to the growing list of vaccinations routinely given to infants. There is some controversy surrounding its use in children (see Vaccination).

IF I HAVE HEPATITIS B, WHAT IS MY RISK OF LIVER DAMAGE?

Hepatitis B is usually a limited, if unpleasant, disease. The flulike symptoms, pain, and jaundice are gone in a month without treatment, although it may take longer to recover your health. Some cases are mild enough to pass unnoticed. Very few cases rapidly progress to liver failure and death.

The real risk of hepatitis B is in chronic infection: sophisticated immunological tests show that a proportion of people who have been infected with hepatitis B carry the virus for years, perhaps for life. They are at increased risk, over the years, of cirrhosis, liver failure, and hepatocellular carcinoma, a cancer of the liver. The risk of liver cancer for a person with chronic hepatitis is seven to ten times higher than for others; in areas where hepatitis B is widespread, it's the leading cause of cancer death, according to an article in *The Lancet* (November 27, 1993).

Infants who are infected with hepatitis B at birth are at extremely high risk of developing chronic hepatitis—about 90 percent. The danger is also heightened in people whose immune system is impaired or suppressed, such as organ transplant recipients or those with AIDS. But for an adult whose immune system is in working order, the chance of developing chronic hepatitis is estimated at less than 5 percent.

Even if you have the chronic infection, the virus may remain inactive, causing no symptoms or liver damage. It can be activated anytime, however, raising the risk of liver disease or cancer.

SHOULD I GET TREATMENT FOR CHRONIC HEPATITIS?

Interferon α, a natural product of the immune system, is the only drug that has been approved for chronic hepatitis B. It is an expensive injectable drug that apparently is effective in eliminating signs of chronic infection in some people and viral activation in others.

A meta-analysis of fifteen randomized controlled studies involving a total of 837 people found that blood tests for chronic infection normalized in 7.8 percent of those treated, compared with 1.8 percent of those who weren't. Viral replication, the sign of dangerous active (as opposed to latent) disease, disappeared in 37 percent of people treated with interferon, compared with 17 percent of the controls (*Annals of Internal Medicine,* August 15, 1993).

Although these hopeful signs should logically mean that interferon will reduce the risk of severe liver disease, the treatment hasn't been around long enough to know whether interferon is effective in this regard. "No study has assessed the effect of interferon therapy on the clinically relevant end points of liver failure, hepatocellular carcinoma, and death as the progression of this disease evolves over decades," the authors wrote.

Nor, for that matter, have follow-up studies been sufficiently extended to say for sure how long the virus remains eradicated, although some data suggest that the benefits last at least seven years.

Side effects with interferon, particularly at the doses that seem more effective, can be quite troublesome, including joint and muscle pain and fever. Up to 20 percent of participants in the trials analyzed in the *Annals* paper required a reduction in interferon dose, and 5 percent had to discontinue treatment.

HOW SERIOUS IS HEPATITIS C?

Most of the hepatitis transmitted by blood transfusion in this country is neither type A nor B; the bulk of this has been identified as caused by a virus called hepatitis C. The disease, like hepatitis B, can also be transmitted sexually or by intravenous drug use.

The acute illness is usually quite mild; often, blood tests are the only sign that infection has taken place. About a more critical question—what are its long-range effects?—less is known.

A substantial number of people who contract hepatitis C have blood tests that show the presence of chronic disease: 60 percent, in one study (*The New England Journal of Medicine,* December 31, 1992). But the implications of this are very much in question. Another article in the same

Journal issue reported an eighteen-year study, which showed no greater mortality among people infected with hepatitis C than those in a control group. There was, however, "a small but statistically significant increase in the number of deaths related to liver disease," the authors said.

Another study, in *Annals of Internal Medicine* (July 15, 1993), followed eighty people who had contracted hepatitis C in the 1970s. Eight had developed liver failure, and it was projected that the chance of symptomatic cirrhosis, after sixteen years, was 18 to 20 percent. "If hepatic failure does occur, it is usually seen only after ten or more years of disease. Before that time, many infected persons die due to other disease processes," the authors wrote—which may be less than comforting.

IS THERE ANYTHING I CAN DO TO HASTEN MY RECOVERY?

Eat a high-protein, high-carbohydrate diet, get plenty of rest, and avoid alcoholic beverages.

HOW CAN I AVOID INFECTING OTHERS IF I HAVE HEPATITIS?

You must assume that your bodily fluids are infectious and take the appropriate precautions, like washing your hands thoroughly after using the toilet.

CAN MEDICATION GIVE ME HEPATITIS?

Acute hepatitis can be caused by a reaction to drugs that carry the small risk of inflaming the liver, such as antibiotics. A study in *Annals of Internal Medicine* (October 1, 1993) looked at 107 people hospitalized for hepatitis for which no cause had been found. The use of erythromycin, sulfonamides, and tetracyclines—three of the most commonly used antibiotics—were all associated with an increased risk of hepatitis.

The risk of hepatitis is not nearly great enough to call the use of these drugs into question. There are an estimated 2.28 cases serious enough to require hospitalization for every million people treated for ten days with erythromycin; 4.8 with sulfonamides; and 1.56 with tetracycline. But since the only effective treatment for drug-induced hepatitis is to discontinue the drug responsible, it's important for doctors to be aware of the possibility.

Other drugs that have been associated with hepatitis are the antituberculosis drugs isoniazid and rifampin; in some cases, this is severe enough to cause death, or require a liver transplant.

Resources

Call the Centers for Disease Control and Prevention, (404) 639-1610, for recorded information on hepatitis (they will send written material by fax if you call and request it).

◆ HERNIA

The supporting structure of the abdominal wall is weakest in the groin area, and our upright posture presses our internal organs against it. Sometimes, a small portion of intestine pushes through the weak point, which is why, along with back problems and hemorrhoids, hernias are a legacy of human evolution.

An estimated 60,600 men have surgery to repair an inguinal hernia each year, making it one of the most common kinds of surgery. Hernias occur at all ages, from infancy through old age.

The protrusion of intestine through the hernia causes swelling and often pain. As long as it can be pushed back into place, and retracts when you lie down, an uncomplicated hernia is likely to be more inconvenient than disabling. But there's always the risk that serious complications will develop. For example, the contents of the intestine might be prevented from moving through.

Hernia can be inborn, but most often it's caused by an activity that raises pressure in the abdomen: lifting a heavy object can do it, but just coughing or straining on the toilet may also be to blame. About 90 percent of hernias occur in men, and it seems to run in families.

IS SURGERY THE ONLY OPTION?

For hernias in infants and children, surgery is the only choice; but for adults, it's usually an elective procedure: you have it when you want, or not at all. You can elect to put off surgery indefinitely and keep the hernia from bulging out at the groin with a truss—a supportive belt.

Surgery is the only real cure for hernia, however. Until you have it repaired, you may have to restrict such activities as heavy lifting.

The risk of complications is not to be taken lightly. The protruding intestine may be trapped in its position outside the abdominal wall (the medical term is *incarceration*). While this isn't life-threatening, it can lead to bowel obstruction or to strangulation—both surgical emergencies.

A strangulated hernia occurs when the blood to the loop of the intestine is cut off. Severe pain, nausea, and vomiting may develop, and the possibility of gangrene makes the situation life-threatening. The risks of the emergency surgery that then becomes necessary are far greater than those of elective hernia repair.

HOW DISRUPTIVE IS THE SURGERY?

Modern hernia repair is a lot less disabling than the surgery of the past. The procedures used nowadays take thirty to sixty minutes, and approximately 70 percent of people have it done on an outpatient basis according to an article in *Surgical Clinics of North America* (June 1993). For the rest, there's usually a two- or three-day hospital stay. Most people can return to work a few days after the surgery, but may have to refrain from strenuous physical activity for three to six weeks.

There's much variation in the way a hernia is repaired. Not only are there different procedures but in some cases there are the options of general, spinal, and local anesthesia. General anesthesia involves a small but real risk of severe complications, including death. Local anesthesia avoids these risks and has the added advantage of allowing the patient to literally walk away from the operating table.

WHAT PROCEDURE WILL BE USED TO REPAIR MY HERNIA?

There are several different operations currently in use, and which one you have will depend largely on your surgeon's preference. The surgery may join the edges of the weakened area of abdominal wall and anchor them to a major ligament. Another technique places a synthetic fiber mesh over the weak place, like a plug or patch on a flat tire.

A recent addition to the options is laparoscopic surgery, which avoids opening the area. The surgeon works with miniaturized instruments through a telescopelike instrument inserted through a tiny incision. As with other laparoscopic procedures, the innovation is designed to cause less trauma, less opportunity for infection, and less postoperative pain.

There are drawbacks to laparoscopy, however. As currently done, it requires general anesthesia, with all its attendant risks. Laparoscopic surgery doesn't seem to hasten recovery time, which after even conventional hernia repair is quite short. The procedure may be more expensive, and it sometimes becomes necessary to switch from laparoscopic to conventional surgery on the operating table, according to an article in *Surgical Clinics of North America* (June 1993). Because the procedure hasn't been in use very long for hernia repair, there are no long-term follow-up data.

Finally, as with any laparoscopic procedure, it's important to know that your surgeon has had adequate training and experience.

Complications of hernia repair, whatever technique is used, are relatively rare. In one series of over fifteen hundred operations using the mesh technique, there were infections in 0.4 percent of cases, and urinary retention in 0.3 percent (*Surgical Clinics of North America*, June 1993). In a small series of twenty-six laparoscopic procedures, there were no wound infections (*Canadian Journal of Surgery*, August 1993).

WHAT IS THE RISK THAT MY HERNIA WILL RECUR?

Hernia recurrence after repair has been a problem. It is estimated that 10 to 15 percent of operations eventually fail, making another operation necessary. Second operations have an even greater failure rate.

About one quarter of recurrences are in the first years after surgery and are caused by tension on the place where the repair itself was made. But 40 to 50 percent of recurrences don't appear until five or more years later, and 20 percent aren't found until fifteen to twenty-five years after the operation. The supportive structure of connective tissue thins and weakens with age, and eventually gives way.

The proponents of various repair techniques generally claim that their method has a lower recurrence rate than others. One paper reported only 0.13 percent recurrences in 759 people treated with a technique that anchored the repaired abdominal wall to a ligament; another, using the mesh technique, reported 0.1 percent. It appears that some surgeons get much lower recurrence rates than others using the same techniques.

It's important to keep in mind that recurrence data are usually subject to error: surgeons lose track of many of their patients, and people who need a second operation often seek a second surgeon. And in the case of laparoscopic surgery, the operation hasn't been done long enough to allow meaningful estimates of long-range success or failure.

✦ HIGH BLOOD PRESSURE (Hypertension)

An estimated fifty million Americans—nearly one adult in three—have elevated blood pressure (hypertension); its treatment is the most common reason for visiting the doctor. There's good reason to take hypertension seriously. It's the principal risk factor for stroke, and an important one for heart attack. Hypertension also increases the danger of heart failure and kidney failure.

Blood pressure—the force with which the heart pushes blood against the walls of the arteries—is expressed in standard terms of how high (in millimeters) it would raise a column of mercury. There are two numbers: the top, or systolic, represents peak pressure at the moment the heart contracts; the bottom, or diastolic pressure, is what is exerted when the heart is at rest.

The treatment of high blood pressure has come a long way from a half century ago, when there were virtually no drugs to lower it or to circumvent the catastrophic events that might follow. Today, there is an ever-proliferating menu of drugs to choose from. The problem is deciding when to use them, and which one to use.

Anything above 140/90 mm Hg is considered high blood pressure. When it is more than mildly elevated—when the diastolic is over 105—there's little question that it should be treated. In the lower end of the spectrum, say, just above 90, controversy begins.

WHAT IS MY RISK OF HEART DISEASE AND STROKE WITHOUT TREATMENT?

High blood pressure is not a disease; it's a biological variable that increases the risk of disease like heart attack and stroke. And the whole idea of treatment is to reduce these risks.

Just a modest reduction in diastolic blood pressure—5 to 6 mm Hg—cuts the risk of stroke by 42 percent. But this means little if that risk was small to begin with. According to the 1993 World Health Organization/ International Society of Hypertension (WHO/ISH) guidelines, each year fewer than one in a thousand young people with mild hypertension and no other cardiovascular risk factors will suffer a serious event like a stroke or heart attack, without treatment. In one large British trial, eight hundred and fifty people had to be treated for a year to prevent just one stroke.

According to a paper in *Annals of Internal Medicine* (August 15, 1993), "provision of hypotensive drugs should depend on absolute risk and potential for benefit rather than on blood pressure level alone." The author points out that a fifty-five-year-old white male with systolic blood pressure of 170 mm Hg and no other risk factors has the same few-year risk of stroke as the same person with a pressure of 136 mm Hg who smokes, and about a one-fifth risk as the same person with normal pressure, but who has a history of cardiovascular disease and diabetes, smokes cigarettes, and has evidence of heart enlargement.

Consequently, a good argument can be made for individualizing treatment, based on your overall risk of heart attack and stroke, taking into account, that is, factors like your age, sex, cholesterol level, lifestyle, and disease history.

CAN OTHER TESTS MORE PRECISELY ESTIMATE MY NEED FOR TREATMENT?

In recent years, tests of biochemistry and heart structure and function have made it possible to predict more precisely who is at increased risk of cardiovascular problems. In an eight-and-a-half-year study of over seventeen hundred people with mild hypertension, those with high levels of a pressure-regulating kidney hormone called renin had five and a half times the risk of heart attack of those with low renin. The 241 people with low renin and no other risk factors had no heart attacks at all in this period.

Another important factor is left ventricular hypertrophy (LVH)— thickening of the main pumping chamber of the heart, a sign that hypertension is actually causing cardiac damage. In a ten-year study of 282 people with mild hypertension, only those with LVH were at increased risk of health problems: they had more heart attacks, needed more bypass surgery, and were ten times as likely to die of hypertension-related illness as those with normal hearts.

In light of such research, blood pressure is only one factor to consider in making decisions about treatment. Some people with "normal" levels may benefit from reducing pressure, while others with "elevated" pressure may have little to gain.

DO I HAVE "WHITE COAT HYPERTENSION"?

To complicate matters further, it's become quite clear in recent years that a significant number of people—perhaps 20 percent—have high blood pressure when measured in the doctor's office but nowhere else. It may be a conditioned response: anxiety in the doctor's office shoots pressure up; being told one has hypertension generates more anxiety, which is triggered every time the doctor measures pressure again. If so, there's not much reason to treat it.

It's possible, however, that if your blood pressure rises in the examining room, it also goes up under other stressful situations, at work and elsewhere. To get a more accurate idea of your real-life pressure, the doctor may recommend "ambulatory blood pressure monitoring": you wear a device for twenty-four hours that takes your blood pressure regularly, as you go about your daily routine.

Many doctors would say that "white coat hypertension" doesn't need to be treated. But the "guidelines for the management of mild hypertension" recently issued by the WHO/ISH point out that "whether the effect is an innocent phenomenon is unknown." A big pressure difference between home and doctor's office pressure could itself mean increased cardiovascular risk, some suggest.

HAVE WE GIVEN NONDRUG APPROACHES
A FAIR CHANCE?

The scientific consensus is that the first response to mildly elevated blood pressure shouldn't be a prescription. The WHO/ISH guidelines, for example, don't advocate drug treatment until diet and lifestyle changes have been given at least a three-month try.

Most doctors would give lip service to that idea. But many tend to be a bit perfunctory in the lifestyle area. They may convey an expectation (or may just assume) that not many people are really going to change the way they eat, drink, or live enough to make a difference, and thus, they go directly to the prescription pad.

In fact, the amount of change needed to bring mildly elevated blood pressure back inside the normal range is well within the reach of many people. The recent "Treatment of Mild Hypertension Study" found that volunteers who were given modest salt-reduction and weight-loss goals (and didn't even do such a great job meeting them) brought their blood pressure down an average of 9/9 mm Hg—enough so that nearly two thirds didn't need any further treatment, even four years later (*Journal of the American Medical Association,* August 11, 1993).

WHAT DIET AND LIFESTYLE CHANGES ARE LIKELY TO MAKE A DIFFERENCE?

Body weight has a marked effect on blood pressure, and a relatively modest loss can have gratifying results. In one study of eight hundred overweight people with mild hypertension, losing ten pounds or more brought an average 12.1 mm Hg drop in diastolic pressure, as great an improvement as achieved with some drugs, according to an article in *Medical World News* (May 28, 1990). It's been estimated that if the whole U.S. population could reduce weight to 100 to 109 percent of ideal body weight, hypertension rates would drop by 70 percent.

Alcohol stimulates the release of adrenaline, which raises blood pressure. Some people are more sensitive to the effect than others; even a drink or two a day could mean 5 mm Hg in a person who is particularly sensitive. The same person who responds to stress with a rise in pressure is likely to react the same way to alcohol, some believe.

Other aspects of diet, particularly potassium, have been shown to have a positive effect on blood pressure. An analysis of data from twenty-seven trials showed that doubling the average intake of potassium (which in this country is quite low) produced an average pressure reduction of 3 mm Hg. Many fruits, such as oranges and bananas, are good sources of potassium.

The effect of exercise has been less consistent in studies, but some have found a regular program as effective as drugs. In one, fifty-two sedentary men with mild hypertension were given drugs or a placebo and placed on a schedule of circuit-weight training and aerobic exercise for fifty minutes, three times a week. Blood pressure dropped as much (about 14/13 mm Hg) in those who simply exercised as in those who also took medication (*Journal of the American Medical Association,* May 23/30, 1990).

Other studies have found improvements, although not as marked, with less vigorous or extensive exercise: half an hour of brisk walking several times a week, for example.

Whatever the effects of weight loss and exercise on blood pressure, they also reduce cardiovascular risk in general. Since staying healthy is the ultimate purpose, weight loss and exercise are important for anyone who is at increased risk of heart disease. The fifth report of the Joint National Committee on the Detection, Evaluation, and Treatment of High Blood Pressure recommends lifestyle change as an adjunct to drug therapy, when it isn't enough alone.

SHOULD I CUT DOWN ON SALT?

The one lifestyle modification idea just about everyone knows about— "take the salt shaker off the table"—is perhaps least likely to make a difference: it's unnecessary for some people, and insufficient for most of the the others.

How salt (more correctly, the sodium in sodium chloride) affects blood pressure is clearly an individual matter. You may have a hefty drop if you cut way down on salt, or it may leave your pressure unchanged. In hypertensives as a whole, a meta-analysis of thirty-three studies found that reducing salt by one third lowered systolic pressure by an average of 7 mm Hg.

Some groups of hypertensives (African Americans, for example) are much more likely than others to be salt-sensitive. There are lab tests that can help predict who will benefit from this approach, but the easiest way to find out whether cutting salt will help you a little, a lot, or not at all is to try it for several weeks and see what happens.

If you do want to reduce your sodium intake, the saltshaker can only be the first step. Estimates of the average salt consumption in this country run as high as nine grams per day—far more than many other places— and the vast bulk (85 percent, some say) is in processed foods. Just one portion of a popular canned soup, for example, has over a gram. Just cutting your salt in half may require quite a bit of effort.

WHAT ARE THE RISKS AND BENEFITS OF THE DRUGS BEING PRESCRIBED?

There are at least five distinct classes (some containing a dozen or more different drugs) of medications for hypertension. All of them seem to do what they're supposed to do: bring blood pressure down, at least in some people.

The Joint National Committee report recommends trying one of two kinds of drugs, beta-blockers and diuretics—first, because only they have been shown to reduce the risk of stroke, heart attack, and death. More recent additions; like calcium channel blockers and angiotensin converting enzyme inhibitors (ACEIs) reduce blood pressure as much as those drugs and have similar effects on heart function, but they haven't been shown to have the same impact on actual disease and death.

There are other differences among the drugs, however. All have side effects, which vary from person to person. Some of the more distressing adverse effects, such as impotence, fatigue, and depression, are more common with beta-blockers and diuretics. And there is some evidence that certain classes of drugs work better for some groups (young men, women, blacks, whites) than others.

Particularly if your doctor prescribes something other than a diuretic or beta-blocker first for hypertension (ACE inhibitors are especially popular because of their side-effect profile), ask about the risks and benefits of that particular drug for someone in your situation.

WILL I HAVE TO TAKE MEDICATION FOR LIFE?

One of the most sobering aspects of being told you have hypertension is the idea that you'll have to take drugs for the rest of your life. But not every doctor would agree that this is always necessary. For some people, it may be possible to use medication intermittently or even stop it altogether. "Most study groups have observed that some formerly treated hypertensive patients remain normotensive after drug withdrawal for months or even years," according to a paper in the *Journal of the American Medical Association* (March 27, 1991).

If medication is suspended, it should be done cautiously, after pressure has been normal for a year or more (some suggest several years), and regular monitoring is essential to detect if it starts going up again.

This approach is most likely to work in people whose hypertension before treatment began was mild, who are young, and who had been treated successfully with a single drug. Making nutritional and lifestyle changes to keep pressure down is particularly important in this situation. One study cited in the *Journal of the American Medical Association* article found that 39 percent of people who stopped medication, simultaneously lost excess weight, and cut back on salt and alcohol kept their blood pressure normal for up to four years.

HOW CAN I PREVENT HIGH BLOOD PRESSURE?

From a public health point of view, it would more effectively reduce the toll of heart disease and stroke to lower *everybody*'s blood pressure by a few points than to treat those who are over an arbitrary standard. It has been estimated that if the whole American population reduced body weight an average of 8 percent, lowered salt use dramatically, and upped potassium intake (by eating more fruit, for example), average blood pressure would drop enough to reduce stroke deaths by 14 percent and heart disease deaths by 9 percent.

For the individual, it certainly makes more sense to prevent your blood pressure from going up than to wait for it to happen and then treat it.

In this country, blood pressure rises continuously with age, but this tendency isn't seen everywhere. Lifestyle factors, over the years, apparently play a role. A study comparing salt consumption and blood pressure in twenty-four different communities—a total of forty-seven thousand people—found significantly lower pressures in places where the salt intake was half of ours. The spread widened with age, which supports the theory that too much salt is in fact responsible for the gradual pressure rise that most people—doctors included—take for granted.

Similarly, limiting alcohol, controlling weight, and staying active while your blood pressure is normal could heighten the odds that it will stay that way.

✦ HIGH CHOLESTEROL

When people talk about food nowadays, they're as likely to mention cholesterol as calories. For well over a decade, there has been a steady drumbeat of exhortations to fight heart disease by cutting down cholesterol.

America's cholesterol has, in fact, declined substantially. From 1961 to 1992, the average serum cholesterol level dropped by 8 percent, from 220 mg/dL to 205. Experts give the decline at least part of the credit for a drop in heart disease rates in the same period. An estimated 25 percent of Americans still have elevated cholesterol (over 240 mg/dL), however.

For all its negative reputation as a major component of the fatty deposits that narrow the arteries (atherosclerosis) in coronary heart disease, cholesterol is no toxic chemical but rather an essential building block of all cell membranes. Not only does your body constantly manufacture cholesterol, you also ingest it in meats, fish, dairy products, and eggs.

WHAT'S THE DIFFERENCE BETWEEN GOOD CHOLESTEROL AND BAD CHOLESTEROL?

Many people find the cholesterol issue confusing, and for good reason. Cholesterol is a fatty substance contained in all animal tissues, and you get far less from food than is synthesized by your own body. Saturated fat is an important dietary factor, because it stimulates your own manufacture of cholesterol. This is why cholesterol-lowering diets are limited in these fats.

Cholesterol is carried through your bloodstream bound to lipoproteins: the fraction bound to low-density lipoprotein (LDL-cholesterol) is apparently available to be deposited on the artery walls, while that bound to high-density lipoproteins (HDL-cholesterol) is being transported out of the body.

The risk of heart disease apparently has less to do with the total concentration of cholesterol in your bloodstream than with the amount and relative proportions of LDL- and HDL-cholesterol. LDL, to put it perhaps too simply, is "bad cholesterol"; extensive studies have found that heart attack risk rises along with its concentration. The risk drops as levels of HDL, protective "good cholesterol," rise.

ISN'T IT TRUE THAT MOST HEART DISEASE RESEARCH IS CONDUCTED ON WHITE MIDDLE-AGED MEN?

The large population studies, most notably the Framingham Heart Study, that have given us our information on the risk factors for heart disease (for example, obesity, smoking, hypertension) have included women. But the studies that have explored the success of interventions, such as drug therapy and smoking cessation, have been conducted primarily on a middle-aged white male population. The U.S. Preventive Services Task Force has acknowledged the uncertainties regarding the magnitude of benefit from lowering cholesterol in the elderly, women, and young men.

WHY SHOULD I SPEND MONEY ON A CHOLESTEROL SCREENING BLOOD TEST IF I'M YOUNG AND HAVE NO HIGH RISK FACTORS FOR HEART DISEASE?

The U.S. Preventive Services Task Force said that the periodic measurement of total serum cholesterol is most important for middle-aged men, but all people can benefit from counseling about lowering dietary intake of fat, especially saturated fat and cholesterol. In the absence of information regarding most of the population, some experts believe the decision to undergo periodic measurement of serum cholesterol should be made on an individual basis after a thorough discussion regarding personal risk factors for heart disease.

IS THERE ANY RISK IN LOWERING CHOLESTEROL?

There's little question that reducing cholesterol lowers the risk (by an estimated 2 percent for each 1 percent of cholesterol) of death from heart attack. But some research indicates that the gain is canceled by more deaths from other causes, so the overall mortality isn't affected. A meta-analysis of six studies that included 25,000 men found that those who lowered cholesterol were less likely to die of heart disease—but more likely to die by suicide, accidents, or violence.

Another study, which followed nearly 351,000 healthy men for 12 years, found that the 6 percent with the lowest cholesterol levels had no heart disease to speak of, but increased rates of stroke, liver cancer, lung disease, suicide, and alcoholism (*Archives of Internal Medicine*, July 1992).

No one has demonstrated a biological mechanism by which low cholesterol might lead to suicide or violent death, particularly in the low-normal range that people strive for. And the associations found in these studies have not appeared in others. One study of 149 men and 156 women, in fact, found that those who consumed a low-fat, high complex-carbohydrate diet (which might be expected to be linked with suicide and violence) showed a significantly reduced rate of depression and aggressive hostility, compared with people who ate the standard high-fat American diet (*Annals of Internal Medicine*, November 15, 1992).

Other factors may be responsible for the effects ascribed to low cholesterol. A study of eight thousand men found that death rates increased with low cholesterol only among those who drank and smoked heavily or had digestive tract disorders (which might themselves produce abnormally low cholesterol).

HOW CAN I IMPROVE CHOLESTEROL?

Heredity has a marked effect on serum cholesterol. A small proportion of people have familial hypercholesterolemia, which makes their blood levels extremely high. The defective gene that is responsible for at least one variety of this disease has been identified. For the rest of us, heredity probably helps determine how well we handle cholesterol. It's why two people eating the same diet may have very different cholesterol levels.

The fat and cholesterol content of our diet is the most widely discussed factor in serum cholesterol. The diet recommended by the National Cholesterol Education Program and various health and medical organizations calls for no more than 30 percent of calories from fat (down from 38 percent in the average American diet), no more than one-third of it from saturated fat, and less than 300 milligrams of cholesterol (down from 400).

Another aspect of diet that has also been shown to influence cholesterol levels is fiber—the indigestible part of plant foods. Oat bran has received most attention in this regard, but the benefit apparently extends to other kinds of fiber, too, and is added to the effect of low-fat diet. A controlled double-blind study of psyllium (a high-fiber seed widely used as a stool softener) found reductions of 4.2 percent in total cholesterol and 6.4 percent in LDL-cholesterol among people already on a low-fat diet (*Annals of Internal Medicine,* October 1, 1993).

The same issue of *Annals* reported a meta-analysis of five randomized, placebo-controlled trials of garlic as a cholesterol reducer. This found that the equivalent of one half to one clove of garlic per day could reduce total cholesterol by 9 percent in people whose blood levels exceed the recommended concentration—an effect comparable to that of some cholesterol-lowering drugs. "The estimate is conservative," the authors wrote.

Other factors influence cholesterol, too. Exercise reduces LDL and raises HDL; smoking reduces HDL. Stress apparently increases cholesterol, and alcohol reduces it, or at least raises HDL.

CAN DIET REALLY LOWER CHOLESTEROL?

Although diet has been the centerpiece of cholesterol-lowering efforts, some studies have called the effectiveness of diet into question. A meta-analysis of sixteen controlled studies that lasted at least six months concluded that the response to the conventional fat-reduced diet (30 percent of calories) was too limited to have a significant effect on truly elevated cholesterol levels (*British Medical Journal,* October 19, 1991).

Other studies have found cholesterol reductions through diet significant, but modest—on the order of 5 percent, for example. Part of the problem is that low-fat diets all too often are not followed; fat is rampant in today's convenience foods, and doctors are notoriously ineffective in teaching people how to cut down their intake.

The other possibility is that the fat reduction in the conventional "prudent diet" is simply not enough to make a meaningful difference. Eating plans that lower fat considerably more—to 20 percent or even 10 percent of calories—generally get a far more robust response. One program that combined a 10 percent fat diet with stress reduction and exercise brought about a 24.3 percent decrease in total cholesterol, and 37.4 percent drop in LDL-cholesterol (*The Lancet,* 1990, p. 226 [8708]:129–133).

Many people have enough trouble managing to reduce their fat consumption to 30 percent of calories; to reduce it much farther will probably require a radical restructuring of how you eat. It's certainly possible, and many people have done it, but it's not the kind of thing your doctor is liable to be much help with. A nutritionist or dietician may be invaluable.

WHEN SHOULD CHOLESTEROL-LOWERING DRUGS BE PRESCRIBED?

When lovastatin (Mevacor) was approved several years ago, it became an immediate best-seller because it was more effective and caused fewer adverse effects than other cholesterol-lowering drugs. As research into and public education about cholesterol have flourished, sales of such drugs have risen steadily, with lovastatin leading the pack. In 1992, more than twenty-six million prescriptions for anticholesterol drugs were dispensed, nearly nine million of them new ones. In addition, an uncounted number of people used niacin, which is available without a prescription (*Statistical Bulletin,* October–December 1993).

All these drugs have side effects, and the downside of lifelong use is uncertain (particularly for lovastatin-type products, which have the shortest history). They lower cholesterol effectively and have been shown to reduce heart attack rates, but no one recommends that they be the first choice for elevated cholesterol. The National Cholesterol Education Program, for example, urges that such drugs shouldn't be prescribed before ''an adequate trial of dietary modification.''

Clearly, not all doctors follow this directive. The effectiveness of drugs, the difficulty many people have changing their diets, and the old habit of writing a prescription rather than settling in for the slow, extended work of behavior change, can mean early recourse to medication. If you're willing to give diet and lifestyle modification a serious try, make sure your doctor knows that you're counting on whatever help he or she can give you—or direct you to.

✦ HYPER- AND HYPOTHYROIDISM

The thyroid became a newsworthy gland several years ago, when then President George Bush and his wife, Barbara, were both diagnosed with Graves' disease, the most common kind of overactive thyroid condition. Among the questions raised was whether the stress of office triggered Bush's illness—or whether the illness affected the president's judgment during the Gulf War. And was the fact that husband and wife developed the same disease a coincidence?

About seven million Americans have thyroid disease. Graves' disease affects about one million, another million have other kinds of hyperthyroidism (overactive thyroid), and five million have hypothyroidism, an underactivity of the gland. Five times as many women as men have thyroid disease.

Both Graves' and Hashimoto's disease (the most common kind of hypothyroidism) are autoimmune disorders: the gland is attacked by the body's own antibodies. Because the thyroid is a key regulator of metabolism (the rate at which the body burns carbohydrates, protein, and fat for energy) throughout the body, its disorders have very diverse symptoms.

CAN STRESS CAUSE GRAVES' DISEASE?

Graves' disease occurs in people who are genetically predisposed to it, but other factors play a role, too (if one identical twin has it, so will the other—half the time). The possibility that stress, "prolonged worry," or "sudden shock" can precipitate the illness has been noted for over a century, according to a review in *The Lancet* (September 4, 1993). But the hypothesis is difficult to prove: increased anxiety or sensitivity to stressors may be *caused* by Graves' disease months before it is diagnosed. Some studies show that Graves' disease increases dramatically when whole populations are under stress (during wartime, for example), but other epidemiological research is inconsistent.

Graves' is an autoimmune disease, and the complex impact of stress on the immune system is a current focus of intense interest; a more defin-itive answer may emerge soon.

Another risk factor for Graves' disease appears to be cigarette smoking. A 1993 study in the *Journal of the American Medical Association* found smokers twice as likely to have Graves' disease as nonsmokers, and nearly eight times as likely to have eye problems linked with the disease.

It's also been proposed that bacteria or virus may trigger Graves' disease in people who are genetically susceptible. Support for this hypoth-esis is its occurrence in husbands and wives (as in the case of President and Mrs. Bush).

HOW CAN I TELL WHETHER I HAVE THYROID DISEASE?

Nearly half of the people with thyroid disease—an estimated three mil-lion—aren't aware of it. If you have the classic symptoms of hyperthy-roidism (bulging eyes, nervousness, rapid or irregular heartbeat); or hypothyroidism (slow pulse, dry skin, lethargy) along with a palpable en-largement of the gland—a goiter—tests of thyroid function are an easy call.

Many cases of over- or underactive thyroid are missed, however, be-cause their symptoms are undramatic problems that can be caused by any number of things. This is particularly true in older people: fatigue and forgetfulness caused by hypothyroidism, or the tremor and weakness of hyperthyroid are all too easily dismissed as "just aging." Change in bowel habits, a consequence of both hyper- and hypothyroidism, can prompt an unnecessary workup for cancer.

If you have elevated cholesterol, hypothyroidism may be a contributing factor.

Thyroid disorders can mimic emotional illnesses, too, and are sometimes attributed to stress. Signs of depression are common in hypo-thyroidism, while Graves' disease can produce a broader range of symp-toms. Rapid heartbeat, tremor, and nervousness can lead to a misdiagnosis of anxiety disorder, or insomnia and weight loss may be mistaken for depression. A less common pattern of euphoria, racing thoughts, and hy-peractivity resembles the manic phase of manic depression.

The drugs prescribed for psychiatric illnesses may be harmful if you actually have thyroid disease. A test of thyroid function should be part of the medical workup before you are diagnosed with depression or other emotional disorders.

It is possible, and not rare, for people with diagnosed psychiatric illnesses to have thyroid problems as well. Treatment requires an endocrinologist with special expertise in these disorders (see Anxiety and Depression).

WHAT TESTS ARE USED TO ASSESS THYROID FUNCTION?

The measurement of thyroid stimulating hormone (TSH)—secreted by the pituitary to regulate the production of thyroid hormone—has been improved in recent years, so it can usually reveal either hypo- or hyperthyroidism. Not all TSH tests are equally sensitive, however.

Some experts also advocate tests that measure the thyroid hormones T3 and T4 to confirm the diagnosis or to detect rare kinds of thyroid disorder that TSH alone will miss (problems caused by a pituitary tumor, for example), or a further evaluation to pin down the cause of the thyroid problem.

Thyroid function isn't always constant, so it's probably best to repeat tests before starting therapy, at least if the symptoms are minor. "The combination of a raised thyrotropin (TSH) and a patient with minor non-specific symptoms is simply an indication for a repeated measurement in 6–8 weeks" suggests a writer in *The Lancet* (June 2, 1990).

WHAT HYPERTHYROID TREATMENT IS BEST FOR ME?

There are three treatments for hyperthyroidism: medication, radioactive iodine, or surgery to partly destroy the overactive gland—and all are "remarkably effective," according to an editorial in *The New England Journal of Medicine* (April 4, 1991). "Nonetheless," the author of the editorial noted, "it is often difficult for patients with Graves' disease and their physicians to choose among these options, not because of major differences in efficacy, but because of concern about the demonstrated and conceivable side effects associated with each type of therapy."

Antithyroid drugs occasionally produce a hypersensitivity reaction; life-threatening side effects like hepatitis or white cell depletion are rare but possible. And while such drugs are effective in the short term, they do not cure hyperthyroidism: remissions are at best lengthy, and you must be monitored regularly for signs of returning illness. The symptoms of hyperthyroidism will often disappear after taking antithyroid drugs for about nine to twelve months. Unfortunately, the symptoms frequently return, requiring another course of drugs.

Radioiodine and surgery (partial removal of the thyroid) are definitive treatments for hyperthyroidism—the illness isn't likely to come back. What does happen (in 40 percent of people by twenty-five years after treatment) is hypothyroidism, which will require lifetime hormone replacement.

Surgery also carries the risk of complications and death, as well as damage to the laryngeal nerve or to the parathyroid (a nearby gland essential in calcium metabolism) "even in the best surgical hands," according to an article in the British Medical Journal (September 26, 1992). Also, there is a small (10 percent) but real possibility that hyperthyroidism will return, for which radioiodine will be the only option.

A persistent concern about radioiodine is the risk of cancer. In addition to being aimed at the thyroid, a radiation dose is also delivered via the blood stream to the gastrointestinal tract, bladder, and gonads. The actual increase in cancer, according to several large studies, is minimal. No relation was found between radioiodine treatment and thyroid cancer, or leukemia, in studies cited by the British Medical Journal article cited earlier.

"No firm evidence links radioiodine treatment with tumors at other sites, although a nonsignificant increase in breast cancer has been described after thirty years of observation," the article went on to say. A Swedish study that followed 10,522 people who received radioiodine therapy for an average of fifteen years found "an overall cancer risk only slightly greater (6 percent) than in that expected in the general population." Their data "are reassuring," the authors conclude (Journal of the National Cancer Institute, August 7, 1991).

The effect of radioiodine on subsequent pregnancy also has been a matter for concern. Although there is less information on this issue than on cancer, the projected risk of genetic abnormality (based on the dose of radiation) is .005 percent, and large studies have found actual rates to be lower. Other studies haven't found impairment of fertility. Radioiodine is absolutely contraindicated *during* pregnancy, however: it can cause hypo-thyroidism and mental retardation in the baby.

When doctors recommend one or another therapy, they generally take factors like age and disease severity into account: medication is more likely to be chosen as a first option than radioiodine for a young person, vice versa for someone who is middle-aged. Surgery is a last resort under most circumstances.

The fact that hyperthyroid treatment isn't solely a matter of science is witnessed by the varying rates of different procedures from one country to another (radioiodine is far more popular in the United States than in Europe or Japan), and even among medical centers.

IF I HAVE HYPOTHYROIDISM, MUST I BE TREATED FOR LIFE?

Sometimes, hypothyroidism is transient. After pregnancy, and after treatment for hyperthyroidism, tests may show low thyroid function for several months, and then spontaneously normalize. In this situation, if symptoms are mild, no treatment or minimal treatment is necessary, suggests an editorial in *The New England Journal of Medicine* (February 20, 1992).

Reversible hypothyroidism can also be caused by too much or too little iodine (in the diet or in medications) or by ingestion of drugs like lithium carbonate, commonly prescribed for manic depression.

The most common kind of hypothyroidism, inflammation of the gland caused by antibodies that inhibit thyroid function, is generally believed to be permanent, and standard therapy is thyroxine (thyroid replacement hormone) indefinitely.

Remissions do occur, however. According to the above *Journal* editorial, various studies have found that 0 to 24 percent of people with chronic autoimmune hypothyroidism will remain normal after thyroxine has been discontinued. Although the author of the editorial doesn't advocate routine withdrawal of thyroxine after several years, he says that a brief reduction or discontinuation of therapy will show if thyroid function has normalized, at little risk.

A study reported in the *Journal of the American Medical Association* (May 12, 1989) found that thyroxine is often prescribed inappropriately, particularly for older people. The approved indications for prescribing thyroxine include hypothyroidism, goiter (thyroid enlargement), and thyroid cancer, but the hormone is also used for nonthyroid disorders including obesity, low blood pressure, high cholesterol, and hair loss. Thyroxine has never been proven beneficial for any of the latter conditions, the authors say.

A survey of 2,575 adults, average age 68.6, found that 10 percent of women and 2.3 percent of men were taking thyroxine, with 12 percent of the women and 29 percent of the men taking the hormone for inappropriate reasons.

ARE THERE ANY THYROXINE RISKS THAT I SHOULD BE AWARE OF?

Hyperthyroidism is well known to accelerate bone loss and is a risk factor for osteoporosis, the bone-thinning disease that often leads to spinal and hip fractures. There are also indications that thyroxine therapy for hypothyroidism can reduce bone mineral density. In a study in the *Journal of the American Medical Association* (May 22/29, 1991), twenty-six premenopausal women who had taken thyroxine for an average of seven and a half years were found to have significantly lower bone mineral density in the hip, arms, and pelvis.

Much of this bone loss has been attributed to the fact that women in the past were taking doses of thyroxine considerably in excess of the dose now deemed appropriate. Today, the appropriate dose is considered to be 1.6 micrograms per kilogram of body weight.

♦ HYPOGLYCEMIA

Hypoglycemia low blood sugar—has two very different meanings. On the one hand, it's a readily diagnosable, potentially dangerous condition associated with diabetes or insulin-secreting tumors, widely recognized by the medical profession.

On the other, it's a collection of symptoms, many of which are similar to those of anxiety or other disorders, that appear related to diet and food scheduling. Standard lab tests are frequently normal in people who have what some call "the hypoglycemia syndrome," or "low blood sugar."

Medical opinion about the syndrome is divided: many, probably most, doctors view it with skepticism at best, and regard the nutritional explanation as a rationalization for what is at bottom an emotional disorder. Others take it seriously and treat it by advising dietary change.

IS HYPOGLYCEMIA A TRUE DISEASE?

Actually, hypoglycemia is a symptom, which can have over a hundred different causes. In diabetics who take insulin, too much blood sugar may be metabolized, leaving levels low; oral diabetic drugs may have the same effect. Much more rarely, the cause is an insulin-secreting tumor, or insulinoma, which takes blood sugar out of circulation too fast.

The existence of another kind of hypoglycemia was first suspected in the early 1920s, when a similar pattern was observed in people who didn't have diabetes. Weakness, hunger, and a constellation of symptoms associated with anxiety was also found: sweating, palpitations, trembling, headaches, confusion, or difficulty concentrating.

CAN I GET HYPOGLYCEMIA FROM MEDICATION?

Many drugs can induce hypoglycemia, including aspirin (in the high doses prescribed for arthritis, for example), quinine (for malaria), and pentamidine (used for *Pneumocystis carinii* pneumonia). Some blood-pressure drugs may lower blood sugar, particularly beta-blockers, and possibly ACE inhibitors as well. Certain cholesterol-lowering drugs, such as clofibrate, may cause hypoglycemia, too. Certain antidepressants, particularly monoamine oxidase inhibitors, may be responsible.

Anyone under treatment for diabetes should discuss with his or her doctor how a new drug might affect blood sugar. The medications above (as well as others) may change the need for insulin or oral diabetic drugs, causing more pronounced and potentially hazardous variations.

One drug whose effect on blood sugar should not be overlooked is alcohol. According to a review article in *Annals of Internal Medicine* (April 1, 1993), "alcohol is the most common cause of disabling hypoglycemia in the United States. It can occur in healthy children, occasional drinkers, and chronic alcoholics." It can also worsen hypoglycemia caused by other drugs.

IS THERE A TEST FOR HYPOGLYCEMIA?

Hypoglycemia in diabetics is readily diagnosed by measuring blood glucose while symptoms are occurring. The same approach isn't always possible with the hypoglycemia syndrome, because the problem rarely coincides with the doctor visit. The glucose tolerance test (in which blood sugar is tracked for hours after taking a measured amount of sugar) seems appropriate, because symptoms attributed to the hypoglycemia syndrome typically occur after meals, rather than after fasting. This has been widely used, but is dismissed by many experts as unreliable.

In people with suspected hypoglycemia who are tested, blood sugar levels are often within normal range, even during an attack. Some doctors propose that "normal" blood sugar isn't optimal for certain individuals; or that the actual cause of symptoms is the body's attempt to keep blood sugar steady, by secreting adrenaline.

An editorial in *The New England Journal of Medicine* (November 23, 1989) stated flatly that "there is no support for hypoglycemia as a cause of postprandial [after meals] symptoms in most patients," and went on to conjecture that abnormal patterns of digestive enzymes may have a role, or that an emotional disorder is actually to blame.

In any case, the bottom line is that for most people, hypoglycemia

can't be proven by a lab test, and the diagnosis will be based on a characteristic pattern relating symptoms to eating. Symptoms can include
sweating, weakness, hunger, dizziness, trembling, headache, palpitations,
confusion, and, occasionally, double vision.

SHOULD I GET TREATMENT FOR HYPOGLYCEMIA?

If you have diabetes, adjusting diet and medication to keep blood sugar
in a healthy range is a first priority. You should have been educated thoroughly to recognize the signs of falling blood sugar, and taught what self-
help measures to take. (Insulin-dependent diabetics experience mild
episodes of low blood sugar that they can handle themselves an average of
twice weekly, according to an estimate in the *British Medical Journal,* March
6, 1993.) Severe hypoglycemia causing unconsciousness or agitation must
be treated as a medical emergency.

Episodes of the hypoglycemic syndrome are not dangerous, but can be
distressing and life-disrupting. If you believe you suffer from this disorder,
there are standard dietary measures to keep blood sugar steady; they are
nutritionally sound—at the very worst, they won't work, but they won't
cause harm.

- Avoid simple sugars (like those in candy, cake, etc.), and include
  lots of complex carbohydrates in your diet (such as potatoes, rice,
  and whole-grain bread) and protein foods (such as meat and eggs),
  which are digested and absorbed more slowly.
- Have a number of small meals daily, rather than three big ones.
- Add fiber to your diet.
- Avoid caffeine, alcohol, and nicotine. All can reduce blood sugar.
- Exercise regularly, and learn to reduce and cope with stress.

If you feel the symptoms that you associate with falling blood sugar,
the best thing to have is a snack high in complex carbohydrates and protein,
such as peanuts. A candy bar can provide quick energy, but after its simple
sugars are metabolized, you may feel worse than before.

◆ HYSTERECTOMY

By the age of sixty, one woman in three has had a hysterectomy, the second most common surgery (after caesarean section) in the United States. Rates have dropped in recent years—to 590,000 in 1990, more than 100,000 per year less than a decade before. How many are necessary?

It's interesting to note the strange connection between hysterectomy (removal of the uterus) and geography. Rates in the United States are up to six times higher than those of other Western countries. Within the United States, you're more likely to have the surgery if you live in the South and Midwest than in the West or Northeast. You're also more likely to have the surgery if your gynecologist is male or if you are black. To prevent the later development of ovarian cancer, many doctors advocate the removal of healthy ovaries (oophorectomy) during a hysterectomy for a woman over age forty-five. The practice has been called into question in recent years, since the ovaries have a significant role in the physical and sexual health of middle-aged women.

After the removal of the uterus, a woman stops menstruating and can no longer bear children. When the ovaries are also removed, the woman goes into an immediate (or surgical) menopause that is more abrupt than natural menopause.

A particularly disturbing study recently appeared in the *Journal of the American Medical Association* (May 12, 1993). Expert examination of records of all nonemergency, noncancer-related hysterectomies at seven HMOs for a year found that 58 percent were done for clearly appropriate reasons; 25 percent for "uncertain" reasons, and 16 percent for *inappropriate* reasons. In one HMO, 27 percent of the surgeries were inappropriate.

Knowledge is power. A ten-year study of hysterectomy rates in Switzerland found a drop of 25.8 percent in one region, a year after a public information campaign in the mass media, as compared with a rise of 1 percent in a neighboring region. For women of ages thirty-five to forty-nine, the rate dropped by 33 percent (*The Lancet,* December 24/31, 1988).

HOW CAN I TELL WHETHER MY HYSTERECTOMY IS REALLY NECESSARY?

A hysterectomy is necessary when there is a diagnosis of invasive cancer of the cervix or uterus. This, however, represents fewer than 10 percent of the hysterectomies. (So-called precancerous, or noninvasive, lesions of the cervix are not an indication for hysterectomy; see Cervical Cancer—Pap Test.) In rare circumstances, an emergency hysterectomy may be necessary after childbirth because of obstetrical hemorrhage. The rest—that is, the overwhelming majority—of hysterectomies are performed for quality-of-life reasons. Hysterectomy is most often recommended by doctors to improve the symptoms caused by several nonlife-threatening conditions, particularly fibroids, prolapsed uterus, chronic pelvic pain, and excessive bleeding that often occurs before menopause. Only you can decide whether a potential improvement in the symptoms is worth the risks of hysterectomy. Fibroids and excessive bleeding often regress with time and no treatment.

IF I HAVE FIBROIDS, SHOULD I HAVE A HYSTERECTOMY?

Benign tumors of the uterus called leiomyomas, or fibroids, are the single largest reason for hysterectomy, accounting for 30 percent of the total. Their cause is unknown. Excessive bleeding, pelvic pain, and symptoms related to pressure on other organs (like the bladder) are often linked to fibroids.

Hysterectomy is often recommended for symptomless fibroids, on the theory that if left alone, they will grow and pose more risk of bleeding and complications if removed then. But that assumption has never been supported by research, and one recent study of ninety-three women found no greater complication rate when fibroids were larger (*Obstetrics and Gynecology*, April 1992). Robert C. Reiter, M.D., and colleagues at the Departments of Obstetrics and Gynecology of the University of Iowa School of Medicine and the University of California, Los Angeles, School of Medicine, state that it is illogical for physicians to recommend surgery to prevent symptoms as the fibroid grows larger. They concluded that surgery can and should be deferred until symptoms develop, thus sparing the risks and expense of an operation for those women whose fibroids will never cause problems.

There is an infinitesimal chance that untreated fibroids will become malignant. But the risk is smaller than the odds of dying as a result of hysterectomy (one in a thousand).

Hysterectomy may be justified when fibroids cause substantial bleeding, pain, pressure, or anemia—in a woman who does not wish to preserve her fertility. However, the most important question is whether pain, bleeding, or other symptoms repeatedly disrupt your important daily activities. Particularly if your fibroids are small, make sure the symptoms are not actually caused by another disorder, like pelvic inflammatory disease (PID).

WHAT ARE THE ALTERNATIVES TO HYSTERECTOMY FOR SYMPTOMATIC FIBROIDS?

Even if fibroid symptoms warrant surgery, hysterectomy isn't the only procedure available. Myomectomy—removal of the fibroids without removing the uterus—has become an increasingly attractive option. The fibroids can be excised during open surgery with an abdominal incision. Or they can be removed through a telescopelike instrument (a laparoscope) inserted through a tiny abdominal incision or the cervix (hysteroscope). Short-term control of excessive bleeding has been reported at 75 to 90 percent with myomectomy, complications at 5 percent, and the need for further surgery at under 20 percent. The procedures haven't been around long enough for long-term follow-up, however.

A nonsurgical approach, injections of gonadotropin-releasing-hormone (GnRH) agonists can shrink fibroids, but they grow back when GnRH is discontinued. This method may be most helpful as a holding action for women who are close to menopause (when fibroids frequently regress spontaneously).

DO I NEED A HYSTERECTOMY FOR EXCESSIVE BLEEDING WITHOUT FIBROIDS?

About 20 percent of hysterectomies are performed for dysfunctional uterine bleeding for which no cause, such as fibroids, endometriosis, malignancy, or infection can be found. Here, too, whether to treat the condition at all (once these potential causes have been ruled out) depends on whether the bleeding is disrupting your activities or causing anemia.

If so, you probably shouldn't think about surgery until medical treatment has been given at least a month's trial, according to a review article in *The New England Journal of Medicine* (March 25, 1993). Nonsteroidal anti-inflammatory drugs (NSAIDs) and hormone replacement or manipulation are the most common approaches.

Even if these don't work, hysterectomy isn't inevitable. Destroying the endometrium—the lining of the uterus—by laser or electrocautery is a far less extensive procedure that has a 70 to 90 percent success rate in halting or markedly reducing excess bleeding. The bleeding recurs, however, in 15 to 25 percent of cases, and long-term outcomes are unknown. Some women have gotten pregnant after endometrium destruction, but doctors advise this option only for women who do not want to preserve their fertility.

One study found that the endometrial resection (destruction of the lining of the uterus) procedure took about half the time of hysterectomy. It was followed by an average hospital stay of one day rather than seven and a recovery time of sixteen days rather than fifty-eight (*British Medical Journal*, November 30, 1991).

CAN SOMETHING OTHER THAN HYSTERECTOMY BE DONE FOR A PROLAPSED UTERUS?

A prolapsed uterus is one that has "dropped." It is sagging within the vagina because supporting ligaments have stretched and weakened as a result of aging, gravity, and/or childbearing. Most women have some degree of prolapse, especially after menopause, when decreasing estrogen levels further weaken the supporting ligaments. Many women feel no discomfort at all; others feel some abdominal pressure or lower backache. A prolapsed uterus does not require treatment.

Rather than removing the uterus altogether, the problem may be resolved with a pessary (a diaphragmlike device to support the organ). The old-fashioned pessary used to be so rigid that it was difficult if not impossible for a woman to apply one or remove it. These days, they are made of plastic or rubber in a wide variety of types. Some are designed to be

inserted and removed by the woman herself; others require insertion by a
health professional.

IS HYSTERECTOMY A VALID TREATMENT FOR ENDOMETRIOSIS OR CHRONIC PELVIC PAIN?

The proportion of hysterectomies done for endometriosis has been increasing, but some experts believe hysterectomy is too drastic a solution. In
fact, it often is not a solution for a significant minority of women with
severe endometriosis. There are many medical and surgical options available for this condition (see Endometriosis), and hysterectomy should be
considered a last resort.

Chronic pelvic pain of unknown origin is a risky reason to undergo
hysterectomy. One study showed that as many as 22 percent of women
who consent to the operation for this problem continue to have chronic
pain following the hysterectomy. High rates of irritable bowel syndrome
(up to 80 percent) have been found among women who undergo testing
for chronic pelvic pain.

IS IT NECESSARY TO REMOVE MY HEALTHY OVARIES JUST BECAUSE I'M OVER FORTY-FIVE?

Many doctors advocate the removal of the healthy ovaries (oophorectomy)
in women scheduled for noncancer-related hysterectomy in order to eliminate the later possibility of cancer. Ovarian cancer is almost impossible to
detect at an early stage and is virtually incurable in most women detected
at later stages. Is it worth having your healthy ovaries removed prophylactically? The ovaries are the principal source of hormones—androgens
(male sex hormone responsible for libido) as well as estrogen. Their loss
causes premature menopause, often with distressing symptoms more
marked than those of natural menopause (see Menopause), even with hormonal replacement. Bone-thinning and an increased risk of heart disease
also are associated with surgical menopause. Though doctors say these risks
are overcome with estrogen therapy, long-term usage (over ten years) is
associated with an increased risk of breast cancer.

Ultimately, a prophylactic oophorectomy is your decision to make.

For a woman of fifty, the probability of developing ovarian cancer is 1.2 percent, and of dying from it, 0.8 percent. If close family members have had ovarian cancer, your lifetime risk is higher: an estimated 5 percent if you have one first-degree relative with the disease; 7 percent if two or more of your relatives have had the disease. Some hereditary syndromes raise the risk to as high as 50 percent.

On the other hand, removal of the uterus alone reduces a woman's risk of ever developing ovarian cancer. An Italian study of over thirty-seven hundred women found that hysterectomy alone, without oophorectomy, cuts the rate of ovarian cancer during the following years by approximately half (the finding had been demonstrated in earlier studies). This may be because hysterectomy alters blood flow to the ovaries, or provides the opportunity to detect cancer at the time of the surgery (*Obstetrics and Gynecology*, March 1993).

The women who should give prophylactic oophorectomy serious thought are those with a family history of ovarian cancer. But removal of healthy ovaries is no guarantee. It is possible to develop ovarian cancer even after the healthy ovaries have been removed. One study followed twenty-eight women with a family history of ovarian cancer who had undergone prophylactic oophorectomy. Three of them subsequently developed a disseminated cancer in the abdominal cavity that was indistinguishable from ovarian cancer.

WHAT ARE THE RISKS OF HYSTERECTOMY?

Like any surgery, hysterectomy has its risks. Mortality rates of about 0.1 percent have been reported, higher when the procedure is associated with cancer or an obstetrical emergency. Complications, mostly fever and infection, have occurred in 24 percent of vaginal hysterectomies (uterus removed through the vagina), and 43 percent of abdominal procedures (uterus is removed through an incision in abdomen), but modern refinements in technique may have reduced them.

As for the long-term aftereffects, sexual dysfunction, adhesions, and chronic pain have been reported. Even without oophorectomy, ovarian failure occurs in as many as 25 percent of women (possibly because of alterations in blood supply), causing symptoms of early menopause.

A decline in sexual function after hysterectomy—reported to occur in

10 to 46 percent of women—depends on the specific population, the circumstances, and the extent of the surgery. About 35 percent experience diminished desire or lack of orgasm. Some of this may reflect hormonal changes, but even hormone replacement does not always restore sexual function. For some women, the contractions of the uterus are an important part of orgasm. For others, the pressure of the penis against the cervix is important to their sexual pleasure.

Androgen, the male sex hormone, is produced by the ovaries and seems related to sex drive in women as well as men. Some studies have found that replacing androgen along with estrogen can restore libido and sexual interest after oophorectomy. The side effects of androgen—excessive facial hair and a deepening of the voice—are unacceptable to many women, however. Dosage can be adjusted to minimize these side effects. Long-term information on the use of androgen replacement therapy is nonexistent.

Whether or not hysterectomy causes depression is controversial. One researcher observed what he called the "occurred syndrome" and noted that 70 percent of women suffered depression after the surgery. Others have reported no increase in emotional distress, and some have found an increase in feelings of well being—possibly related to relief of symptoms and worry.

Resources

The HERS Foundation provides phone counseling to women who have been told they need hysterectomy, and may be able to refer you to a doctor knowledgeable in surgical techniques that preserve the uterus.

HERS Foundation
422 Bryn Mawr Avenue
Bala Cynwyd, PA 19004
(610) 667-7757

♦ IMPOTENCE

The inability to have an erection is a situation that virtually all men face now and then. When it occurs more than 25 percent of the time, it's described as erectile dysfunction, or "impotence."

The problem is apparently more widespread than previously thought: one study found that half of American men over forty (about nineteen million) suffer at least mild erectile dysfunction, roughly double earlier estimations. Its causes run the gamut from relationship difficulties to illness to injury.

This diversity is no surprise, considering the complexity of the process that culminates in erection. The brain, the nervous system, hormones, and circulation all come into play. Generally initiated by erotic stimulation, nerve impulses induce muscles in the penis to relax, allowing blood to engorge that organ. Pressure on veins keeps the blood from leaving, and maintains the erection long enough to have sexual intercourse.

COULD MY IMPOTENCE BE PSYCHOLOGICAL?

Until fairly recently, experts thought that was almost always the case. Estimates of psychogenic causes ran as high as 95 percent. Better methods of evaluation and diagnosis, however, have shown that medical illness and other physical problems are involved in perhaps 75 percent of erectile dysfunction.

But it's not simply a matter of "either/or." Even when organic abnormalities can be found, anxiety, depression, or relationship complexities may compound their impact. Conversely, physical treatment may help men whose impotence seems psychological.

HOW CAN I DEAL WITH EMOTIONAL PROBLEMS THAT CAUSE OR CONTRIBUTE TO IMPOTENCE?

Anxiety prevents the muscle relaxation necessary for erection. This may have its origin in psychological conflicts about sexuality or may relate to a current situation in a relationship.

One common scenario involves the man who has had what would otherwise be an isolated inability to have an erection (perhaps due to alcohol or fatigue). The next time, his worry about a repetition of the problem becomes a self-fulfilling prophecy. It's a vicious cycle: the longer impotence continues, the harder it is to stop.

Anything that distracts a man from the erotic experience itself—preoccupation with performance, money problems, or work, for example—interferes with the chain of thoughts, feelings, and physical events that produce an erection.

Anger at one's partner, jealousy, guilt, or sexual conflicts deeply rooted in childhood may be involved. A man who was brought up to think of sex as something illicit or nasty may be impotent with his wife, but not with other women.

Sexual dysfunction is one of the classic symptoms of depression. In the same way that depression disrupts sleep and interferes with normal appetite, its physiological and emotional changes can stifle erections.

Whatever the cause of erectile dysfunction, its psychological impact is rarely insignificant. For most men, sexual adequacy is closely tied to the sense of self. Feelings of guilt, worthlessness, and shame are common consequences of impotence. Even when erectile dysfunction has an identifiable physical cause, psychological counseling or therapy is generally indicated both to help ameliorate the problem and to deal with the emotional fallout.

WHAT KIND OF THERAPY IS BEST FOR ME?

If a disorder like depression, generalized anxiety, or substance abuse is identified, it must be treated. Performance anxiety is typically approached with behavioral therapy that teaches how to focus comfortably on the experience of physical intimacy without distraction or pressure. More extensive psychotherapy may be indicated to address emotional issues like guilt or shame, and to alleviate some of the distress caused by impotence.

Whenever possible, treatment includes both sexual partners. Couples therapy may aim at improving communication and conflict resolution, as well as airing problems that have developed around the erectile dysfunction itself.

According to a National Institutes of Health (NIH) consensus conference (*Journal of the American Medical Association,* July 7, 1993), the effectiveness of psychotherapy and behavior therapy in treating impotence hasn't been well documented, but it seems that results are best when both partners are included.

IS IMPOTENCE INEVITABLE WITH ADVANCING AGE?

Although the ease of achieving an erection, its rigidity, and other parameters of sexual performance do decline with age, there's no reason to expect that the years (until the eighties, anyway) should rob a man of his sexual ability.

Erectile dysfunction does, however, become increasingly common with age. According to a survey of seventeen hundred men in Massachusetts, 5 percent reported complete impotence at the age of forty, compared with 15 percent at seventy. If you add moderate dysfunction, the numbers are about one quarter at forty, and one half at fifty.

Responsible, perhaps, is not aging, per se, but illnesses that grow more common with the passing years, and the medications used to treat them (e.g., antihypertensives). "Age appears to be a strong indirect risk factor in that it is associated with an increased likelihood of direct risk factors" is how the NIH consensus conference summarized the connection.

HAVE DISEASES THAT CAN CAUSE IMPOTENCE BEEN RULED OUT?

Anything that impairs the circulatory or nervous system may be involved. Diabetes, which can do both, is held to be responsible for one out of four cases of impotence in older men, and in a significant proportion of younger men as well. Atherosclerosis, which blocks arteries to the heart in coronary heart disease, may also reduce blood flow to the penis. High blood pressure, neurological disorders (such as Parkinson's disease or multiple sclerosis), kidney disease, endocrine disorders (e.g., diabetes), and liver disease are among other possible causes.

If not previously diagnosed, any of these diseases should be treated, of course. This will sometimes resolve the erectile dysfunction, but if irreversible anatomical damage has already taken place, further measures will be necessary.

WHEN ARE HORMONES PRESCRIBED?

A hormonal imbalance is involved in as many as 30 percent of cases of impotence, by some estimates (but far less by others). A man's level of testosterone, the principal male hormone, may be too low; estrogen, the female hormone, may be too high (as occurs with liver disease, for example); or elevated amounts of a pituitary hormone, prolactin, may block the process necessary for erection.

Testosterone declines after about age forty, but for the majority of otherwise healthy men, it remains high enough to maintain normal erections.

Testosterone injections may alleviate impotence in men whose levels are abnormally low—but this kind of treatment will have no advantage if the level is normal. There are treatments to normalize excessive prolactin and estrogen, too.

DOES LIFESTYLE MAKE ANY DIFFERENCE?

Smoking has a very negative effect on erectile ability. It's not only a risk factor for atherosclerosis, but it also directly impairs the delicate circulation to the penis. Because nicotine constricts blood vessels, just a cigarette or two may bring about an immediate decline in erectile function.

Heavy drinking disrupts the normal balance of male and female hormones, which can lead to impotence. And because alcohol depresses the nervous system, a few drinks can interfere with erections, particularly in older men.

High LDL-cholesterol and low HDL-cholesterol appear to be risk factors for erectile dysfunction; it's another reason to follow a prudent diet that limits saturated fats. Obesity (which affects hormones) can also be a factor.

MIGHT DRUGS THAT I'M TAKING
CAUSE IMPOTENCE?

Some estimate that two hundred different medications—both prescription and OTC—have sexual dysfunction as a side effect. This includes such unlikely suspects as antihistamines and decongestants.

The NIH consensus conference estimated that one quarter of erectile dysfunction is caused by medications taken for other conditions. Common among them are antidepressants, antianxiety drugs, and medications used for ulcer.

Cardiac drugs are perhaps most frequently responsible. Beta-blockers (e.g., Inderal), which are used for high blood pressure and heart disease, are implicated most often, but other antihypertensive medications have this side effect, too. Some of the newer blood pressure and heart medications— ACE inhibitors and calcium channel blockers—appear less likely to cause erectile problems.

When discussing impotence with your doctor, it's vital to mention *all* drugs, prescription or OTC, that you are using. Often, an alternative can be tried that has the same therapeutic effect without the drawbacks.

UNDER WHAT CIRCUMSTANCES IS
SURGERY ADVISED?

Vascular surgery is intended to alleviate impotence by rebuilding the arteries that supply blood to the penis by tying off some of the veins that remove blood from the penis.

The track record of vascular surgery is uneven. Arterial surgery (which may graft a vessel from elsewhere in the body) appears to be helpful when there is a focused blockage in circulation, usually due to a congenital abnormality or an injury, but is less effective when the blockage is widespread (as it is when caused by atherosclerosis). Some experts doubt that venous surgery is worth doing at all. According to the NIH consensus conference, "decreased effectiveness of this approach has been reported as longer-term follow-up periods have been obtained."

Probably, the NIH report suggests, vascular surgery for erectile dysfunction should be considered experimental, and should be done in a medical center by experienced surgeons. A thorough evaluation of the blood vessel system in the penis is a vital prerequisite before such surgery is even considered.

HOW WELL DOES INJECTION THERAPY WORK?

This is a widely used treatment for impotence resulting from physical causes. Men are taught to inject substances directly into the penis to dilate the arteries and produce an erection; papaverine and phentolamine are most often used. In one study, about half of men instructed in the technique were still using it eight years later.

Most side effects are minor—pain, ulcerations, or hard nodules—but occasionally, prolonged, painful erections occur that require urgent medical attention.

A synthetic version of a chemical messenger called prostaglandin E, used alone or with a reduced amount of papaverine, appears to have fewer side effects, according to a panel of experts convened by the American Medical Association (*Journal of the American Medical Association,* June 26, 1991). All of these drugs have been approved by the FDA for other indications, but none for treatment of impotence.

ARE THERE NONDRUG ALTERNATIVES?

There's a vacuum constriction device that is placed over the penis; air is pumped out, which draws blood into the penis. A band is then placed at the base of the penis to maintain the erection until intercourse is over.

The device works for more than 90 percent of men, with few side effects. But the method requires proper instruction, manual dexterity, and time (about three to five minutes), and some find the lack of spontaneity distressing. Training both sexual partners may be an important key to the satisfactory use of this device, suggests the NIH consensus committee.

WHAT ELSE IS THERE?

Penile implants are either semirigid rods placed in the shaft of the penis to produce a permanent erection, or an inflatable alternative: a saline solution pumped into the rods produces an erection that can be reversed at will.

Many men have used this approach satisfactorily, but mechanical failures (especially with the pump) may require reoperation. Because this treatment is irreversible—a natural erection will never again be possible—it's usually considered a last resort and only after a very thorough evaluation.

SHOULD I SEE A SPECIALIST?

Given the complexity of erectile dysfunction and the wide range of possible causes, a thorough diagnostic workup is often required to distinguish between psychological and physical factors. A workup typically involves monitoring the occurrence of erection during sleep, and testing the ability to have an erection by injecting a single dose of artery-dilating chemicals.

While any good physician who understands impotence well may be able to assess the role of medical diseases, drug side effects, and the like in causing problems, further investigation is best conducted by a urologist. A mental-health professional may be needed to evaluate the role of psychological factors.

Anything more invasive than the vacuum constriction device should be left to a specialist, many think—although thorough training and experience in the field may qualify some primary care physicians to do injection therapy.

The NIH consensus statement noted that medical education in erectile dysfunction is, for the most part, inadequate, and that discomfort with the subject—both on the part of men and their physicians—often proves an obstacle to treatment. You may have to take an active role to get the help you need.

Resources

Association for Male Sexual Dysfunction
320 East 72nd Street
New York, NY 10021
(212) 794-1616

Provides the latest information about testing and treatment and will refer you to specialists and local support groups.

◆ INCONTINENCE

The involuntary passing of urine—incontinence—is by no means rare: an estimated ten million suffer from the problem in this country, three times as many women as men. Urinary incontinence becomes much more common with age: it affects an estimated 15 to 30 percent of older people living independently, and at least half of those in nursing homes, according to a 1988 National Institutes of Health consensus statement.

Incontinence is not something people like to talk about. Only a minority of those who suffer from it seek professional help, and many wait for years before taking that step. When they do, they may not get the care they need. A 1993 report by the Agency for Health Care Policy and Research cited evidence that many physicians hesitate to discuss incontinence or fail to treat it properly.

WHAT CAN BE DONE ABOUT INCONTINENCE?

Unfortunately, the only public attention to incontinence seems to be the television ads for adult diapers, which fosters the notion that there's nothing much else you can do for it—a misconception that keeps many from getting help. Contrary to common belief, incontinence is not a normal, inevitable part of aging: it's a symptom of many underlying disorders, most of which are treatable.

Behavior modification, special exercises, medication, and surgery all have their place in treating incontinence. With the help of one or a combination of approaches, 90 percent of people can cure the condition or substantially relieve symptoms.

WHAT CAUSES INCONTINENCE?

Controlled urination is a complex mechanism that requires nerves, muscles, and the bladder to work in harmony; things can go wrong at any number of points. Urinary tract infections, anatomical abnormalities, or weakness in pelvic muscles stretched by childbirth may be responsible. So can any number of diseases that affect the nervous system, such as stroke or multiple sclerosis. The decline of estrogen after menopause may weaken the muscles necessary for bladder control.

Damage to nerves or muscles after surgery such as hysterectomy in women, or prostatectomy in men, also can be to blame. And sometimes no cause can be identified.

Over-the-counter and prescription drugs affect the urination process in various ways and can cause or aggravate incontinence. Some common culprits are antihistamines and decongestants (both are often in OTC cold remedies), antidepressants, antipsychotics, and some blood pressure medications.

WHAT KIND OF INCONTINENCE DO I HAVE?

The different kinds of incontinence require different treatment. In *stress incontinence,* the muscles that normally keep the urethra closed aren't strong enough, so when abdominal pressure is increased by sneezing, lifting, coughing, or laughing, some urine leaks out. This is far more common in women, possibly due to damage to pelvic muscles by childbirth or changes during menopause, but it also affects men after prostate surgery.

People with *urge incontinence* find it difficult, if not impossible, to suppress the muscle contractions that initiate urination. Once the bladder fills past a certain point, it contracts involuntarily, and often there's no time to get to the toilet.

Overflow incontinence is, paradoxically, the result of difficulty urinating. The bladder doesn't empty completely, because it's blocked (by an enlarged prostate, for example) or because essential nerves or muscles aren't working properly. Eventually, it becomes too full and urine escapes.

Many people have a combination of these types.

A doctor who does a thorough office examination can often diagnose fairly accurately what kind of incontinence is involved without more extensive tests. A very specific description of your symptoms, perhaps documented in detail by a "urination diary," along with a medical history, physical examination, and perhaps a stress test (you cough with a full bladder), often supplies enough information to plan treatment.

If the basic evaluation can't diagnose the incontinence or if standard treatments don't work, you may be referred to a urologist for tests that measure how the muscles and nerves that control urination are functioning. A urologist's workup is also indicated if symptoms and lab tests, such as blood in the urine or recurrent urinary tract infections, suggest an underlying condition that complicates matters.

WHAT TREATMENT DO YOU USE FIRST?

Both nondrug approaches and medication, as well as surgery are quite effective if used appropriately. As a rule, the Agency for Health Care Policy and Research (AHCPR) guidelines urge that the safest and least invasive option should be tried first. This generally means behavioral treatment, which has no adverse effects or complications, and which cures or improves symptoms in 70 to 87 percent of people with stress or urge incontinence. The downside of this approach is the commitment of energy it demands from you (and your doctor). Also, results take time: it may be months before you see a difference.

There are two basic behavioral methods: exercise and bladder training. Exercise aims to strengthen the pelvic floor muscles that control urination. These, typically, are Kegel exercises, where you identify the specific muscles that stop urine flow, and contract them many times daily.

Bladder training aims to reestablish voluntary control over urination. It consists of following a rigid schedule—going to the bathroom at gradually lengthening intervals (whether you need to or not), and refraining from urinating in between, using relaxation and muscle strengthening to help control the urge.

CAN BIOFEEDBACK OR OTHER DEVICES HELP?

Biofeedback uses technology to help you identify the muscles involved in urination, and learn how to strengthen and control them. It's used in combination with exercise and bladder training. Studies of its effectiveness are inconsistent: some show no benefit, while in another, women who used it to supplement Kegel exercises achieved a 76 percent reduction in incontinence, compared with 51 percent for women who used the exercises alone.

Another recent innovation for women is vaginal weights. Small cones of gradually increasing weight are placed within the vagina for fifteen-minute sessions, twice a day, and this stimulates the contraction of pelvic muscles—the same ones that control urination—to hold them in place.

Devices to stimulate pelvic muscles and nerves electrically have also been used. The AHCPR guidelines urged caution with this method until its effectiveness has been documented.

WHEN IS MEDICATION PRESCRIBED?

The use of drugs requires an accurate diagnosis of the incontinence problem. Medications that increase the contraction of the sphincter that controls urine flow, for example, are appropriate for stress incontinence, but very wrong for urge incontinence, while those that suppress bladder contractions responsible for urge incontinence would make overflow incontinence worse.

Studies of medication effectiveness vary widely: at best, according to the AHCPR guidelines, their results are comparable to those with behavioral techniques. Depending on the drugs used and the people who use them, they cause side effects in 0 to 70 percent of cases. Estrogen has been used for stress incontinence in women after menopause, but studies of its effectiveness have been inconsistent.

Medications can be helpful for people who prefer them to the steady effort and slow results of strengthening or bladder training, when these methods haven't worked, or when the specific condition requires them. Often, combining behavioral and drug therapy achieves much better results than either modality used separately.

WHEN IS SURGERY ADVISED?

Surgery is usually the last option, and it demands a thorough, detailed evaluation of the problem. There are a number of different procedures, depending on the cause of incontinence and the steps necessary to correct it. For stress incontinence, surgery may tighten the pelvic muscles and realign the bladder and urethra, or put in an artificial sphincter. If an obstruction is causing overflow incontinence, it can then be removed.

According to the AHCPR report, the most common procedures for stress incontinence have good cure and improvement rates (upward of 80 percent cured) but a high rate of complications as well (20 to 30 percent). It has been suggested that most studies do not follow up for a long enough period after surgery, and that symptoms more frequently return over time. In one study, 27 percent of 131 women who had Burch colposuspension, a common procedure for stress incontinence, suffered genital prolapse and needed more surgery (*American Journal of Obstetrics and Gynecology,* August 1992).

Prior abdominal surgery, including hysterectomy, may affect the outcome of surgery to correct incontinence. In one series of eighty-six women, those who had previously had a hysterectomy were significantly less likely to have relief of symptoms than those who had not (*Journal of Reproductive Medicine,* February 1988).

A less ambitious approach for people with urethral sphincter insufficiency involves injecting collagen or a Teflon paste around the urethra in order to increase urethral compression. The collagen procedure appears to have a somewhat higher success rate, according to the AHCPR report, but complications are few with both methods. An expert panel of the American Medical Association evaluated the Teflon procedure and found it "promising" for the treatment of stress incontinence in women and postprostatectomy incontinence in men, but added that its safety in women hasn't been demonstrated with the appropriate clinical trial.

Resources

Call Help for Incontinent People at (800) BLADDER. This is a nonprofit organization that may refer you to specialists in your area and offers educational materials about incontinence.

✦ INFERTILITY

Infertility appears to be on the rise because many more couples are now waiting to have their first child at an older age; but in fact, the so-called epidemic of infertility in the United States is—if you will forgive the pun— a misconception. "There is no more infertility today than there was thirty years ago," said Anjani Chandra, Ph.D., of the Family Growth Survey Branch of the National Center for Health Statistics (NCHS). The national surveys conducted periodically by the NCHS show that the overall infertility rates within age groups have not changed since 1965.

Several years ago a widely publicized—and misleading—study published in *The New England Journal of Medicine* showed that one in six women are infertile. Dr. Chandra said that the true figure is one in twelve. Contributing factors include sexually transmitted diseases, postponed parenthood, and environmental pollution. Some infertility is doctor caused, such as genital abnormalities in men and women born of mothers given synthetic estrogen (DES) during their pregnancies, pelvic inflammatory disease associated with certain intrauterine devices used for birth control, the overtreatment of cervical abnormalities (see Cervical Cancer), and, ironically, the adhesions caused by surgical treatments for infertility. In most cases, however, the cause or causes of infertility are unknown.

Infertility treatment has become a two-billion-dollar-a-year industry, offering a menu of high-tech treatments with low success rates. In-vitro fertilization, in which the egg is removed, brought together with sperm in the laboratory, and then implanted in the uterus, is increasingly used. The procedure has been around for close to twenty years. Relative newcomers are gamete intrafallopian transplant (GIFT), which unites sperm and egg in the fallopian tube, and elaborations on IVF that treat the egg to make it easier for sperm to penetrate or even inject the sperm directly into the egg.

The baby chase can be exhausting, both physically and emotionally, and expensive. The workup that precedes high-tech fertilization can cost three thousand dollars, and the procedures themselves, which often must be repeated, go for upward of eight thousand dollars. A single IVF procedure, ordinarily the least expensive of the high-tech options, is between seven thousand and fifteen thousand dollars, with an additional two thousand dollars for medications.

ARE WE TRULY INFERTILE?

A couple is deemed infertile, by the World Health Organization definition, after two years of unsuccessful attempts to conceive. But in the United States and Canada, many doctors start to talk about interventions after just one year, particularly for couples who are over thirty. The fact that a fair number of couples diagnosed as infertile eventually conceive without treatment suggests that science still has a way to go in defining the problem precisely. Contrary to conventional medical wisdom, the overwhelming majority of women who want to start childbearing in their thirties will be successful, according to John Bongaarts of the Population Council (*Family Planning Perspectives,* March/April 1982).

WHAT IS THE CAUSE OF INFERTILITY?

The treatment of infertility depends on the cause, and high-tech, high-cost interventions should never be the first approach. Difficulties may reside in the man, the woman, or both.

Only in the last two decades has it been appreciated that one third or more of infertility cases are attributable to male dysfunction. Doctors have been alert to low sperm counts for years, but today, it's possible to examine for more subtle abnormalities—in shape, movement, and sperm anatomy—that can take a toll on fertility. The sperm-producing function of the testicles is extremely sensitive to heat; a deterioration of sperm quality in the summer may be responsible for lower birth rates in the spring, according to an article in *The New England Journal of Medicine* (July 5, 1990). An anatomical defect (varicocele) that brings too much blood to the testicles may keep them too warm constantly; correction by surgery (or with water-cooled underwear) has been shown to improve sperm production.

Among women, some common causes of infertility that should be thoroughly evaluated and addressed early in the treatment process are anatomical—obstruction of the fallopian tube, often due to prior infection (see Pelvic Inflammatory Disease)—and hormonal imbalance.

HOW LIKELY ARE WE TO BENEFIT FROM IN-VITRO FERTILIZATION?

In view of the physical demands, emotional depletion, and expense of IVF, you'd want the effort to substantially increase your chance of conception. This isn't necessarily the case, however.

For one thing, many "infertile" couples conceive while waiting to get into high-powered programs, or otherwise without treatment. A review article in *The New England Journal of Medicine* (December 2, 1993) noted that "a surprising number of pregnancies" occur independently of medical help. The difference in outcome between those who do and don't participate in the $2 billion-a-year fertility industry is simply not large.

How large? A study that for two to seven years followed 1,145 couples diagnosed as infertile found that pregnancies occurred in 41 percent of those who had been treated, and 35 percent of the untreated (*The New England Journal of Medicine*, November 17, 1983).

Things have changed a lot since 1983—new treatments, techniques, and technologies have been developed—but the 6 percent spread apparently has not. A recent study by the same researchers of two thousand couples found that state-of-the-art medicine still makes the same small difference. "Treatment has developed in almost miraculous ways," researcher Dr. John A. Collins, professor of obstetrics/gynecology at McMaster University, Hamilton, Ontario, said in an interview, "but this has not changed the basic likelihood of a couple succeeding."

WHAT IS THE AVERAGE CENTER'S "TAKE-HOME BABY RATE" FOR COUPLES LIKE US?

Making it harder to know just what you stand to gain from "assisted reproductive technology," its practitioners have been conspicuously lacking in candor about their results. False information has been so widespread, in fact, that congressional hearings, held in the late 1980s, led to a 1992 bill (the Fertility Clinic Success Rate and Certification Act) that will require every infertility clinic to report its track record annually.

A lack of truth in advertising hasn't been limited to small, shady enterprises. Even the prestigious Mount Sinai Medical Center was threatened with legal action by New York City's Department of Consumer Affairs. Its overall success rate for IVF, it seemed, was half of what was claimed in a promotional brochure.

What is "success" in the fertility game? Fertilizing an egg in the laboratory may swell a clinic's batting average, but it's many steps away from a live birth. When considering an infertility clinic, make sure you ask the bottom-line question: the "take-home baby rate." And make sure you get it specific to your age and diagnosis.

WHAT ARE THE RISKS OF IVF?

Although IVF has been around for nearly two decades, relatively little is known about long-term risks to mother or child.

One possible consequence of the drugs given to induce ovulation (a central part of most infertility treatments like IVF) is ovarian hyperstimulation syndrome. According to an article in the *British Medical Journal* (January 19, 1991), this occurs in 3 percent of cycles: when severe, the syndrome causes fluid retention, vomiting, and coagulation abnormalities. It may require hospitalization.

The risk of ovarian hyperstimulation syndrome is greatest for young, thin women. It is best prevented by keeping careful watch over estrogen levels induced by the treatment and by making sure the drug should have been prescribed in the first place. Misuse of hyperstimulation drugs is widespread. A review of the medical records of 3,837 women who underwent infertility treatment between 1974 and 1985 in Seattle showed that 52 percent of the infertile women given Clomid had normally functioning ovaries (*New England Journal of Medicine*, September 22, 1994). The practice stems from the "misguided notion that if [Clomid] makes a subfertile woman more fertile, then surely it can only make a normal woman more fertile," according to Robert Nachtigall, M.D., and Elizabeth Mehren, authors of *Overcoming Infertility* (New York: Doubleday, 1991).

The same review of the medical records of Seattle women showed an increased rate of ovarian cancer among those who took Clomid. Of the more than three thousand women treated for infertility, eleven cases of ovarian cancer were identified. Nine of the women with ovarian cancer had taken Clomid, and five of the nine had taken the drug during twelve or more monthly cycles. Normally, about four cases of ovarian cancer would be expected in a similar cohort of infertile women who did not take infertility drugs.

IS THE RISK OF OVARIAN CANCER ASSOCIATED WITH CLOMID OR WITH ALL HYPERSTIMULATION DRUGS?

The Seattle study period ended in the mid-1980s. Few women in this study were taking more powerful drugs like Pergonal and Lupron, which are standard protocol for in-vitro fertilization. The true extent of infertility drug-caused ovarian cancer will not be known for many more years. The average age of the women at the end of the Seattle study was the early forties, whereas ovarian cancer is overwhelmingly a disease of older women.

WHAT ARE THE RISKS TO THE BABY?

The principal risk to the baby comes from the fact that assisted reproductive technologies greatly increase the incidence of multiple births: the rate with IVF is 27 percent, compared to 1 percent in the general population. This in turn is primarily responsible for an excess of preterm deliveries (24 percent, compared with an expected 6 percent) and deaths around the time of childbirth (twenty-seven among eighteen thousand IVF babies followed, compared to an expected ten). Other complications, such as cerebral palsy, are also more common in multiple births.

One way to reduce these risks is to limit the number of implanted embryos, which has become more feasible with the development of technology to preserve fertilized eggs by freezing some for later implantation if needed. In the United Kingdom, legislation limits the number of embryos that can be implanted simultaneously to three.

When an IVF program in Vancouver assumed a similar limit (no more than three embryos implanted, or in exceptional circumstances, four), the multiple birth rate dropped from 26 percent to 8 percent, while the rate of successful pregnancies rose from 19.5 to 25 percent.

On the positive side, babies conceived by IVF thus far seem no more likely to have birth defects. But a registry to track such children has yet to be established. Until then, we do not know about long-term effects.

HOW CAN WE DEAL WITH THE STRESS OF INFERTILITY?

Stress is known to impair fertility, through its effect on hormone production. And infertility, to say nothing of the effort demanded by treatment, can cause great stress. The resulting spiral makes conception harder than ever.

According to an article in *Fertility and Sterility* (March 1993), the stress response probably reflects an evolutionary strategy to suppress conception in perilous times. A study of thirty-eight women found the greatest levels of stress among those whose infertility had no anatomical explanation, and that social support—a well-known protector against stress—was low in this group.

"Findings in this study suggest that psychosocial therapy directed at strengthening the individual's social support network may prove to be among the more valuable treatments for some forms of infertility in women," the authors concluded.

Resources

Guidebooks based on self-reported data provide success rates at various infertility clinics. One, published by the Society for Assisted Reproductive Technologies (SART), includes reports from 247 clinics in the United States and five in Canada. Write SART for prices and an order form:

Society for Assisted Reproductive Technologies
1209 Montgomery Highway
Birmingham, AL 35216
(205) 978-5000

In Vitro Fertilizations Clinics: A North American Directory of Programs and Services by Mary Partridge-Brown lacks a breakdown of success rates by age and diagnosis, which the SART directory includes, but offers information on cost, drugs used, and anesthesia, which the SART book doesn't. It's available for $28.50 from:

McFarland and Company, Inc.
Box 611
Jefferson, NC 28640

Call or write for information about quality of care and outcome information:

New England Patients' Rights Group
P.O. Box 141
Norwood, MA 02062-0002
(617) 769-5720
fax (617) 769-0882

This organization provides a physician referral service, medical call-in hours (nurse counselor available for members), a telephone helpline, a national newsletter, and support groups ($35 annual membership):

Resolve, Inc.
1310 Broadway
Somerville, MA 02144
(617) 623-0744

◆ INFLAMMATORY BOWEL DISEASE

Between one and two million Americans suffer with inflammatory bowel disease (IBD). Whites are more likely to get the condition than blacks, and Jews, four times more likely than anyone else.

The inflammation in IBD can be anywhere in the gastrointestinal tract, with symptoms also possible in other parts of the body (such as arthritis and skin rashes). Most often, the focus of disease is the large intestine or ileus (the far end of the small intestine). The two most common kinds of IBD, ulcerative colitis and Crohn's disease, have similar symptoms: diarrhea, pain, and weight loss. But they affect different parts of the bowel in different ways, and their courses, complications, and treatments are different.

If a parent, brother, or sister has Crohn's or ulcerative colitis, your risk goes up markedly. Most often, IBD begins in childhood or adolescence, and can have a serious effect on growth. It's a lifelong condition, and your goal shouldn't be just keeping the disease under control, but maintaining a rewarding quality of life.

WHAT CAN I EXPECT OVER THE LONG TERM?

People with either Crohn's disease or ulcerative colitis live about as long as anyone else. IBD is a condition that remains quiescent for a time, and then flares (both with and without obvious triggers), and the goal of drug treatment may be to maintain remission, as well as putting out the immediate fires.

Surgery may be in the future if you have ulcerative colitis, and it is a strong likelihood with Crohn's disease.

Complications like infection, intestinal constriction, and other structural damage are more common with Crohn's, but the risk of cancer is increased substantially more by ulcerative colitis. Regular examinations, such as colonoscopy for early signs of bowel cancer, may be mandatory, and the risk of cancer is likely to influence decisions about surgery.

Taking care of IBD can involve diet, learning about your disease, and getting psychological support as well as drugs and possibly surgery.

ARE THERE DRUGS THAT WILL WORK WITH FEWER SIDE EFFECTS?

The classic drug for IBD is sulfasalazine, an anti-inflammatory: frequently, it can both induce and maintain remission. Corticosteroids are often pre-scribed for acute relapses, although there's a limit to how long they can be safely used. Powerful drugs to suppress the immune system (azathio-prine and cyclosporine, for example) may also have a role, depending on the location and severity of the disease.

All of these drugs can have adverse effects (which are sometimes severe enough to limit their use). New versions, however, can sometimes provide the same benefits at a lower price.

More than 10 percent of people with ulcerative colitis can't use sul-fasalazine because of allergy, and more have troubling side effects like headache, nausea, stomach upset, and malaise. These can sometimes be avoided with new drugs that take the active part of the sulfasalazine mol-ecule (salicylic acid, which is very similar to aspirin), without the "sulfa" part that causes most of the trouble. According to an article in the *British Journal of Hospital Medicine* (April/May 1992), these work as well as sul-fasalazine for maintenance.

Side effects of corticosteroids can be emotional (depression), physical (osteoporosis), and sometimes dangerous, such as increased susceptibility to infections, blood clots, high blood pressure, and cataracts. So, although these drugs are effective for IBD, they can't be used for very long. New medications are said to minimize the risk, and possibly extend their use. They are administered locally, by enema, and thus cause no body-wide symptoms, or in a form that's broken down rapidly soon after it leaves the digestive tract.

A double-blind study found one such compound (fluticasone) less ef-fective than a standard steroid (prednisolone) for active ulcerative colitis, but also less likely to raise blood hormone levels, and thus, presumably, to cause side effects.

WHAT CAN DIET DO FOR ME?

It's not surprising that diet plays an important role in a digestive illness like IBD. Just how important depends on the specific nature of your illness, and is the subject of some debate.

Most basically, a nutritionally adequate diet is essential, but can't be taken for granted, because IBD symptoms often discourage healthy food consumption, and the disease process interferes with absorption. If diarrhea or abdominal pain lead you to eat poorly and lose weight, increased inflammation and infection may follow. People with Crohn's disease, in particular, often find that particular foods can trigger exacerbations, and learn to avoid them. If so, you may need help in planning a diet and taking supplements to maintain good nutrition.

For young people with IBD, optimal nutrition is vital. Growth may be severely hampered by inadequate intake of calories and nutrients.

Your diet may need to be changed as particular symptoms come and go. If diarrhea is a problem, it may help to limit your intake of fruits, vegetables, fatty foods, and caffeine. Constipation ordinarily responds well to increasing fiber (perhaps with a psyllium-containing product), but if it is caused by intestinal narrowing, or strictures—a complication in Crohn's—you may have to limit roughage instead.

More than 10 percent of the population can't digest lactose properly, and suffer from gas and cramping when they consume dairy products. For people with IBD, lactose intolerance worsens symptoms that are already burdensome. Avoiding dairy and rearranging your diet to make it up nutritionally could help you feel better.

The role that nutrition can play in actual treatment of IBD is the subject of some disagreement. A special "elemental" diet, which provides all nutrients in simple chemical form that's very easily absorbed, seems effective in treating new cases of Crohn's disease. In theory, it allows the bowel to heal by letting it rest, but experts disagree on whether it simply redresses poor nutrition or is actually therapeutic.

A recent study reported in *Gut* (1993, no. 34) found that people with active Crohn's, both new and longstanding, improved as much on the elemental diet as with steroids. They stayed in remission significantly longer after drug treatment, however.

This approach would avoid steroid side effects, and seems especially promising for young patients, in whom even relatively low, limited courses of the drug may interfere with growth. The elemental food preparations are not terribly pleasant, however, and quite a few people (nine of twenty-two, in the *Gut* study) are intolerant of the diet.

Fish oil supplements are an attractive approach to IBD; the fatty acids abundant in certain fish oils are said to temper the biochemical chain reaction that results in inflammation. Although studies haven't shown a dramatic effect on symptoms, one did find that the supplement made it possible for people with ulcerative colitis to lower their steroid dose (*Annals of Internal Medicine*, 1992, no. 116).

WHEN SHOULD I CONSIDER SURGERY? WHAT CAN I EXPECT TO GET FROM IT?

It's estimated that one third of people with ulcerative colitis, and two thirds of those with Crohn's disease, will need surgery at some point.

The standard operation for ulcerative colitis, removal of the colon (colectomy), generally cures the disease. Today's surgery usually spares the rectum, avoiding the need for an ileostomy (a created opening in the abdomen to allow elimination of wastes) and ostomy bag that was common in the past.

Colectomy is commonly considered for severe complications, such as hemorrhage, for extensive inflammation that apparently can't be controlled with drugs, or when cancer or a premalignant condition has developed. In young patients, the operation may be advised when growth is seriously impaired or complications occur.

In weighing surgery, the risk of colon cancer needs to be taken into account. Nearly half the people who have ulcerative colitis before the age of twenty will develop cancer in the next thirty-five years, and colectomy will effectively eliminate the danger. Alternatively, careful, regular monitoring will detect colon cancer at a stage when it may be curable—if you do it faithfully.

In Crohn's disease, the most common surgery is removal of seriously inflamed parts of the ileum and large intestine. It relieves symptoms but doesn't cure the disease: half of people will have recurrences in ten years. According to an article in *International Surgery* (January–March 1992), half of those who have Crohn's disease surgery have a second operation during the next fifteen to twenty years; 30 percent have three; 10 percent, four; and 5 percent, five.

The surgery is apparently far safer if done before serious complications of Crohn's disease have developed. In some reported series of operations, mortality is as high as 4 to 5 percent, but in medical centers where it is done earlier in the illness, the rate is 1 percent or less, according to the *International Surgery* paper.

HOW CAN I GET THE PSYCHOLOGICAL SUPPORT I NEED?

A lifelong disease that causes distressing symptoms, that needs regular medical care, and is subject to serious exacerbations, IBD can take a significant toll on emotional well-being, work, and family. In the case of Crohn's, in particular, stress may worsen symptoms and trigger flares. Many people find support groups particularly helpful in coping with the stress of their illness.

Resources

This foundation will provide you with brochures and other educational information about IBD and will put you in touch with local chapters and support groups:

Crohn's and Colitis Foundation
444 Park Avenue South
New York, NY 10016-7374
(212) 685-3440 or (800) 343-3637

This association will provide education and support for people who need to use an ostomy bag after surgery:

United Ostomy Association
36 Executive Park, Suite 120
Irvine, CA 92714
(714) 660-8624

◆ INSOMNIA

Can't sleep? You're not alone. About 35 percent of your fellow Americans share this debilitating problem. Insomnia—an inability to get enough restful sleep despite ample opportunity—is the most common sleep disorder. It's not a disease, but a symptom (most often of physical illness, emotional illness, stress, or an unhealthy lifestyle).

About half of those who have insomnia call it serious, and 4 percent are taking prescription medications for it. There are also a host of do-it-yourself strategies that may help. But then again, they may not: for truly intractable and distressing sleep disturbances, there are high-tech labs to identify just what's going wrong with the sleep process, attempting to point the way to a solution.

JUST HOW MUCH SLEEP DO I NEED?

The need for sleep is one of those basic biological facts that varies widely. The average person does best with seven and a half to eight hours, but some people need nine or more to feel rested, and others get by fine every night on five. That's why the definition of insomnia is essentially subjective: you aren't getting enough sleep to feel fully rested and alert the next day.

Generally, we need less sleep as we age, and some older people who report difficulty sleeping simply may not have adjusted their lifestyle to the change. True insomnia is increasingly common in the aged, however. The test, again, is whether a person feels fully rested.

WHAT HAPPENS IF I MISS A NIGHT'S SLEEP?

Less than you would think. Physical and mental performance declines remarkably little. Your mood is likely to take a serious hit, however. The pessimism many people feel after too little sleep makes the impairment seem a lot greater than it is. One mental faculty that suffers is creativity.

Researchers have found spontaneity, flexibility, and originality to decline markedly after a single sleepless night. You'll probably be able to do familiar tasks at work, but you may find it difficult to respond to an emergency.

The impact of two night's sleep loss is considerably greater. Even familiar jobs and basic problem solving become harder. Insomnia's effects are cumulative, and sometimes insidious. People who remain competent at work are likely to let their social lives languish from fatigue.

Although, again, individual differences may vary widely, most people seem to be virtually unaffected as long as they get five hours or so of restful sleep: less than that, and they feel it.

WHAT CAN BE DONE FOR ME?

Many of the possible causes of insomnia are medical, and they can't be treated until they're diagnosed. Illnesses that cause pain, like headache or arthritis, can obviously impair sleep, and so can anything that interferes with breathing, like allergy or sinusitis. Infections, diabetes, tumors, kidney failure, and thyroid disease may also disturb sleep. Inability to get enough restorative sleep is a key to the diagnosis of fibromyalgia, a disease which is also characterized by widespread musculoskeletal pain, fatigue, and tenderness when mild pressure is applied to various cites between the neck and the knees (see Fibromyalgia).

According to a review article in *The Lancet* (June 5, 1993), twice as many people attending hospital clinics complain of sleep disruption than in the general population.

HOW CAN I FIND OUT IF IT'S BECAUSE OF STRESS?

Pressure at work, turmoil at home, anything that has your mind aroused can keep you awake (or make whatever sleep you get less restful). The problem is likely to continue until the stress is relieved or resolved.

In addition, insomnia is common in more serious emotional disorders. Sleep loss—early morning awakening, in particular—is a cardinal symptom of depression. It's also frequent with anxiety disorders. For this reason, it's important to detect and treat psychological problems, which may require psychotherapy or medication.

According to a review article in *The Lancet* (June 12, 1993), 80 percent of insomnia that brings people to their doctors is related to anxiety or depression.

ARE DRUGS CAUSING MY INSOMNIA?

Sleep disturbance is a common side effect of some over-the-counter and prescription medications, and many others can affect a minority of individuals this way. Decongestants like pseudoephedrine and phenylpropanolamine are common culprits; they may be in a combination cold remedy (check the label).

Often, sleep disturbance can be minimized by adjusting the dose schedule. If you need a cold pill at night, for example, make sure it contains no decongestant.

Recreational drugs can severely impact sleep, especially stimulants like cocaine. And the role of our most popular drug, alcohol, isn't always appreciated. Substance abuse, most commonly alcohol abuse, is responsible for about 10 to 15 percent of chronic insomnia.

Even one or two drinks at dinner may disrupt sleep. You may fall asleep more readily, but the sleep is liable to be fragmented—you're likely to awaken during the night—and less restorative.

COULD MY LIFESTYLE BE CAUSING INSOMNIA?

Late, heavy meals can make it more difficult to sleep soundly. And the effect of caffeine, not surprisingly, is profound. Individuals differ: for some, a cup of coffee after an early dinner, or even in late afternoon, is enough to cause a restless night.

You may be getting caffeine without knowing it. In addition to coffee and tea, cola beverages contain appreciable amounts of caffeine. Some painkillers have enough caffeine to keep you up if you take them late in the day (read the label). If you're especially sensitive to caffeine, you may be affected by the small amounts that occur naturally in nuts, chocolate, and other foods.

Exercise helps you sleep soundly. If you're sedentary, insomnia may improve substantially when you start a regular exercise routine. But its immediate effect is physically arousing, so exercise early in the day if you can, and avoid it in the evening.

Generally, you'll have less trouble sleeping if you arrange your schedule to allow an hour or two to wind down before bedtime. Working late may keep your mind in overdrive when you want it to slow down.

WHEN ARE SLEEPING PILLS PRESCRIBED?

Sleeping pills (also called *hypnotics*) are never a lasting solution to insomnia. At best, they become less effective after being used regularly for several weeks or so, as the body adjusts to them, and prolonged use apparently reduces the deepest, most restful stages of sleep. When you stop taking them, "rebound insomnia" is common. Some cause daytime grogginess.

Although it's surely more pleasant to sleep than to toss and turn, the bottom line, for most people, is alertness and performance the next day. "In this role, hypnotic agents fare poorly," says a review article in the *Mayo Clinic Proceedings* (June 1990). "None has systematically improved subsequent daytime functioning, either directly or as a result of improved sleep."

The sleeping pills most often prescribed nowadays are benzodiazepines (chemical cousins of Valium), which metabolize quickly and cause less hangover than heavier drugs like barbiturates. But these are not free of problems either, as recent experiences with Halcion made quite clear. Some of the newest drugs are said to pinpoint the part of the brain that affects sleep, and so cause fewer side effects, but their advantage isn't proven.

Perhaps the best use of sleeping pills is to help you through a time when sleep is essential (after surgery, sleeplessness can retard healing), or for a day or two when anxiety about tomorrow's demands keeps you tossing and turning. (Don't take a sleeping pill for the first time when you have something important the next day, however.)

OTC sleep aids (they contain antihistamines) make you drowsy: they won't put you to sleep, but might make it easier to drift off. Don't use them for too long, however. Some people find that an aspirin or two at bedtime helps them to sleep, and there is some evidence that this approach is as effective as some prescription drugs.

SHOULD HALCION BE PRESCRIBED?

Triazolam (Halcion), a short-acting benzodiazepine, promised to give sound, natural sleep while causing no drowsiness the next day. By the late 1980s, it was the most widely prescribed sleeping pill in this country and abroad.

But there were problems. People reported amnesia and confusion after taking the drug. And that was just the beginning. Much more bizarre side effects began to surface: paranoia, hallucinations, suicidal and homicidal behavior. Among Halcion's alleged victims were author William Styron (he became clinically depressed) and former President George Bush (he vomited during a state dinner in Japan). A woman in England was acquitted of murdering her eighty-three-year-old mother, on grounds that Halcion had made her temporarily insane.

A Scottish psychiatrist who reviewed research claimed that the manufacturer, Upjohn, had suppressed data that revealed serious psychiatric side effects. Upjohn sued the doctor for libel.

British authorities were impressed enough by the risk to take Halcion off the market; France restricted its use to a lower dose. Despite the clamor, the FDA decided to leave it on the shelves, with a stronger warning about possible adverse effects, and ordered further tests.

At best, Halcion may cause severe problems for some people (especially those over the age of sixty-five), none for others. But there are other sleeping pills available, whose safety is a lot less questionable. It makes sense, if you must take something, to take one of those.

CAN I USE NONDRUG METHODS?

Behavioral strategies—changing how you live and sleep—have none of the drawbacks of sleeping pills. And according to a small National Institutes of Health study, they work *better*: chronic insomniacs who used behavior change for eight weeks reduced their tossing and turning time from two hours to an average of fifty minutes, compared with seventy-five minutes for those who took pills.

A self-help program to fight insomnia should include the lifestyle changes described here. In addition:

- Make your bed a place to sleep. Don't read, eat, or watch television there. Don't go to bed until you're sleepy; if you stay awake for more than fifteen minutes, go to another room and do something quiet and relaxing, like reading a dull book. Don't go back to bed until you're sleepy again.
- Keep a regular schedule: get up at the same time each morning (including weekends) no matter how much sleep you didn't get.
- Learn a relaxation technique like meditation. Not only will this ready your body for sleep, it will take your mind off worries that otherwise would keep you up.
- Try a warm beverage, like milk or herb tea, at bedtime. This stimulates a nerve (the vagus) in your stomach that naturally slows down your whole nervous system.

SHOULD I BE TESTED IN A SLEEP LABORATORY?

Sleep-disorder centers have an arsenal of high-tech (and high-priced) instruments to monitor brain and body activity during the night, and to pinpoint just what's going wrong with the sleep cycle. They may find a correctable problem that has made your insomnia resistant to all the usual treatments.

According to a 1991 report by the Agency for Health Care Policy and Research of the U.S. Public Health Service, the effectiveness of these methods in insomnia hasn't been proven. In any case, they are not for garden-variety sleeplessness. Those who do the testing save it for insomnia of at least four nights a week that has lasted for six months or longer, isn't caused by medical or psychiatric illness, and hasn't responded to behavioral treatment or medication.

◆ IRRITABLE BOWEL SYNDROME

Can a condition that affects an estimated 15 percent of people in the United States and other Western countries, with symptoms as logically incompatible as constipation and diarrhea, actually be called a disease? However you define it, irritable bowel syndrome (IBS) can cause a lot of grief. In addition to recurrent diarrhea, which may alternate with or be replaced by constipation, IBS typically involves abdominal bloating and pain, often severe.

IBS is a "functional disorder," which means that no anatomical abnormalities are seen in the digestive tract of those who suffer from it. What appears to be disturbed is the motility of the gastrointestinal system—the muscular contractions that move the process of digestion along. Some researchers suggest that nerves in the intestine are unusually sensitive, predisposing a person to IBS pain.

SHOULD I SEE THE DOCTOR IF I HAVE SYMPTOMS OF IBS?

Most people with these symptoms—80 percent, by one estimate—don't seek medical attention. Whatever distress it causes, IBS is never fatal and will not permanently damage your health, and there's no real cure. If symptoms impair the quality of your life, however, you may get some control over the disorder with a doctor's help.

A more compelling reason to seek medical advice is to make sure that what you have *is* IBS. Diarrhea, constipation, and abdominal pain are also the symptoms of many other diseases, some more treatable than IBS, and some not nearly as benign. Among the disorders that may cause similar symptoms are food intolerance, infections with parasites like *Giardia*, inflammatory bowel disease, and malignancy. A visit to the doctor to allay your anxieties about serious illness is *not* a waste of time or money.

IS IBS PSYCHOSOMATIC?

The connection between emotions, mental health, and IBS is fascinating if confusing. People who come to medical centers to be treated for IBS have been found to have more emotional disorders, including depression and anxiety, and respond more strongly to stress than the average person.

On the other hand, community surveys have found that people who have IBS but who are *not* seeking treatment are no different psychologically from those with healthier digestion. This suggests that psychological problems, stress, and the like do not *cause* IBS. They may, however, strongly affect how distressing you find its symptoms and how readily you seek medical help for them. What's more, stress and emotional turmoil can produce digestive symptoms in anyone, with or without IBS—as you well know if you've ever had "butterflies in the stomach" or suffered from cramps or diarrhea when feeling under pressure. If you have IBS, stress can make it worse.

The digestive system has the second-highest number of nerve cells (after the brain) in the body, making it particularly responsive to stress. Some studies have found that the gastrointestinal tract of people with IBS reacts, physiologically, more strongly to the stress of stimuli like loud music or driving in traffic. This doesn't mean that people with IBS are particularly sensitive to stress per se, but that their digestive tracts are generally more reactive—they also respond more strongly to drugs and food.

Perhaps the most important thing to keep in mind is that whatever may trigger IBS symptoms, the pain is real.

DOES DIET AFFECT IBS?

Although studies are inconsistent in pinpointing the role of diet in IBS, many people find that what they eat affects their IBS. Depending on your individual biology, certain foods may seem to produce or exacerbate symptoms: most commonly, lactose in dairy products, fatty foods, alcohol, sorbitol-containing gums and candies, and caffeine. If you are prone to allergies, it is possible that your IBS will improve if some foods are eliminated from your diet.

Whether you go through an elaborate testing procedure or just keep a food diary and avoid the foods that seem to cause you trouble, make sure you maintain an adequate intake of all the essential nutrients.

An ample supply of fiber is important. Controlled trials have not supported the effectiveness of fiber against all the symptoms of IBS, but it clearly seems to help constipation and (less clearly) abdominal pain. Whole grains, beans, and fruit contain fiber, as do supplements like bran and psyllium. If your diet is low in fiber, don't increase it too quickly, or you may worsen the bloating and diarrhea of IBS. (One gradual approach is to start with one tablespoon of bran per day, and work up to a tablespoon three times a day with meals.) Furthermore, make sure you drink plenty of water.

WILL DRUGS HELP?

The drugs used to treat IBS are as diverse as its symptoms: antidiarrheals, laxatives, antispasmodics, antidepressants, and antianxiety drugs, to name the most popular ones. By and large, the drugs don't treat the disorder as a whole, but whatever symptoms predominate. Antidepressants have been found helpful in chronic pain, including that of IBS.

Many drugs have been tried for IBS, but a review of research in the area concluded that just about all the trials have been flawed. The bottom line is: no drug is of proven benefit in IBS.

One thing that makes it difficult to prove the efficacy of drugs is that people with IBS are unusually likely to respond to placebo: the placebo rate in various trials has been 40 to 70 percent. Don't be too quick to assume that if you take medication and feel better, the drug is responsible and you should take it indefinitely. All the drugs used for IBS have side effects.

SHOULD I TRY HYPNOSIS?

The strong connection between bowel function and the nervous system suggests that relaxation exercises might help IBS. Studies have found that techniques like meditation, relaxation training, hypnosis, and biofeedback can reduce the symptoms of IBS, whether used alone or in combination with medical therapy.

In one such trial, thirty-three people with IBS who had not responded to medical treatment received four sessions of hypnotherapy (and were taught to do self-hypnosis twice a day) over a seven-week period. Twenty improved, eleven of whom lost almost all their symptoms. They were still better three months later, and some had improved still more. The same approach is just as effective in group therapy (*The Lancet,* February 25, 1989).

Another trial used psychotherapy. Fifty-five people whose IBS symptoms remained despite drug and diet therapy were given seven sessions of a simple kind of psychotherapy in which their symptoms, feelings, and emotional problems were discussed. After three months, their average symptoms, particularly diarrhea and abdominal pain, had improved. Symptoms were unchanged in a control group of forty-nine people who continued medical treatment.

Generally, self-hypnosis, relaxation, and the like are only effective in people who find the approach congenial and who are motivated and willing to put in the work required for success.

Resources

International Foundation for Bowel Dysfunction
P.O. Box 17864
Milwaukee, WI 53217
(414) 964-1799

This nonprofit organization provides relevant educational materials on request.

◆ KIDNEY STONE

People often describe the pain of a kidney stone as the worst they've ever experienced. Yet by and large, the acute condition passes within days—sometimes abruptly—and it rarely causes serious or lasting problems.

The stone, usually made of calcium but sometimes of other substances, forms when chemicals in the urine become so concentrated that they crystallize out of solution. Pain develops when the stone lodges in a place that obstructs urine flow, in the kidney itself or in the ureter, the tube that connects the kidney with the bladder. Eighty percent of the time, the stone eventually works its way out of the body, through urination, all by itself.

About 10 percent of men develop at least one kidney stone in their lifetime, and about one third as many women. Most often, it first happens when they're in their thirties to their sixties. Almost everyone who has had one stone develops another, some studies say, within the following twenty years. According to an article in *Clinics in Laboratory Medicine* (March 1993), the incidence of kidney stones has increased by 60 to 75 percent over the last twenty-five years.

MUST I HAVE SURGERY?

Acute kidney stones are generally given the opportunity to leave the body spontaneously, through urination, usually with a prescription of potent painkiller to ease the experience. Between 20 and 45 percent of people are hospitalized (usually if pain is severe enough to require intravenous painkillers; or if infection, urinary obstruction, or dehydration are possibly involved).

One stone out of five needs to be removed surgically. The size of the stone (on X ray) or worsening symptoms often lead to this decision. This used to mean major surgery, but nowadays, the usual methods are less invasive and require little (or no) hospitalization, and a much briefer recuperation period.

The most common method is extracorporeal sound wave lithotripsy

(ESWL). You lie in a bath, while a device generates shock waves that pass through the water and your soft tissues. When they converge on the stone, they pound it into fragments, which eventually pass out through the urine. The treatment itself lasts sixty to ninety minutes, and many people are out of the hospital within a day and back to work within several.

ESWL has complications about 1 percent of the time: bleeding, urinary obstruction (by the fragments), severe pain, and infection. Whether or not it's an option depends largely on the size of the stone and its location. About one time in ten, some further procedure will be necessary, according to an article in *Patient Care* (August 15, 1990).

In percutaneous nephrolithotomy (PCNL), a tubelike instrument is introduced into the kidney through a small incision in your side: the stone is brought into view and removed with a forceps or tiny basket, or fragmented by a device that produces ultrasonic or hydraulic shock waves.

Because it is more invasive and has twice the complication rate of EWSL, PCNL is usually saved for instances where ESWL isn't likely to work because the stone is too large or in a difficult location. Sometimes, the two are used together. Hospital stay for each procedure is one to three days and recuperation takes less than a week in most cases.

Uteroscopy is something like PCNL, but the stone is approached from below, through the urethra. It can be successfully used for nearly all stones in the lower end of the ureter. The complication rate for this procedure is 5 percent.

Open surgery, which was once just about the only option for kidney stone, is now used only in unusually complicated situations, or when other methods fail—about 5 percent of the time.

CAN THE STONE JUST BE DISSOLVED?

The majority of stones (about 75 percent), are composed of a calcium compound that won't dissolve. For many of the rest, which are made up of uric acid or cystine, dissolution therapy may be an option, particularly if pain is manageable and there are no signs of obstruction.

Potassium citrate, either in tablets or by IV infection, makes the urine less acid, which dissolves uric acid stones. It must be done carefully: system alkalosis, congestive heart failure, and elevated blood pressure are possible complications.

IF I HAVE A STONE THAT'S CAUSING NO SYMPTOMS, DO I NEED TO DO ANYTHING?

Sometimes a kidney stone is discovered "incidentally" in the course of an X ray for something else. If it's causing no trouble, you can usually leave it alone. Such stones can grow, shift position, and cause sudden, acute symptoms, however. Removal may be a good idea if you're planning to spend time in the wilderness or abroad, far from medical care that you may need in a hurry, or if you're had previous disabling attacks.

The wait-and-see approach may be ill-advised if you have only one kidney, or if you expect to become pregnant (at which time an acute episode would be hard to treat).

HOW CAN I KEEP STONES FROM COMING BACK?

Six retrospective studies have shown that a person with a kidney stone has a 14 percent chance of another within a year, a likelihood that rises to 35 percent at five years and 52 percent at ten, according to an article in *Annals of Internal Medicine* (December 15, 1989). Some people may be destined to have no more than one stone, with or without therapy, but it is impossible to predict in whom there will be recurrences.

Neither drug therapy nor extensive evaluation is usually advised for people who have had one stone. About as many people would have side effects from treatment as would be spared the pain of a second attack. The stone will probably be analyzed (you may be asked to urinate through a strainer to catch the stone when it is passed), and a battery of routine blood and urine tests ordered to see what may have caused its formation.

Often, the preventive advice is to drink abundant water (an eight-ounce glass of water every waking hour) to keep urine so dilute that stones won't form. People who ordinarily lose a lot of fluid through perspiration (because of high heat or occupation) or are physically very active should take special care to drink enough water. Also, make sure you do not have a high intake of animal protein, which is directly associated with the risk of stone formation.

Another standard piece of advice, limiting calcium intake, has been contradicted by a study that followed over forty-five thousand healthy men without kidney stones, ages forty to seventy-five years, for four years (*The*

New England Journal of Medicine, March 25, 1993). It found that a high dietary intake of calcium actually reduces the risk of symptomatic kidney stones. Increased calcium intake appears to rid the body of excess calcium oxalate, the component of the majority of kidney stones.

This study contradicted another standard bit of dietary advice to people who have formed recurrent calcium oxalate stones. Such people are usually told to limit their intake of foods high in oxalate, which include certain nuts and vegetables, chocolate, cocoa, and tea. The four-year study also showed that consumption of these foods was not associated with the risk of kidney stones. On the other hand, potassium supplementation reduces calcium excretion in healthy adults, which the study found to be associated with decreased risk of stone formation.

If tests show a high level of uric acid in the urine, you may be advised to avoid foods that are high in purines, such as organ meats and red meat. They should also avoid vitamin C supplements, which the body metabolizes into oxalate. It must be noted, however, that there have been no large prospective, controlled studies of diet modification of sufficient length to determine what changes in the diet would reduce the rate of recurrence among people with first kidney stones.

◆ LOW-BACK PAIN

Perhaps reflecting the strain of standing upright on an elaborate construction of bones, ligaments, and muscles, back pain is one of the most common health problems. An estimated four people out of five have significant back discomfort at some time. It disappears within days, weeks, or months for 90 percent, but usually recurs later.

The other 10 percent aren't so lucky: they suffer severe, persistent pain that interferes with life and work. In seeking help, they're confronted by an array of solutions ranging from relaxation to major surgery. To further cloud a confusing situation, there's an unsettling tendency for new treatments to arouse great enthusiasm (and convincing research support), only to fall out of favor several years later.

In an editorial in *The New England Journal of Medicine* (October 3, 1991), Richard A. Deyo, M.D., M.P.H., of the Veterans Administration Medical Center, Seattle, wrote of "fads" in the field. "The history of medical care for low back pain—one of the most common causes of morbidity and absenteeism in the United States—involves serial fashions in diagnosis and therapy," he wrote. "Such fads are not innocuous; they may lead to unnecessary morbidity and costs . . ."

If you have serious back problems, it's essential—but may not be easy—to find a doctor who will help you get the treatment that's best for your particular condition.

HOW CAN I TAKE THE ROLE OF STRESS SERIOUSLY AND ADDRESS IT?

Stress is a contributing factor in most conditions involving back pain, although it is rarely solely responsible. Tension tightens muscles, making them more prone to injury, and it reduces blood flow to sensitive areas, causing pain. Even when an anatomical defect (like a herniated disk) appears to be involved, stress may make a substantial difference in your experience of pain, and how much or little it interferes with your life.

Even today, with the impact of stress widely accepted and understood by much of the public, not all doctors take it as seriously as they should. Some tend to overlook the possible contribution of stress and rely too quickly on medications and expensive, high-tech diagnostic procedures, or dismiss problems with no obvious anatomical cause as "all in your head."

The modern arsenal of techniques to reduce stress ranges from meditation to biofeedback to family counseling. Although ultimately they come down to work you must do yourself, expert, professional guidance is often invaluable. Few doctors are trained or inclined to do much in the area of stress reduction, but they should be able to direct or refer you to a qualified practitioner. At the very least, they should support your efforts.

HOW LONG MUST I STAY IN BED WITH SEVERE PAIN?

It wasn't so many years ago that extended periods of bed rest were routinely advocated for back pain, to give injured tissue a chance to heal. But in 1986, an important randomized study showed that people who were assigned to two days of bed rest missed 45 percent fewer days of work than their counterparts who were told to stay in bed for a week. Both groups did equally well in terms of pain and ability to function.

Today, "early ambulation" is widely accepted as a sound principle for many health problems, including back pain. It's recognized that *disuse* often causes more problems than "rest" can resolve. When back muscles are immobile for more than a few days, they tighten and stiffen, which makes them weak, painful to move, and prone to further injury.

Just how long you need to rest an injured back, and how rapidly you can return to normal function and to work depends on the nature of your particular problem (whether nerve function is impaired is important, for example), but "less is more" is a good general concept when it comes to bed rest.

DO I NEED MEDICATION AND FOR HOW LONG?

According to a review article in *Annals of Internal Medicine* (April 15, 1990), the effectiveness of nonsteroidal anti-inflammatories (NSAIDs) for back pain in general has been suggested by some well-designed clinical trials. Stronger narcotic painkillers may be necessary for acute pain—for short-term use only.

Muscle relaxants such as diazepam (Valium) and cyclobenzaprine (Flexeril) are widely prescribed for back pain, but evidence supporting their effectiveness is "limited," the review article said, and it isn't certain that they're any better than NSAIDs alone. "Like narcotic analgesics, their use should be strictly time-limited, with one week being a general guide," the authors wrote.

If your doctor thinks you should be on anything stronger than NSAIDs for more than a brief time, find out why. In the case of chronic pain (pain that has lasted more than three months), overuse of medications can become a significant part of the problem.

Among drugs often prescribed long-term to alleviate chronic pain (in the back and elsewhere) and promote sleep are tricyclic antidepressants. Results of randomized trials have been mixed; the evidence supporting their use is "suggestive," but not definitive, according to some experts.

WHAT EXERCISE AND LIFESTYLE CHANGES WILL HELP MY BACK?

Although health professionals may have an important role in treating acute back pain, in the long run, you're on your own. "Strategies to manage low-back pain must be long term and preventive," a review article in the *British Medical Journal* (April 3, 1993) concluded, "and the responsibility to keep fit, maintain an exercise program, and remain relaxed so as to avoid physically stressing the spine is that of the individual, not of the professionals."

Your doctor can teach you ways to strengthen and protect your back, or (more likely) can direct you toward professionals or programs where you can learn them.

The place of exercise in back rehabilitation has become well established, but although evidence supporting its value has grown, it's still far from overwhelming. For one thing, many studies have been poorly designed; a review of sixteen randomized controlled trials of exercise therapy found that only four were free from "major flaws in their methods" (*British Medical Journal,* June 29, 1991).

Even among people who advocate exercise, there's no consensus about which kinds are best: some favor exercises that bend the back forward (flexion), others backward (extension). Stretching and strengthening have their proponents, and many programs combine both. Aerobic exercises, particularly swimming and walking, are frequently recommended to prevent future back pain, in addition to the usual reasons.

Especially if your back problems have been persistent or severe, exercise should be tailored to you and your particular physical condition, preferably by a physical therapist or other professional who is skilled and experienced in this area.

Learning to sit, stand, and move properly can protect your back against injury and cumulative strain. Anyone with back problems should know body mechanics for safe lifting, reaching, and sitting. A firm chair to sit in, a firm mattress to sleep on, a well-designed desk to work at may do more to keep pain away than the best doctor and strongest drugs.

A doctor, physical therapist, occupational therapist, or other health professional with special competence in this area can teach you proper posture and movement, tips to guard against strain, and ways to work safely. A relatively new development in this area is "back school," an organized program where you learn the principles of back anatomy, mechanics and dynamics, and how to put them into practice.

HOW WILL THE RESULTS OF DIAGNOSTIC TESTS AFFECT TREATMENT?

The physical problems that can cause back pain are diverse and not always well understood. It has been estimated that 80 percent of back pain is the result of soft-tissue injury not revealed by X ray or other diagnostic procedures. If such procedures are used, it's generally to see if an anatomical defect, such as a herniated disc, spinal stenosis (narrowing of the space through which the spinal cord passes), or osteoarthritis is involved.

Most modern diagnostic techniques are less painful and invasive than older ones. Magnetic resonance imaging (MRI), perhaps the most widely used follow-up to a simple X ray, supplies a detailed look at the spine without radiation (it uses a strong magnetic field), but it is quite expensive and many people find the experience—you must spend over half an hour almost enclosed in a narrow tube—highly anxiety-provoking.

What will the procedure show, and might treatment change as a result? If not, why have the test done at all? These are reasonable questions that aren't always asked by doctors—or those they treat.

The interpretation of test results isn't always a cut-and-dried one. Disk herniation, for example, is quite common in the general population, and finding it on MRI or X ray doesn't necessarily mean it is responsible for your pain. A proper diagnosis takes into account the history of the problem and the physical examination as well as the test findings. If the distribution of pain corresponds to the place where the disk is herniated, for example, it suggests a connection between one and the other.

COULD MANIPULATION HELP?

About one person in twenty goes to a chiropractor each year, often for back pain, and generally without a doctor's blessing. Historically, physicians have considered chiropractors quacks, not colleagues. In 1987, the chiropractic profession won a lawsuit against the American Medical Association and other medical organizations for "systematic long-term wrongdoing and the long-term intent to destroy a licensed profession."

What manipulation of the spine can do for the wide range of ills for which it is prescribed is difficult to say, but there are indications that for back pain at least, it is often as good or better than what medicine has to offer.

In a randomized controlled trial of 741 people with low-back pain, those who were sent to chiropractors did better on tests of pain and impairment than the group who had standard outpatient clinic care. The difference was most marked among those with chronic or severe pain, and became more evident through two years of follow-up.

"For patients with low back pain in whom manipulation is not contraindicated chiropractic almost certainly confers worthwhile, long-term benefit in comparison with hospital outpatients management," the researchers concluded (*British Medical Journal,* June 2, 1990).

A review article and meta-analysis in *Annals of Internal Medicine* (October 1, 1992) was considerably less enthusiastic. Analyzing data from the nine of twenty-five controlled trials that met quality criteria, the researchers concluded that "spinal manipulation is of short-term benefit in some patients, particularly those with uncomplicated, acute low-back pain. Data are insufficient concerning the efficacy of spinal manipulation for chronic low-back pain.''

Although chiropractors do 94 percent of spinal manipulations in this country, similar treatment is also done by some osteopaths, physical therapists, general practitioners, and orthopedists.

Can manipulation cause harm? The *Annals* review article noted that complications of spinal manipulation therapy have not been systematically tracked, but that none were reported in clinical trials involving more than fifteen hundred people. Reviewing 135 case reports of serious complications (including eighteen deaths) showed that manipulation of the lower back was far less likely to cause harm than treatment of the cervical (upper) spine, and that misdiagnosis of a serious condition such as tumor was a greater danger.

The risk of causing severe nerve damage by lumbar manipulation was estimated, using this data, at less than one case in a hundred million manipulations.

WHAT ARE THE RISKS AND BENEFITS OF BACK SURGERY?

Surgery for low-back pain—most often removal of a herniated disk, possibly with fusion of disks—is not an option to take lightly. It is mandatory when symptoms (like loss of bladder control, impotence, and loss of sensation) indicate the danger of serious nerve damage, and might be worth considering if pain has remained seriously disruptive for a month or longer, despite conservative therapy, and where an anatomical defect has been identified that is amenable to correction.

It is important to realize that surgery is most helpful when pain is caused by pressure on the nerve. But even when sophisticated tests show such pressure, and when your pain is where the nerves travel, it is never certain that correcting the first will cure the second.

Most surgery is for disk herniation, in which the inside of the cushioning disk between the spinal vertebrae bulges or leaks out, pressing on a nerve and causing back pain, leg pain (sciatica), and muscle weakness.

The advantages of surgery for this condition are apparent at first, but disappear over time. One year after treatment, 90 percent of people who have had surgery report good overall results; 80 percent have relief of leg pain; and 70 percent show improvement in muscle weakness—compared with 80 percent, 50 percent, and 50 percent, respectively, after nonsurgical treatment. Ten years later, however, results are identical: 90 percent in both groups report good overall results; 98 percent, leg pain relief; and 85 percent, increase in muscle strength.

According to data from studies of more than forty-three thousand people who have had lower back surgery, the risk of serious complications (including heart attack and pulmonary blood clot) ranges from .2 to 3 percent, depending on age; and of less serious complications (infection or thrombophlebitis), 4 to 7 percent. Mortality risk is under 1 percent, at any age, and the chance that nerve impairment will occur or worsen is 2 percent.

The other principal indication for surgery, narrowing of the channel through which the spinal cord passes (spinal stenosis), has not been studied as thoroughly as disk surgery; there are no randomized controlled trials comparing it to nonsurgical treatment. An analysis of seventy-four reports found a "good or excellent overall result" in 70 percent, one year after treatment. This compares with 10 percent in people who have had non-surgical therapy. The risk of serious and less serious complications is somewhat greater than with disk surgery: 2 to 5 percent, and 10 to 13 percent, respectively.

Surgery is sometimes considered for people who have severe and incapacitating back pain, for which no clear anatomical explanation can be found. The results here are less promising, and the advantage over non-surgical treatment is questionable. One study reported relief of back pain in 43 to 55 percent of people, depending on what underlying condition was found during the operation.

The rate of back surgery in this country is eight times what it is in most European countries, and twice as high in the American West as in the Northeast.

WHAT IS THE SAFETY AND EFFECTIVENESS OF SURGERY?

If treatment for low-back pain is a changing, inexact business, it's not because data aren't available. Lumbar fusion, for example, is often added to other procedures. A review of articles on the subject concluded that "for several low back disorders no advantage has been demonstrated for fusion over surgery without fusion, and complications of fusions are common. Randomized controlled trials are needed to compare fusion, surgery without fusion, and nonsurgical treatments in rigorously defined patient groups" (*Journal of the American Medical Association,* August 19, 1992).

Transcutaneous electrical nerve stimulation (TENS) has been shown to be effective in 30 to 50 percent of low-back pain by some studies, but no better than placebo by others. But the risk of TENS is negligible, an article in *The Lancet* (February 23, 1991) points out, and "what is important is that TENS can produce some relief in over 30 percent of patients with intractable back pain."

Acupuncture, the ancient form of Chinese medicine that involves inserting very thin needles into specific areas of the body, has gained acceptance among Western physicians, especially for chronic pain. A review of the medical literature showed that acupuncture can provide at least short-term relief to 50 to 80 percent of people suffering acute or chronic pain due to a variety of causes, including back pain.

Injections of a chemical, chymopapain (also known as chemonucleolysis) to dissolve part of the herniated disk was a popular approach in the 1980s, but later trials found it less effective than surgery. Side effects can occasionally be severe, including serious allergic reactions, paralysis, and death, so the procedure is far less often done today. Yet a review of forty-five published studies exploring the efficacy of chymopapain come to this conclusion: "Chemonucleolysis, though somewhat less effective than open disectomy, can be successfully and safely used in about four of five carefully selected patients without the trauma, risks, and subsequent fibrosis associated with lumbar disc surgery" (*Spine,* December 1994).

◆ LYME DISEASE

Fifteen years ago, no one had ever heard of Lyme disease. Now, the illness inspires headlines like TICK TERROR. Lyme disease isn't very common (about ninety-seven hundred cases in forty-five states in 1992), but in areas of concentration, particularly parts of the Northeast (such as Block Island, Rhode Island), as many as 5 percent of the population get it each year. Reported cases have increased almost twentyfold over the past decade (but it's uncertain to what extent this just reflects more accurate diagnosis).

Lyme disease has probably occurred for centuries, but it wasn't fully described until 1968, when a rheumatologist looked closely at a cluster of childhood arthritis cases near Lyme, Connecticut.

As it's currently understood, Lyme disease has three stages. The first is a rash surrounding a bite by the tiny deer tick that carries the organism. The disease is caused by a coiled bacterium—a spirochete called *Borrelia burgdorferi* (named for its discoverer, Dr. Willy Burgdorfer). Within weeks comes a flulike siege of fever, muscle pain, and fatigue. There may be neurological symptoms, such as temporary paralysis of one side of the face (Bell's palsy), or chest pain. If untreated, more severe problems like arthritis or encephalitis will appear several months after that in about 80 percent of cases, and may persist indefinitely.

SHOULD I BE TESTED FOR LYME DISEASE?

The diagnosis of Lyme disease isn't always easy. The characteristic rash (a reddened circle with the tick bite in the center) is absent in 20 to 40 percent of cases, and is too subtle to notice in others. The lab test currently in use, which detects antibodies produced to fight the disease, isn't terribly accurate. Other antibodies can also produce positive test results, and the test can't distinguish between a currently active infection and one that ran its course years before. Conversely, the test may remain negative for the first few weeks after infection.

It's been estimated that even in a population where Lyme disease is

common, screening with the antibody test would yield twenty false positives for every genuine infection. What's more, standards at various lab-
oratories are extremely inconsistent. In one study, more than half of
forty-five labs failed to identify Lyme disease in one batch of positive serum,
and false positives ran from 2 to 27 percent (*Journal of the American Medical
Association,* August 19, 1992).

Some experts think that Lyme disease testing is used too extensively
in this country (in Wisconsin in one recent year, there were 545 cases
reported, and 94,000 serum samples tested), and urge that it be done only
when a history (of a tick bite or at least exposure to woodsy areas where
the ticks are found) and relevant symptoms justify it. The distribution of
the tick should be kept in mind.

Assuming that a positive antibody test means Lyme disease can lead to
lengthy, unnecessary, unsuccessful treatment.

HOW EFFECTIVE IS TREATMENT?

The treatment for Lyme disease—heavy doses of antibiotics to kill the
organism responsible (a spirochete, related to the germ that causes syphilis)—is effective most of the time when begun early, when the rash or
flulike symptoms appear. Unfortunately, a small number of people continue to have symptoms of fatigue, headaches, and progressive paralysis,
despite prompt and extensive treatment with antibiotics.

Once the disease has reached the later stage of arthritis and other
complications, intravenous antibiotics (which are given in the hospital) may
be required. They work in an estimated 90 percent of cases. In the others,
the disease lingers on.

Some experts believe that Lyme disease is incurable in many people.

IF I'VE BEEN BITTEN BY A DEER TICK, ARE
ANTIBIOTICS ADVISED?

This has been the center of some controversy. Antibiotics are costly and
can cause side effects such as diarrhea and yeast infections, and they
shouldn't be used unless necessary. The question is: do the benefits outweigh the risks?

This is largely a question of geography. If you live in a place where many deer ticks are infected with Lyme disease bacteria (in Westchester County, New York, it's as high as 50 percent), a bite may mean enough exposure to justify giving antibiotics preventively (though some experts would question this). In other areas where the disease is common (Northeast, Middle Atlantic States, and parts of the northern Midwest and West), it's more of a judgment call. Pockets of infection can make a bite in one town substantially riskier than in another.

Elsewhere, risk of the disease may be sufficiently lower to justify a wait-and-see approach. After all, antibiotics not begun until the rash develops or an antibody test turns positive are still effective (*The New England Journal of Medicine,* August 20, 1992).

HOW IS CHRONIC LYME DISEASE TREATED?

Virtually all experts agree that a few—some say very few—people with Lyme disease stay sick despite antibiotics, or have symptoms like arthritis that improve during treatment but return when treatment stops. But what of the more substantial number who develop chronic, life-disrupting illness (that may include severe joint pain, memory and thinking impairment, and prostrating fatigue), but who test negative for active Lyme? This is another area of disagreement.

Uncertainty is almost guaranteed about an illness whose symptoms resemble those of others, whose mechanism is poorly understood, and for which tests are not entirely reliable. To make things more complicated, it may be that some chronic symptoms, like arthritis, are caused not by the infection itself but by the body's reaction to it.

Tests like analysis of cerebrospinal fluid (which requires a spinal puncture) can show whether the infection continues. But certain proteins on the *Borrelia burgdorferi* bacterium apparently resemble human proteins closely, and the antibodies produced to fight the infection may continue to attack joints and other tissues after all signs of infection have disappeared.

Misdiagnosis, some say, is common. One study found that of 788 people referred to a special clinic by physicians who thought they had active Lyme disease, only one quarter actually did. Among the others, the true diagnosis was most often fibromyalgia (which can be triggered by Lyme disease but then has a life of its own) or chronic fatigue syndrome. "The most common reason for lack of response to antibiotic therapy was mis-diagnosis,'' the authors concluded (*Journal of the American Medical Association,* April 14, 1993).

On the other hand, some experts believe that current methods are simply inadequate to diagnose Lyme disease in many people who have persistent symptoms. Some in this predicament believe their diagnosis of Lyme disease is questioned by researchers purely because they have not responded to the standard antibiotics regimen. Because the disability is often severe, and the treatment (high doses of intravenous antibiotics) extreme, the need for better tests and a better understanding of the illness is clear. Research funds administered through the National Institutes of Health have increased nearly tenfold (to $1.4 million annually) in the years from 1987 to 1994.

HOW CAN I PROTECT MYSELF?

You won't get Lyme disease if you avoid the tick that carries it. The deer tick (or black-legged tick on the West Coast) lives on deer and small rodents and is found in woodsy sections. Development has driven deer into suburban areas in increasing numbers, so it's as possible to be bitten in your backyard as while hiking through the underbrush. In the Northeast, in fact, it appears that far more people are exposed to Lyme disease in residential areas than in recreational settings like state parks.

Cover yourself (and your children) well, with long sleeves and pant cuffs tucked into socks, when you go hiking during tick season (April through October in the Northeast). Apply a tick repellent containing DEET (not for children who are likely to suffer toxic reactions even at low concentrations). Stay on trails and don't romp through the underbrush.

Keep out of woodsy parts of your own property, and keep lawns clear of leaf waste and underbrush.

Inspect yourself (and your children) for ticks after you've been ex-posed. The deer tick is tiny (about the size of a poppy seed, in the stage when it can carry Lyme disease) and hard to spot. But if you see one and remove it before it's been attached for twenty-four hours, it can't transmit the disease. Grasp the tick with tweezers and pull firmly but gently; don't touch it, but keep it for identification later.

IS THERE A VACCINE?

Not yet. There is one for dogs (whose lifestyle puts them at considerably greater risk of tick bites than people), but its effectiveness hasn't been proven. A vaccine using a protein from *B. burgdorferi,* but not the bacterium itself, is currently being tested on people in high-risk areas.

Even if a vaccine were found to be effective, it's unclear how widely it would be used. For most people treated early, Lyme disease isn't terribly dangerous, and any vaccine can have adverse effects. Possibly, immunization would be reserved for those who have substantial exposure to woods or underbrush in areas where many ticks are infected.

Resources

There are many support groups for people with chronic Lyme disease, particularly in parts of the country where the disease is widespread. A local hospital or chapter of the Arthritis Foundation can help you find one. Call the U.S. Centers for Disease Control and Prevention for the latest information about Lyme disease at (404) 332-4555.

✦ MALIGNANT MELANOMA

"Skin deep" is misleading when it comes to malignant melanoma. About thirty-two thousand Americans develop this most serious kind of skin cancer annually, and sixty-seven hundred die of it. The incidence of malignant melanoma has tripled in the last forty years—a faster growth than any other kind of cancer. By the year 2000, according to a review article in *The New England Journal of Medicine* (July 18, 1991), it's estimated that one American in ninety will develop the disease.

Melanoma, a malignancy of pigmented skin cells, can spread throughout the body. As opposed to many other cancers that mostly strike older people, it can occur anytime in adulthood. The average age at diagnosis is fifty-three. It is the most common cancer among whites in their late twenties, and among white men in their late thirties.

Although five-year survival has improved dramatically in recent decades (from 49 percent in the early 1950s to 81 percent in the early 1990s), increasing incidence has meant a rise in overall mortality from melanoma of 150 percent during this period.

DOES EARLY DETECTION MAKE A DIFFERENCE?

Unlike some other cancers, the stage at which melanoma is diagnosed literally may mean the difference between life and death. If the lesion is found when still confined to the skin, an estimated 79 percent of people will still survive five years later; if it has already spread throughout the body, all but 5 percent will be dead, most within a year.

Melanoma grows downward before it spreads. If it is removed while less than .75 millimeter thick, your chance of five-year survival is 96 percent; if it is 1.5 to 2.5 millimeters, the five-year survival is 75 percent. For a person with a lesion that hasn't spread beyond the skin, but is 4 millimeters or thicker, five-year survival is less than 50 percent.

Since melanoma is a cancer on the surface of the skin, the detection strategy is low-tech and noninvasive: visual inspection. A 1992 National

Institutes of Health (NIH) consensus conference on diagnosis and treatment of early melanoma advised regular whole-body examinations by a dermatologist or primary care physician, to detect lesions that should be biopsied to see if they are malignant.

No randomized trial of screening (compared to no screening) has been done.

CAN I EXAMINE MYSELF?

Self-examination is another key to early detection, but you have to know what distinguishes a possible melanoma from an ordinary freckle or mole that it resembles.

- Be aware of new lesions you haven't noticed before, or moles that have grown or changed perceptibly. And remember "ABCD": Asymmetry; Border irregularity; Color variety; and Diameter.
- A suspicious lesion is asymmetrical—it isn't round or oval, and one half is different from the other half. Its edges are notched, scalloped, or indistinct. Its color isn't uniform, but may mix shades of brown, black, red, blue, or white. The possibility is greater if it's wider than the diameter of a pencil eraser, although smaller lesions can be malignant, too.
- A melanoma may itch, burn, or bleed, but most often, it doesn't.

Melanomas aren't necessarily concentrated in the usual sun-exposed areas, but can also arise on the genitals, between the buttocks, on the scalp, and in the spaces between your fingers and toes. The type of melanoma most common in dark-skinned people, acral lentiginous melanoma, is typically found on the soles or palms, or under the fingernails.

WHAT IS MY PERSONAL RISK OF MELANOMA?

Light-skinned, blue-eyed people who sunburn easily and tan poorly are most likely to develop melanoma. If a close relative has had it, your risk is also increased. Although blacks and Asians have a far lower rate of melanoma, they are *more* likely to die of it if they do get it: possibly because the type that they are prone to (acral lentiginous melanoma) spreads more quickly, and is more easily overlooked.

Having moles (melanocytic nevi) doesn't necessarily increase your chances of melanoma, but a great number (over fifty) or several unusually large ones (two inches plus) does mean your risk is greater. And a certain type, once called "dysplastic nevi" but now called "atypical moles," requires vigilance: the atypical mole itself may turn malignant, or melanoma may develop elsewhere.

How great your risk of melanoma depends on personal and family history. If neither you nor anyone in your family has had melanoma, the lifetime risk for a person with atypical moles is 6 percent (compared with about 1 percent for the general population). If one family member has had melanoma, your risk is 15 percent; if two or more have had it, your risk rises to 50 percent.

After you've had a melanoma removed, you're more likely than average to have another. According to the NIH consensus statement, at least 3 percent of people develop a second lesion within three years. In certain melanoma-prone families, one third will have a repeat melanoma within five years.

If you fall into any of these elevated risk categories, you should have a whole-body exam by a dermatologist. Optimal frequency for such examinations has not been established.

DOES SUN EXPOSURE CAUSE MELANOMA?

Sunlight is the most important environmental risk factor for melanoma. The incidence of malignancy rises in white populations that live closer to the equator, and falls in higher latitudes where sunlight is weaker. Increasing leisure-time exposure to sunlight, a trend toward wearing less clothing, and the increase in ultraviolet exposure caused by the depletion of the ozone layer have been held responsible, in part, for increasing melanoma rates.

But the connection between sun exposure and melanoma isn't as direct as for other skin cancers. The people at highest risk, some suggest, are those whose exposure to sun is intermittent, rather than habitual, and substantial sunburns, particularly early in life, seem a particular danger.

A Dutch study of 141 people with melanoma and 183 controls found that melanoma risk was greater among indoor than outdoor workers, and that the effect of sunbathing, sunburns, and vacations in sunny places were more marked in those who worked indoors (*Environmental Health Perspectives,* August 1993).

DO I NEED MAJOR SURGERY FOR MELANOMA?

In melanoma that's confined to the skin, removal of the lesion itself is usually all that's necessary, and recent evidence has shown that smaller surgical margins (the benign tissue that's removed along with the tumor) than had been customary are generally safe. According to the NIH consensus statement, a margin of 1 centimeter (compared with the older practice of 5 centimeters) is now considered adequate for melanomas less than 1 millimeter thick. Wider excisions—up to 3 centimeters—are generally advised for thicker melanomas, but ongoing prospective randomized trials are investigating the effectiveness of less extensive surgery.

It is possible that the malignancy has spread to nearby lymph nodes, even if metastasis (spread to distant organs) isn't evident, and some suggest that removing the nearby lymph nodes will improve the outlook. It appears that this prophylactic measure doesn't benefit people with very thin (under 1 millimeter) or thick (4 millimeters or over) melanomas. Although some studies suggest therapeutic value for those in between, randomized prospective trials haven't shown that immediate lymph node removal will improve survival any more than waiting until symptoms of actual spread appear.

If the malignancy has spread to the lymph nodes, they are typically removed, and the surgery is followed by chemotherapy, various kinds of immune-boosting therapy, or radiation, but "none of these strategies have definitively improved survival," the 1991 *Annals* review article said. There is no point in risking the infection, numbness, and lymphodema (permanent fluid retention of the affected limb) that can occur when lymph nodes are removed from the groin area (in the case of melanoma) or the leg or armpit area (melanoma on the arm).

Once melanoma has metastasized more widely, chemotherapy, radiation, or surgery are used to reduce symptoms and lengthen survival. But no agent or combination yet found can achieve more than short-term, partial improvement in most cases.

WILL MY PAIN BE TREATED AS AGGRESSIVELY AS MY CANCER?

This question should be asked by all people choosing an oncologist (cancer specialist) following a diagnosis of any type of cancer. Studies consistently show that people with terminal cancer pain are undertreated. Ask whether your oncologist is affiliated with a hospital that has a pain management program. This shows an active commitment to alleviating pain.

Resources

Have your doctor contact the Armed Forces Institute of Pathology to arrange for a second pathology opinion (see Breast Cancer). Malignant melanoma is a rare cancer and mistakes can occur in diagnosis. Contact the National Cancer Institute's CancerFax (see Breast Cancer Resources).

♦ MENOPAUSE

Usually in her late forties or early fifties, a woman's body slowly begins what will ultimately become a sharp decrease in the production of the sex hormones estrogen and progestin, and she undergoes menopause. It's more than a physiological event in the life cycle: menopause has psychological, cultural, and even political meanings, all of which can affect the experience for individual women.

The greatest controversy surrounds hormone replacement therapy. Estrogen relieves some of the discomforts associated with menopause, particularly hot flashes and vaginal dryness. Short-term estrogen use during menopause was, and still is, the most common scenario. But in recent years, doctors have begun advocating long-term use to reduce the risk of later-life illnesses like heart disease and osteoporosis. The bone thinning of osteoporosis accelerates in the years after menopause, causing bone fractures not likely to occur until old age.

Earlier generations of women who took estrogen showed a higher than normal incidence of endometrial cancer (uterine). To reduce this risk, doctors now prescribe another hormone, progestin, to women with an intact uterus. There is also an increased incidence of breast cancer shown among long-term users of estrogen.

IS MENOPAUSE ALWAYS DISTRESSING?

Not long ago, conventional wisdom was that "the change of life" was invariably a time of trial, with depression and mood swings compounding physical suffering. In a popular book of the mid-1960s, *Feminine Forever,* Robert Wilson, M.D., used terms like "the horror of living decay" to anatomize menopause (and prescribed hormones as an antidote). Modern research and a more thorough sharing of the experience of women have come up with a very different picture.

In a study of twenty-five hundred menopausal women in New England, for example, only 3 percent expressed regret about the physical changes they experienced, and the rate of depression was 10 percent—similar to community studies at all ages. Over time, their feelings about menopause brightened: negative attitudes mellowed and positive ones stayed that way (*Journal of the American Medical Association,* June 24, 1988).

Nearly three quarters of the women reported two or more physical symptoms associated with menopause (predominantly hot flashes, cold sweats, and menstrual problems) but these exerted at most a slightly negative effect on attitudes. On the other hand, women who were depressed before menopause were more than twice as likely to report distressing symptoms.

And what correlated more strongly than menopause itself with both physical and mental problems were "life changes"—the stressors that cause trouble at any age, like recent divorce or death of a spouse, or caring for an aged parent.

One possible reason for this brighter than usual picture, the researchers suggested, was that the women in the study were surveyed out in the community, whereas most menopause research has focused on women who come to see the doctor—and are presumably experiencing more than the usual distress.

Another study confirmed that menopause has no discernible effect on emotional health. Researchers at the University of Pittsburgh followed 541 women near the time of menopause, for three years. In this time, 101 passed through menopause. Comparison with 101 age-matched controls found little difference: anxiety, depression, anger, stress, and job dissatisfaction were close to equal (*Journal of Consulting and Clinical Psychology,* 1990, no. 58).

SHOULD I TAKE HORMONES?

The original indication for hormone therapy—alleviating physiological effects of menopause (most prominently, hot flashes)—is still fairly straightforward. If these problems distress you sufficiently, relatively *short-term* therapy may make you more comfortable (although some women continue to have hot flashes despite estrogen therapy).

Estrogen can also reverse the thinning and drying of vaginal tissues that may make sex painful after menopause. Results appear as good with a topical cream, which introduces far less hormone into the system than pills and may require application as infrequently as once a month. Estrogen can also be delivered in a transdermal skin patch, which has the advantage of requiring only a twice-a-week application, and the disadvantage of potential skin irritation.

As for long-term use of hormone, the research leaves much to be desired. Virtually all of our information on estrogen comes from population studies, as opposed to carefully controlled clinical trials. (There is virtually no long-term information regarding the addition of progestin.) Population studies take a backward look at large groups of people, in this case, to correlate estrogen use with lower rates of disease. Many population studies, for example, show a major reduction in heart disease among estrogen users that is not shown among nonusers. The rub is this: upper-income women tend to be estrogen users, and women in the upper-income bracket tend to have lower rates of heart disease whether they take estrogen or not. Furthermore, women with a predisposition toward stroke and heart disease were advised not to take estrogen, because the drug increased the risk of stroke. In summary, the women who took estrogen in these population studies were healthier to begin with.

What we need is a well-designed clinical trial to answer the many questions regarding estrogen's—and progestin's—long-term benefits and risks. Unfortunately, answers are a long way off because just such a trial began in 1990. It's called the PEPI, Postmenopausal Estrogen/Progestin Interventions, and is sponsored by the National Institutes of Health. Over eight hundred women, aged forty-five to sixty-four, have been followed for three years. When preliminary results were published in 1994, they showed that the women taking estrogen alone and the women taking estrogen combined with micronized progesterone showed reduced risk factors for heart disease. The question of whether estrogen and the combination lowers the rate of heart disease will not be answered for over ten years, if additional funding permits this study to continue.

HOW CAN I MAKE A DECISION ABOUT LONG-TERM HORMONE THERAPY?

To decide whether to embark on a long-term drug regimen, you need a good idea of your personal chances of developing heart disease and suffering a hip fracture. Unfortunately, there are many gaps in our research knowledge. Virtually all the existing research has looked at women who took estrogen alone, and only white women at that. Progestin would not be offered to women who have had a hysterectomy.

(Much of the data in the answers to the next two questions comes from a risk assessment analysis published in *Annals of Internal Medicine,* December 15, 1992. The analysis is based on assessing the risks of heart disease and hip fracture in a fifty-year-old white woman who does or does not take estrogen.)

WHAT IS MY PERSONAL RISK OF HEART DISEASE?

Although there is no abrupt acceleration in coronary heart disease (CHD) after menopause, there is a gradual increased incidence as a woman ages. Heart disease is the leading cause of death among women, and estrogen depletion appears to be a contributing factor.

Just how much of a difference will estrogen therapy make? A fifty-year-old white woman has a 46 percent probability of developing CHD in her lifetime, and a 31 percent chance of dying from it, at a median age of seventy-four years. Estrogen replacement (with or without progestin) reduces the risk of developing the disease to 34 percent.

If, however, the same woman already has CHD or a number of risk factors (such as smoking, high cholesterol, or a strong family history of heart disease), her risk of recurrent or new CHD is 84 percent, and her life expectancy is six and a half years shorter than her healthier counterparts. Estrogen therapy is predicted to reduce the risk to 76.4 percent and extend her life expectancy by 2.1 years.

The greater your risk of heart disease, therefore, the better the argument for estrogen therapy.

WHAT ARE THE ODDS THAT I WILL SUFFER A HIP FRACTURE?

Bone density declines after menopause, often leading to loss of height and posing the risk of fracture. Hip fracture (three quarters of which occur in women over seventy-five) can have the most serious consequences, including significant pain, disability, loss of independence, and death.

It seems quite clear that estrogen therapy slows the rate of bone loss, but the effects on fracture are less certain.

How likely are you to suffer a hip fracture? For a fifty-year-old white woman, the lifetime risk is 15 percent, and the probability of dying from it is 1.5 percent. Hormone replacement reduces the risk of fracture to about 13 percent.

If you have low bone density or other factors that put you at increased risk, however, your chance of hip fracture is considerably higher: 36 percent. Estrogen therapy reduces this to 31.4 percent and will extend life expectancy by a full year. (Small-boned women are at higher than average risk of fracture; Asian women at higher risk than whites, who are at higher risk than blacks.)

But the current advice—take estrogen for five to ten years after menopause—may not bring even these limited benefits. According to a study of 670 elderly women in the Boston area, those who took estrogen for seven years or longer indeed had higher bone density. But by the time they reached seventy-five years—hip fracture country—there was little difference in bone density from nonusers.

Taking estrogen for the first five years after menopause, when the most rapid bone loss occurs, will not protect you years later when you need it most, the study suggests. Other research confirms that when estrogen is withdrawn, at whatever age, bone loss kicks in at the accelerated postmenopausal rate.

To prevent hip fracture, then, estrogen replacement has to be a lifelong commitment. An alternative approach is to begin hormone therapy around the time of maximum risk—or wait until a fracture has already occurred, to prevent subsequent ones.

(For unknown reasons, 15 percent of women who take estrogen will lose bone density anyway.)

HOW SAFE IS HORMONE THERAPY?

Overall, estrogen replacement increases the risk of cancer. Unquestionably, estrogen alone markedly increases the risk of endometrial (uterine) cancer—from 2.6 to 19.7 percent, after the age of fifty. The addition of progestin protects against endometrial cancer and apparently brings the risk back down to untreated levels.

Things are less clear for breast cancer. Short-term estrogen replacement seems to have little effect on breast-cancer risk. Population studies have provided contradictory results for long-term usage. Some showed no risk of breast cancer and others indicate a risk only after ten years of use. A 1991 meta-analysis by the Centers for Disease Control and Prevention combined the results of the best studies that explored the relationship between estrogen use and breast cancer. "For women who experienced any type of menopause, risk did not appear to increase until after at least five years of estrogen use. After fifteen years of estrogen use, we found a 30 percent increase in the risk of breast cancer," wrote the researchers (*Journal of the American Medical Association,* April 17, 1991). "Among women with a family history of breast cancer, those who had ever used estrogen had a significantly higher risk than those who had not."

Even the addition of progestin raises questions. While some studies show no added risk of breast cancer when progestin is taken with estrogen, others find an alarming rise. A 1989 Swedish study, for example, found a fourfold rise in breast cancer with the combination of estrogen and progestin (*The New England Journal of Medicine,* August 3, 1989).

The Swedish research has been criticized because the group studied was quite small and the estrogen used for the most part was different from the formulation prescribed in this country. Perhaps the safest thing to say is that experience with combined estrogen and progestin is quite short, definitive studies have yet to be done, and that women who take it now are participating, in a sense, in a vast experiment.

In addition, estrogen therapy makes fibroids (benign tumors in the uterus that normally shrink after menopause) grow, and triples the risk of gallstones. Both conditions may require surgery. Common side effects with estrogen are fluid retention, high blood pressure, weight gain, and susceptibility to yeast infections. Progestin may cause vaginal bleeding, acne, depression, and breast tenderness.

WHAT ARE ALTERNATIVES TO HORMONE THERAPY?

A nonhormonal drug, Bellergal (which contains the sedative phenobarbital) has been approved by the FDA for hot flashes, night sweats, and the insomnia induced by menopause. But it works for only some women, and may be addictive. Natural remedies such as vitamin E, vitamin B_6, and the herb ginseng, have their proponents, but these have never been tested scientifically. Vitamin E is safe up to 800 IU daily (and appears to have other health benefits, including protection against cancer), but megadoses of vitamin B_6 (over 150 milligrams per day) can be toxic.

Biofeedback trains people to regulate physiological processes such as body temperature, and may be helpful to some women in quelling hot flashes. The approach hasn't been tested rigorously, however.

The dryness and thinning of vaginal tissues that often accompany menopause may be redressed by regular sexual activity (with or without a partner), and by ordinary lubricants like K-Y jelly or vegetable oil. Don't use petroleum jelly (for example, Vaseline) because it is not water soluble and thus could lead to an irritation or promote infection in the vagina or urethra.

As for bone loss, weight-bearing exercise like walking will maintain bone mineral density. Calcium (1,500 milligrams per day), in dairy products, green leafy vegetables, or supplements, appears to strengthen bones, although its effect is smaller than estrogen. Excess dietary protein, alcohol consumption, and smoking appear to hasten the loss of calcium from the body, and should be avoided.

Whether or not you take estrogen, you should adopt a lifestyle that reduces heart attack and cancer risk. Exercise regularly, eat a low-fat, high-fiber diet, stop smoking, and take steps to reduce stress.

If you want to go the nonhormonal route to postmenopausal health, you'll probably be on your own: a Gallup survey found than less than 2 percent of women ages forty-five to sixty had gotten any substantial information on these approaches from their doctors.

Resources

Suggested reading:
Menopause Without Medicine by Linda Ojeda, Ph.D. (1989)

Hunter House Inc., Publishers
P.O. Box 847
Claremont, CA 91711

Menopause Naturally by Sadja Greenwood, M.D. (1992)

Volcano Press
P.O. Box 270
Volcano, CA 95689

◆ MITRAL VALVE PROLAPSE

Mitral valve prolapse (MVP) is the most common heart problem in young people, and the second most common valve disorder in the population at large. But just how common is difficult to say. Depending on diagnostic criteria, estimates of its prevalence range from 3 to 20 percent.

The disorder, caused by a malfunction in the valve between the receiving and pumping chamber on the left side of the heart, can be entirely unnoticeable (and often discovered in the course of a routine examination), or associated with a variety of symptoms that are generally more troubling than burdensome; including weakness, fainting, palpitations, and chest pain. Most people with MVP needn't restrict their activities at all, or suffer any adverse consequences.

For a minority, however, MVP is a far more serious business. According to an article in the *British Medical Journal* (April 10, 1993), 3 to 10 percent of people with MVP develop such life-threatening complications as congestive heart failure, infective endocarditis (an infection of the heart lining), or cerebral thrombosis. In this country, an estimated four thousand deaths yearly can be attributed to MVP.

HOW IS MVP DIAGNOSED?

The first indication of MVP is an abnormal sound when the doctor listens to your heart: a click added to the usual "lub-dub" of the heartbeat, as the valve shuts. A murmur after the click indicates that blood is leaking back after the valve is supposed to have closed, which is more serious. Because the behavior of the valve varies in the same person, experts suggest doing the examination on several different occasions.

The diagnosis is usually confirmed by echocardiogram, which uses ultrasound to provide a picture of the heart's workings. The echocardiogram can also supply useful details about the valve that can help in planning treatment and preventing complications. There is no real consensus on echographic criteria to diagnose MVP, however, so it is important for the test to be interpreted by someone with experience and expertise.

WHAT CAUSES MVP?

The vast majority of MVP (98 percent, by some estimates) is primary— that is to say, not caused by anything else—and genetics clearly plays an important role. Family studies show that half of the younger (under the age of fifty) female relatives of people with MVP also have the disorder, as do 10 to 30 percent of male, older female, and juvenile relatives. If you have MVP, it's a good idea for your close family members to be examined, too.

In a minority of cases, MVP is secondary—caused by something else, most often a more general connective tissue disorder such as the Marfan syndrome, which also affects skin, bones, and the aorta.

HOW CAN I BE SURE MY SYMPTOMS ARE CAUSED BY MVP?

While MVP is most often symptomless, in some people it is accompanied by some or all of what's called "the MVP syndrome": anxiety, shortness or breath, fatigue, and palpitations. Chest pain is the most common part of the syndrome, affecting 60 percent of people who have it.

Whether these problems are actually caused by MVP is not clear. Many of the symptoms are similar to those of panic disorder, but "a recent controlled study suggested a high rate of co-occurrence but no cause and effect relation between mitral valve prolapse and panic syndromes," according to the 1993 *British Medical Journal* article.

Some researchers have found that people with MVP syndrome have an abnormally responsive autonomic nervous system, which could cause the symptoms. But people who have the same symptoms without MVP display the same nervous system hyperreactivity, suggesting that MVP has nothing to do with it.

In some cases at least, the symptoms of "MVP syndrome" may well be caused by something else. Studies have found esophageal disorders or bronchospasm in a high proportion of people with MVP and chest pain, for example. For this reason, it is essential to have a complete series of tests to see if cardiovascular, pulmonary, digestive, thyroid, or diabetes are actually responsible for what is blamed on MVP.

WHAT DRUGS ARE PRESCRIBED?

Beta-blockers (drugs like Inderal and Tenormin, also used for high blood pressure) are thought to be helpful for the MVP syndrome; they improve chest pain 25 to 50 percent of the time, and often help palpitations as well. Some suggest using them only in high-stress situations. Their effectiveness, however, has never been confirmed in placebo-controlled randomized trial.

Treatment for other conditions uncovered by examination may help, too.

HOW CAN COMPLICATIONS BE AVOIDED?

People with MVP are at increased risk of bacterial endocarditis, a life-threatening infection of the heart lining, deterioration of the valve that requires surgery to replace it, and stroke. But it has become clear that not all MVP carries equal risk. A study of 456 people with the condition found that such complications were considerably more likely in one group: those who had a thickening of the tough, fibrous substance of the valve. This accounts for just 18 percent of people with the disorder (*The New England Journal of Medicine,* April 20, 1989).

Other studies have found complications more common among men, people over forty-five, and those who have a heart murmur caused by blood flowing back after the valve should be closed.

"Our feeling—although we can't say for sure—is most people with MVP, perhaps as many as 90 percent, will probably never be affected by it," says Andrew R. Marks, M.D., of Massachusetts General Hospital, Boston, who authored the report.

To protect against infectious endocarditis, people with MVP have been routinely advised to take prophylactic antibiotics whenever they have surgery, a skin infection, or any procedure that may release bacteria into the bloodstream, including relatively minor dental work. Is this necessary even for people with minor MVP that doesn't carry as great a risk? Dr. Marks thinks so. Endocarditis is an extremely serious disease, and the side effects of antibiotics are relatively mild. Moreover, no definitive studies have shown that people with the minor form of MVP are entirely without risk of endocarditis.

If your MVP involves a systolic murmur or thickening of the valve, you may need to take antibiotics more regularly, and have your doctor check your heart thoroughly every several years, to make sure things haven't deteriorated. Blood-pressure medication or drugs to regularize your heart rhythm are sometimes protective. Eventually, you may need surgery to replace the valve.

◆ MULTIPLE SCLEROSIS

Multiple sclerosis (MS) is a frightening diagnosis. It's the most common cause of disability, other than injury, among young adults in the United States. Yet its extremely variable course means that a substantial number of people with MS will live fairly normal, lengthy lives.

In MS, an autoimmune disease of the central nervous system, the myelin sheath covering nerve cells is apparently attacked by the body's immune system. The reported frequency of MS has markedly increased: from 46 per 100,000 in 1915, in one county in Minnesota (where extensive studies have been done), to 108 in 1978 and 173 in 1985. To a great extent, this probably reflects more accurate diagnosis, but the actual incidence has probably also risen. Today, an estimated 250,000 people in the United States suffer from MS, and there are 8,000 new cases each year.

IF THERE IS MS IN MY FAMILY, AM I AT RISK?

It appears that genetics and environment both play a role in MS. The inherited predisposition apparently involves several genes. If one identical twin has MS, the risk to the other (who has exactly the same genes) is 26 percent; among fraternal twins of the same sex, the risk is 2.4 percent. This suggests that even if the genetic risk is heightened, whether or not you develop MS depends in large part on environmental factors, according to a paper in *Current Opinions in Neurology and Neurosurgery* (April 1992).

Women are about twice as likely to develop MS as men, and some studies suggest that the risk is higher for same-sex relatives of people with the disease. If a brother or sister has it, however, it appears that your risk is somewhat elevated, regardless of your sex.

WHAT FACTORS IN THE ENVIRONMENT CAN TRIGGER MS?

Geography appears to influence the rate of MS. Generally, the disease is significantly more common in northern than southern latitudes. Although a number of studies have found that people who migrate take on the MS rate of their new homes, there are weaknesses and ambiguities in the research that make it hard to determine what this finding actually shows about the contributions of genetics and environment to incidence of MS (*Canadian Journal of Neurological Sciences,* February 1993).

What specifically triggers MS remains a mystery. The occurrence of clusters and outbreaks of cases supports a role for infection. But it seems unlikely that a single virus or bacteria is to blame, although "It is conceivable that infection in general may act as a non-specific trigger for the immune system by initiating the onset of MS or by triggering a relapse," according to the *Canadian Journal* paper.

Stress, both physical and emotional, has been associated with the appearance or worsening of MS, but whether there's actually a cause-and-effect relationship hasn't been shown. An association with diet, exposure to heavy metals, surgery, exertion, and heat have also been suggested, but have little scientific support.

IS IT CERTAIN THAT I HAVE MS?

The diagnosis of MS is often quite difficult in its early stages. Since the disease can affect diverse parts of the nervous system, its symptoms are extremely variable. Tingling in one or both arms or legs is common, as is some visual impairment, particularly double vision. Dizziness, clumsiness, and weakness may occur. The sense of touch may become blunted, making it difficult to tie your shoes or sort change. A change in urinary habits—increased frequency and urgency—is not uncommon.

All these symptoms are "nonspecific"—virtually any combination of them may occur as a result of other diseases. Typically, MS comes in episodes of such symptoms that worsen and then go away. The diagnosis can't really be made until several episodes (perhaps with changing symptoms) have occurred.

Age can give a clue. On average, MS develops in the early thirties, but it's not rare to see it anytime between fifteen and fifty. In younger or older people, MS is unlikely, but still possible.

The ability to detect MS has been greatly sharpened in recent years by the widespread use of magnetic resonance imaging (MRI), which can show areas of abnormal tissue in the nervous system. MRI is not foolproof, however. There are false negatives (in an estimated 5 to 10 percent of people who clearly have MS), and positives, particularly in people older than their fifties. This and other tests can only be interpreted properly together with symptoms and physical examination, according to an article in *Patient Care* (September 30, 1989).

WILL I BE DISABLED?

Episodes of MS can occur frequently or rarely, with little residual impairment in between, or the illness may progress without a break. Overall, just 15 to 20 percent of people with the disease will have an exacerbation each year. Half the cases of the disease that at first seem chronic and progressive will stabilize within two years, according to an article in the *Cleveland Clinic Journal of Medicine* (February 1992). Generally, attacks are less frequent with the passage of time.

Disability from MS is not inevitable, or may be very gradual. In one study of 672 people, 37 percent had no restrictions on their activities ten years after the diagnosis, and 8 percent were disabled at that time. About one person in four is confined to a wheelchair twenty-five years after MS develops. Over half can continue to lead relatively normal lives for decades.

Despite fears to the contrary, significant impairments in mental ability are rare, at least until late in the illness. Difficulty remembering, concentrating, or thinking may reflect depression—a common reaction to any chronic illness—rather than the MS itself, and should respond well to treatment.

Although the course of MS is extremely hard to predict, the outlook is better if, during the first five years after diagnosis, your episodes are infrequent (one or two a year) and fairly brief. Men, people who developed MS in their teens or after forty, and those whose first symptoms involved movement rather than sensation, are likely to become disabled more quickly.

WILL MS SHORTEN MY LIFE?

Again keeping in mind the diverse symptoms and progression of MS, for the most part, the disease won't markedly reduce life expectancy. In one study, 76 percent of one group of people with MS were still alive twenty-five years after their disease began—85 percent as great as a matched group without MS. Even in studies that show a more significant impact, there is often little effect on survival for the first ten years.

Several studies have found that half of deaths among people with MS can be attributed to the disease, while other causes of death are much like those in the population at large. Suicide is a significant factor: it accounts for nearly 30 percent of deaths, more than seven times the general rate, according to an article in Current Opinions in Neurology and Neurosurgery (April 1992). While depression, a major risk factor for suicide, is understandable in the face of a progressive disease, it shouldn't be accepted as inevitable. An untold number of these suicides are preventable with the help of antidepressant drugs.

WHAT DRUGS CAN HELP FIGHT THE DISEASE?

The only really established drug therapy in MS is for the acute exacerbations. Corticosteroids shorten episodes and induce new symptoms to remit more quickly (probably by reducing inflammation surrounding nerve cells), but there's no evidence that they slow the disease process.

In addition, various drugs and nondrug therapies can help ease symptoms, including baclofen for muscle spasticity, and physical therapy. Appropriate exercise may help maintain strength and energy. Limiting excess weight will not only help to maintain function but it will also reduce fatigue.

Medication to slow the progression of MS or prevent exacerbations is still experimental. Azathioprine, which suppresses immune function, has seemed promising in a number of controlled trials, although the advantage has not always been statistically significant. Other candidate drugs are cyclosporine and interferon. But all "show only minimal or modest benefits and are at times associated with troublesome or severe toxicity," according to the Cleveland Clinic article.

WHAT CAN I DO TO HELP MYSELF?

It's important to maintain as active a life as possible, while avoiding excesses. Muscle-training exercises and massage can be beneficial.

Resources

Your local chapter of the National Multiple Sclerosis Society or contact headquarters for information:

National Multiple Sclerosis Society
733 Third Avenue
New York, NY 10017
(800) 344-4867   (212) 986-3240

◆ ORAL CONTRACEPTIVES

When oral contraceptives (OCs) containing hormones first became available in the 1960s, they were given an imposing sobriquet—"The Pill"—and simultaneously hailed as the key to women's reproductive freedom and damned as a door to promiscuity. The passing years have put the development in perspective, but issues surrounding OCs (in particular, the safety of regular, long-term hormone use) retain the capacity to arouse passionate debate.

OCs are an extremely popular means of birth control, currently used by eighty to one hundred million women worldwide. The effectiveness of different formulations vary, but they remain the most reliable in preventing pregnancy of all popular contraceptive methods except sterilization.

In recent years, OCs have been joined by several new systems for delivering the same hormones over a longer period of time, notably the progesterone implant.

SHOULD I USE OCs?

The choice of a birth control method has always been an intensely personal one, and never more so than today. Among the principal advantages of OCs are their effectiveness (when taken conscientiously), and the comfort factor: they don't intrude on the spontaneity of intimacy the way inserting a diaphragm or putting on a condom would.

Leaving aside questions of long-term risk, the choice of contraception today has definite health implications. OCs provide virtually no protection against sexually transmitted diseases, while condoms substantially lower the risk of most, and the diaphragm plus spermicide appears to have at least some effect.

WHAT KIND OF OC WOULD BE BEST FOR ME?

There are three basic kinds of OC available today. The combination pill contains a fixed dose of two hormones, estrogen and progestogen, and it's taken twenty-one days a month. The triphasic pill contains varied amounts of the two hormones, designed to approximate the natural cycle more closely, and is taken every day. The progestogen-only pill (also known as "minipill") has only the one hormone, and is also taken every day.

According to a review article in *The New England Journal of Medicine* (May 27, 1993), triphasic pills "offer little if any advantage over the monophasic pills." Between combination and progestogen-only pills, however, there is a good deal to choose from.

The combination pill actually prevents ovulation by short-circuiting the sequence of hormones that normally leads to it, while the progestogen-only pill allows the egg to be released, but slows its descent down the fallopian tube, thickens cervical mucus to prevent sperm from fertilizing it, and makes the lining of the uterus inhospitable for the egg, should it be fertilized.

The combination pill is somewhat more effective than the progestogen-only formulation (more than 99 percent effective, compared with 97 percent), and the latter is often reserved for women who are not at the peak of their fertility—who are over thirty-five, for example—or who, for various reasons, can't take the combination pill. Fewer than 8 percent of American women who use contraception take the minipill route. There are differences in side effect and health-risk profiles, which may make one kind of pill or another more attractive to you.

In addition, different OCs use different variations on the same basic hormones, in a range of doses and proportions. It may take some trial and error to find the formulation that works best in your individual case.

WHAT SIDE EFFECTS CAN I EXPECT?

Today's OCs are very different from those of thirty years ago. The types of hormones are different, and the doses are far smaller. Combination pills have as little as one fifth as much estrogen and one sixth of the amount of progestogen as the original formulations, according to an article in the *Journal of the National Cancer Institute* (March 5, 1993).

Side effects, accordingly, are reduced, but they still occur. With the combination pill, they are largely a result of the estrogen component, and they vary as widely as women's individual responses to that hormone. Weight gain, increase in breast size and tenderness, nausea and vomiting, increased appetite, dizziness, and headaches have been reported.

Some women feel great when taking the pill, but others become significantly depressed. Diminished sex drive has been seen—in one placebo-controlled study with the triphasic pill, it was quite marked, according to an article in *New Scientist* (September 29, 1990).

The side effects of the progestogen-only pill are far fewer (which is one reason for its use), particularly with the development in recent years of newer varieties of the hormone. The most common distressing adverse effect is menstrual irregularity. Periods are shortened and erratic in about 40 percent of women who use the progestogen-only pill, and 20 percent have spotting or amenorrhea.

WILL OCs INCREASE MY RISK OF HEART DISEASE?

The health effects of OCs—which are, after all, hormones, often taken for quite a number of years—have been a persistent concern. The risk of cancer and of heart disease has been particularly debated.

It's important to remember, again, that today's OCs use vastly lower doses of hormones than those of a generation ago, and that data from the past must be interpreted with caution. This is especially dramatic in the case of heart disease. A 1977 study found a nearly fivefold increase in the risk of death from heart disease among women taking high-estrogen OCs. But recent studies of women who are taking pills with a fraction of the old estrogen dose have a very different picture. In at least one large study, the risk was *lower* than for women who had ever used OCs.

"There is no evidence that formulations containing low doses of estrogen are associated with an increased risk of cardiovascular disease," *The New England Journal of Medicine* 1993 review article concluded.

Progestogen-only pills should, in theory, be at least as safe, and probably safer, but there is little data on long-term risks.

Some OCs apparently do increase the risk of cerebral thrombosis—stroke caused by a blood clot. In a Danish study of over fifteen hundred women, those who used older OC formulations with a high dose of estrogen had about three times as many strokes as women who used no OC, while those who used modern low-estrogen pills had about twice the risk. Progestogen-only pills had no substantial effect on stroke rate.

The study found that a woman's age or the length of time she had used OCs had no effect on the relative risk (*British Medical Journal,* April 10, 1993).

WILL OCs INCREASE MY RISK OF CANCER?

This is a knottier problem, and there's no simple answer that applies to all pills and all kinds of cancer. It appears, in fact, that OCs may protect against some cancers, while increasing the danger of others.

There's ample evidence that combination OCs offer some protection against cancers of the ovary and endometrium. After using them for ten years, women had one fifth the expected risk of ovarian cancer, and the effect lasted for fifteen years after they stopped taking the pill, according to a study cited in *The New England Journal of Medicine.*

A study of women over age fifty found that those who had used OCs at some point, even as briefly as a year, had half the risk of endometrial cancer of matched controls who never took the pill. The effect was still seen in women who hadn't taken OCs for twenty years (*Obstetrics and Gynecology,* December 1993). These women, for the most part, took earlier versions of the pill that contained high doses of estrogen; whether today's OC would have the same protective effect is difficult to say.

Although the issue is a complex one, it seems that estrogen-containing pills may indeed increase the risk of breast cancer, at least for younger women. A study of women under forty-five that analyzed data from twelve studies found the rate of breast cancer increased by 42 percent among those who had taken OCs for periods ranging from over five to over twelve years. Commenting on this and other research, the 1993 *Journal of the National Cancer Institute* article concluded that "a true increase in risk of breast cancer in young women" was a likely consequence of prolonged OC use.

To some extent, it appears that this risk is most marked among women who take OCs before having children. A meta-analysis of a number of studies, reported in *Cancer* (1990, no. 66, pp. 2253–63), found the increase predominantly among those who had taken OCs for at least four years before a term pregnancy.

IS THERE ANYTHING THAT MAKES MY RISK PARTICULARLY HIGH?

The risk of blood clots associated with OCs appears significantly higher for women who smoke, and smoking has long been considered a contraindication for their use. With the lower-estrogen modern pills, however, current thinking is a bit more flexible, especially if there are no other factors that increase your cardiovascular risk.

Smoking is an even poorer idea than usual, however, if you take OCs. Aside from the heart disease issue, there's at least some evidence that smoking increases the danger of cervical cancer among women who use the pill, by making DNA more vulnerable to mutations (*New Scientist,* January 8, 1994).

Age and blood pressure are similarly less rigid contraindications than they once were. The lower-dose combination pills are safer than the older products for women over thirty-five. The effect on blood pressure varies from one individual to another. Combination OCs cause hypertension in 4 to 5 percent of women and increase it further in 9 to 16 percent of those who already have high blood pressure. Your doctor may suggest a careful trial to see how you react. Progestogen-only pills do not raise blood pressure and may actually reduce hypertension risk.

CAN OCs BE USED AS A MORNING-AFTER PILL?

The hormones in a combination OC can effectively prevent implantation, if taken within seventy-two hours after unprotected intercourse. Higher than the normal dose must be taken; however, it may be necessary to take them more than once, and the side effects, particularly vomiting, may be distressing. If done properly, the method is quite successful—it works in about 97 percent of cases, according to an article in *Contemporary OB/GYN* (January 1994). Both for safety and effectiveness' sake, however, it should be attempted only under the supervision of a doctor who knows how to do it properly.

HOW SAFE ARE INJECTED OR IMPLANTED HORMONE CONTRACEPTIVES?

These work much like OCs, but the drug is implanted just beneath the skin, injected once monthly, or put in a vaginal ring. In either case, implanted contraceptives release a daily amount of progesterone only or progesterone plus estrogen, equivalent to what you'd get in a pill. Failure rates are similar to those with OCs.

These devices haven't been used long enough, however, to give any clear idea of long-term health risks. The side effects with the progestogen-only devices in any case can be a problem. Within three years, half of the women who have had Norplant progestogen-only implants have had them removed, for the most part because of menstrual irregularities.

♦ OSTEOARTHRITIS

An estimated sixteen million Americans have osteoarthritis severe enough to cause some symptoms; it is the most common kind of joint disease. Actually, 80 to 90 percent of people over forty have some evidence of the condition on X ray, although they often do not have symptoms.

In osteoarthritis, the cartilage that lines and cushions the joint begins to crack and fray. If degeneration progresses, pain, swelling, and stiffness develop. Eventually, bone may rub directly on bone and the joint itself deteriorates, causing disability and deformity.

Although it becomes more common and severe with advancing years, osteoarthritis is not simply the result of the wear and tear of aging. As with other kinds of arthritis, some people appear to be genetically more susceptible than others. Their cartilage may be especially prone to breakdown, or very slight imperfections in how certain joints fit together may make them unusually vulnerable.

There is no cure for osteoarthritis and no drug to halt or reverse its progression. The course of the disease is usually quite gradual, however, and you can do a lot to minimize the damage and disability.

(Note: Many of the same approaches that are helpful for rheumatoid arthritis are also helpful for osteoarthritis. Read both sections for a full description.)

IF I HAVE OSTEOARTHRITIS IN ONE JOINT, WILL I GET IT ELSEWHERE?

Not necessarily. Osteoarthritis may affect a single joint, several, or many. The hands, back, neck, and the weight-bearing joints, particularly knees and hips, are most commonly affected. A joint that has been traumatized earlier in life is more likely to develop osteoarthritis. A football injury to the knee, for example, may lead to arthritis in that joint later on.

Habitual use of a joint in your job, however, is not believed to increase the risk of osteoarthritis. People who frequently type on keyboards are not especially prone to get arthritis in their hands, for example. If you do have osteoarthritis, though, overuse of the joints in which it has developed may exacerbate the condition.

When running first became a popular exercise, there were concerns that the repeated pounding could lead to osteoarthritis of the knees or other weight-bearing joints. Repeated studies have pretty much laid this fear to rest. In one (*Rheumatology*, March 1993, no. 20, pp. 461–68), joint X rays of thirty-three runners, ages fifty to seventy, and thirty-three non-runners found that osteoarthritis of the knee and spine did not progress more rapidly over a five-year period among the runners.

DO I NEED TO TAKE MEDICINE?

No drug alters the course of osteoarthritis, but drugs are often necessary to relieve the pain. Although the disease process itself is not well understood, it appears that inflammation does *not* play the significant role it does in some other kinds of arthritis, and several recent studies have shown that high doses of anti-inflammatory drugs are no more effective than painkillers alone.

A 1991 study found 4,000 milligrams per day of acetaminophen (Tylenol) to be a more effective pain reliever with fewer side effects, compared with high doses of ibuprofen, in a study of 126 people with chronic knee pain due to osteoarthritis (*The New England Journal of Medicine*, July 11, 1991).

Narcotic pain relievers such as codeine or Percodan are fraught with side effects and the danger of dependence. They can and should almost always be avoided in chronic illnesses like osteoarthritis.

Drugs are not the only way to deal with pain. Applications of heat or cold are also quite helpful. Acupuncture and massage can provide considerable relief. And it is certainly worth learning some relaxation techniques, like meditation. Not only does stress make pain more distressing, tense muscles actually make it worse. A physical therapist can help you learn to use nondrug pain remedies effectively.

CAN I STILL EXERCISE?

Exercise is actually one of the most important ways you can help yourself. Inactivity makes the joint stiffer and more painful; muscles weaken and give the joint less support. A sensible exercise program will prevent this vicious cycle.

A specific exercise prescription will keep arthritic joints flexible and strengthen the muscles that support them. Particularly if your arthritis is moderate or severe, the guidance of a physical therapist or physician is strongly recommended. If you start gradually and work carefully, there's little danger of injuring even badly damaged joints.

Regular aerobic exercise can also help arthritis, along with providing the usual fitness benefits. If your back or weight-bearing joints are affected, running is a poor choice, but swimming is ideal. It stretches and strengthens muscles and joints throughout the body, the water relieves joints of the stress of weight, and the warmth is soothing. Walking, treadmill exercise, and a bike (moving or stationary) are also possibilities.

A study in *Annals of Internal Medicine* (April 1, 1992) enrolled ninety-two persons with osteoarthritis of one or both knees in a program of fitness walking. After eight weeks, they could walk nearly 20 percent farther than when they began. Their ability to function increased by more than one third, and they suffered 27 percent less pain. Similar changes were not seen in a control group who did not exercise.

SHOULD I CHANGE MY DIET?

There is some evidence that certain nutrients (fish oils) and food allergies may play a role in easing or exacerbating rheumatoid arthritis. Organ meats and excess alcohol can trigger attacks of the kind of arthritis called gout. But nothing of this sort has been documented for osteoarthritis.

What clearly can make a difference, however, is weight. According to 1988 data from The Framingham Study, people who were in the heaviest quintile were one and a half times (men) or twice (women) as likely to develop knee osteoarthritis than those in the lightest three quintiles. Further data from the same study found that weight loss of about twelve pounds over the previous ten years decreased the risk by 50 percent.

If you already have osteoarthritis of the back, knees, or hips, obesity can make it worse, and a diet to keep weight under control should be part of your self-help program.

WHAT ELSE CAN I DO TO HELP MYSELF?

Quite a bit. Your posture, your sleep position, how you move, the way your desk is arranged at work—all these things can minimize the strain on arthritic joints and the fatigue that makes osteoarthritis more disabling. A physical therapist or occupational therapist can be an invaluable "coach" to help you help yourself. (Take the time to find one who is experienced in working with arthritis—not all are.)

If your arthritis is at all severe, consider a self-help course available at local hospitals, YMCAs, and the local chapter of the Arthritis Foundation. There is good evidence that people (with any kind of arthritis) who take such a course function better, experience less pain, and see the doctor less frequently than others (see Rheumatoid Arthritis).

WILL I NEED SURGERY?

Surgery to replace joints severely damaged by arthritis has become increasingly popular as techniques have been refined and encouraging results have accumulated. More than 150,000 total joint replacements are performed in the United States each year. Osteoarthritis and rheumatoid arthritis are principal reasons. A Mayo Clinic study showed these diseases are the cause for 90 percent of knee replacements.

Joint implants don't last forever, although they last longer than was earlier believed. A Mayo Clinic study found that fifteen years after hip replacement, 88 percent were still functioning and 78 percent were satisfactory. Results with knee replacement, a newer procedure, were somewhat less impressive. After five years, 91 percent were still in place, with 80 percent in place after ten years, and 69 percent in place after fifteen years. (If an artificial joint fails, it is usually replaced with another.)

Like any major surgery, joint replacement carries risk of blood clots, infection, and other complications. Should you have it done? The sole reason for joint replacement is relief of severe pain and disability, so you alone can be the judge. Although an artificial hip or knee is not nearly as good as nature's own, it can make normal life possible again for people who have been sidelined by pain.

Resources

The Arthritis Foundation is a source of information and guidance. It offers a booklet, "Coping with Pain," that will help you design your own pain management program. Write to:

Arthritis Foundation
P.O. Box 19000
Atlanta, GA 30326
(800) 283-7800

The foundation also publishes the *Guide to Independent Living for People with Arthritis,* which includes descriptions, pictures, and ordering information for over six hundred helpful devices ($9.95 plus $2.00 for shipping and handling).

Local chapters of the foundation sponsor the Arthritis Self-Help Course: six weeks of about two-and-a-half-hour sessions that teach the essentials of pain control, exercise, medication, and nutrition, and deal with the psychological difficulties of arthritis. Call for details on where the course is offered in your area.

♦ OSTEOPOROSIS

The loss of bone mass is an inevitable consequence of aging in both men and women. Bone builds up until about the mid-thirties and then declines. The average woman will lose 50 percent of cancellous bone (the fracture-prone bone concentrated in the spine and at the end of long bones) during her life; the average man, 30 percent. When bone mass drops low enough to make fracture a risk, you have osteoporosis.

While osteoporosis is associated with advanced age, it can also be the result of drug therapy (with corticosteroids, in particular) or disease (such as hyperthyroidism).

Whatever its cause, osteoporosis reflects an imbalance in the normal process of "remodeling" by which bone is constantly renewed. Early in the remodeling cycle, cells called osteoclasts sculpt tiny depressions in the bone; then osteoblasts fill it with new bone. If more bone is resorbed than is replaced, osteoporosis eventually results.

Although hip fracture is often portrayed as an inevitable result of osteoporosis and osteoporosis as an inevitable consequence of aging, most elderly people will never suffer hip fracture. Consequences for the minority who will fracture in old age, however, can be severe. Of the one and half million fractures due to osteoporosis that occur yearly in the United States, many lead to disability, loss of independence, or death. (For more information about osteoporosis and its prevention, see Menopause.)

WHAT CAN I DO TO PROTECT AGAINST OSTEOPOROSIS WHILE I'M YOUNG?

Building bone mass early in life is like putting money in the bank against your retirement years: the more you squirrel away, the more you'll have later, when you need it most. Although at least half of your peak bone mass is determined by genetic factors, environment and behavior are responsible for the other half. Diet and exercise are the keys.

When it comes to exercise, weight-bearing activities such as walking and running appear to be critical, perhaps because the stress on bone stimulates it to replace itself (the same way that exercise builds muscle). Even among children ages six to fourteen, you can see a difference. One study found that physically active children (more than two hours a day) had 10 percent more bone density (measured in the spine, wrist, and hip) than those active for less than an hour daily. A randomized controlled trial in young women also found that exercise increased bone density, according to a paper in the *British Medical Journal* (May 22, 1993).

Calcium is the most critical part of the diet for bone building, but here, evidence is less compelling. Some studies do show that calcium supplements increase bone mass in children and adolescents, and that the advantage remains in adulthood. A placebo-controlled trial found that members of twin pairs who took 1,000 milligrams of calcium daily had greater bone gain than those who had placebo.

Whether or not supplements can help, there's little question that you should at least get the Recommended Daily Allowance of calcium. And there's every chance you're not: it's 800 milligrams daily for adults, and 1,200 for adolescents, but the average American gets only 300 milligrams. Milk products are the most concentrated source (one cup of skim milk contains about 300 milligrams), but some green vegetables, notably spinach, kale, and collard greens, are rich in the mineral, too.

Avoid habits that rob your body of calcium. Smoking is among the worst: a University of Wisconsin study of women in their twenties and thirties, for example, found significantly lower bone density in the spines (a frequent site of osteoporotic fracture late in life) of smokers than nonsmokers. High consumption of salt, protein, caffeine, and phosphate (contained in many carbonated soft drinks) also hastens the excretion of calcium.

Young women who train intensely (such as long-distance runners) may have disturbed menstrual periods or lose them altogether, which has been associated with loss of spinal bone. If you're a serious athlete, this is something to discuss with your doctor.

AM I AT RISK FOR OSTEOPOROSIS?

Generally, women with smaller bones are at increased risk; Caucasian and Asian women are more likely to suffer from the condition than African-American women. Heredity also plays a role: if your mother suffered a hip fracture after age fifty, you're likely to have lower bone mass. Another high-risk factor is the surgical removal of the ovaries in a woman of reproductive age; this drastically reduces the primary source of estrogen which is crucial to strong bones.

Since bone loss is a lifelong process, the older you are, the greater your risk of fracture from osteoporosis. Weight apparently has a strong bearing on bone strength, too. A study of nearly ten thousand women older than sixty-five found that those who weighed more had greater bone mass (measured at the wrist and heel). Weight loss after fifty had "a substantial and adverse effect on bone mass," the authors wrote (*Annals of Internal Medicine,* May 1, 1993).

The study found that smoking (past, but especially present), caffeine consumption, and lack of weight-bearing exercise was associated with reduced bone mass, too.

SHOULD MEN WORRY ABOUT OSTEOPOROSIS?

Despite its reputation as a woman's disease, bone-thinning strikes men, too. In fact, the incidence of osteoporosis-related fractures in elderly males seems to be increasing, according to a paper in the *British Medical Journal* (May 26, 1990). Thicker bones, slower loss of bone mass, and shorter life expectancy make such fractures far less common than among women, but if men live long enough, they can run into problems.

Building bone is a lifelong process, for men as well as women, and the same exercise and diet advice holds for them, too. The *British Medical Journal* study examined forty men, ages twenty-one to seventy-nine, and found that at all ages, those who consumed the most calcium had the strongest bones.

HOW CAN I PROTECT AGAINST OSTEOPOROSIS AFTER MENOPAUSE?

Although there is a rapid loss of bone density in the years after menopause, most women will never suffer a hip or wrist fracture. The minority who will are not likely to experience pain or fracture due to osteoporosis until advanced age. For example, the median age of first hip fracture is seventy-nine years.

As more researchers begin to explore the question of why elderly people fall, it has become clear that osteoporosis is not the only explanation for hip fracture. Many elderly people fall and break their hips because of impaired vision, environmental factors (e.g., scatter rugs), inappropriate prescription drugs (e.g., Valium, barbiturates), wearing high heels, and neurological conditions. The most commonly cited factor for an increased risk of hip fracture is a fall; yet fewer than 5 percent of all falls among elderly people result in a hip fracture. Clearly, more research is needed.

If you are considering estrogen therapy specifically to prevent osteoporosis, consider the fact that researchers have yet to demonstrate that it reduces the rate of fracture. What has been demonstrated is that estrogen preserves bone density—while the woman is taking the drug. Unfortunately, the density disappears by the time a woman reaches advanced age, according to one study. David T. Felson, M.D., and colleagues at several Boston medical centers found that the current medical advice to women—take estrogen for five to ten years after menopause—does nothing to reduce the rate of hip fracture in old age (*The New England Journal of Medicine*, October 14, 1993). In this groundbreaking osteoporosis study, the first to include elderly women (ages sixty-eight to ninety-six), those who had taken estrogen in the years after menopause showed no greater bone density by the time they reached age seventy-five than those who never took estrogen. "Osteoporosis is unlikely to be prevented by taking estrogen for just a decade or so after menopause," wrote Drs. Bruce Ettinger and Deborah Grady in an editorial that accompanied this study. They described two options physicians can offer to women who want to prevent osteoporosis with estrogen therapy. Women can start taking estrogen at menopause and never stop, or they can begin estrogen therapy only after the first fracture.

(For more information on postmenopausal hormones, see Menopause.)

ARE THERE ALTERNATIVES TO ESTROGEN?

Whether calcium can slow bone loss in the few years after menopause is open to question: studies that used supplements as high as 2,000 milligrams per day have been inconsistent. But for many older women, a supplement does seem beneficial. In a study published in *The New England Journal of Medicine* (September 27, 1990), a calcium supplement slowed bone loss in women who were six or more years past menopause but only those who were consuming 400 milligrams or less before the study started. (The average daily calcium intake in this country, remember, is 300 milligrams.)

The study also found that calcium citrate malate, a form of the mineral in fortified citrus juices, worked better than calcium carbonate, which is used in many supplement pills.

Weight-bearing exercise appears to help older women preserve bone, in the same way that it helps younger women store it. According to at least one study, low-impact exercise (which carries a lower risk of injury) is as effective in this regard as high-impact workouts. Improvements were seen with as little as three twenty-minute walking sessions per week (*Medicine and Science in Sports and Exercise,* vol. 24, no. 11.

Only one other drug besides estrogen has been approved for the prevention and treatment of osteoporosis: calcitonin, a hormone that tips the balance toward bone strength by slowing the rate at which old bone is broken down. Injections of the hormone calcitonin have been shown to increase bone mass in women who already have osteoporosis, and intranasal (inhaled) doses of the hormone can slow the loss of certain kinds of bone, but not others.

Calcitonin apparently has few side effects, but it is expensive (treatment with the injected form costs about twenty-five hundred dollars yearly), and the intranasal preparation is not yet available in this country. Whether the hormone actually prevents fractures hasn't yet been shown.

Another type of drug, biphosphate, has been the focus of intense interest. These drugs inhibit bone resorption to the extent that new bone formation can actually strengthen bone already weakened by osteoporosis. Typically, the drug (etidronate is most commonly used) is taken for two weeks, then a calcium-rich diet or supplement is taken for thirteen weeks.

In a study of 423 postmenopausal women who had already suffered at least one vertebral fracture due to osteoporosis, those who took the drug for two years had less than half as many new fractures as those who took a placebo (*The New England Journal of Medicine,* July 12, 1990). A study with a smaller number of women found an even more pronounced reduction in fracture rates, over a three-year-period (*The New England Journal of Medicine,* May 3, 1990).

Etidronate has been approved as a treatment for a different bone disease (Paget's disease), but not for osteoporosis.

Vitamin D also plays a role in healthy bone metabolism, and some research suggests that an inadequate supply may be a factor in osteoporosis. A study of 138 women, ages forty-five to sixty-five, found that bone density correlated significantly with blood levels of one form of vitamin D; those with the highest levels had 5 to 10 percent more bone mass, at various sites, than those with the lowest (*British Medical Journal,* August 1, 1992).

Vitamin D is quite toxic in excess, and supplements aren't advised. You can safely ensure an adequate intake by drinking milk (each cup is enriched with one quarter of the Recommended Daily Allowance), or by getting at least half an hour of sun exposure on your face, arms, and legs every day.

SHOULD ALL WOMEN HAVE PERIODIC BONE DENSITY TESTING AFTER THEY REACH MENOPAUSE?

No. The U.S. Preventive Services Task Force recommends against the routine use of tests that measure bone density. They are expensive and time-consuming, and their usefulness in predicting fracture has not been fully assessed. As noted earlier, hip fracture is about much more than thinning bones.

◆ OVARIAN CANCER

Ovarian cancer is the fourth leading cause of cancer deaths among women (after lung, breast, and colorectal cancer). Each year, about twenty-two thousand women are diagnosed with the disease, and thirteen thousand die from it. With that said, ovarian cancer is actually an uncommon disease. One woman in seventy will develop ovarian cancer in her lifetime, but, like the more common cancers, ovarian cancer is most likely to strike in the later years. Furthermore, this much-quoted one-in-seventy statistic from the National Cancer Institute must be put in perspective. It is based on a woman's lifetime risk of developing ovarian cancer—if the woman lives to be ninety-five. The average lifespan of an American woman is seventy-nine years.

Despite considerable research and some advances in evaluation and treatment of ovarian cancer, the overall outlook hasn't improved much in recent years. According to an editorial in *Cancer* (August 15, 1991), five-year survival of women with ovarian cancer was 39 percent in 1990—compared with 36 percent in 1975. During the past decade, deaths from the disease have actually increased each year.

With such frightening statistics and the death of a high-profile personality like Gilda Radner, ovarian cancer has garnered substantial media attention. This has caused many women to overestimate their risk of developing ovarian cancer and to seek screening tests that have been judged inappropriate by a panel of experts.

HOW CAN I REDUCE MY RISK OF OVARIAN CANCER?

Women who have given birth show a lower rate of ovarian cancer, and the risk drops with each child (and, to a lesser degree, with each failed pregnancy).

Oral contraceptives, like pregnancy, allow the ovaries to "rest," which reduces the risk of developing ovarian cancer. According to a review of twenty studies in *Obstetrics and Gynecology* (October 1992), the ovarian cancer rate among women who had used the pill for five years was 46 percent lower than others.

Reduce your intake of saturated fats, which are found in meat and dairy products. Dietary fats seem to play a role in development of hormone-fed cancers like ovarian cancer. Increased intake of fibrous vegetables (but not fiber from fruit or cereals) will also cut your risk. A predominantly vegetarian diet decreases the body's level of circulating estrogens, which may reduce your chances of developing ovarian cancer.

Some researchers have implicated certain dairy foods like cottage cheese and yogurt in the development of ovarian cancer, because they contain large amounts of lactose. A Harvard study found that women with ovarian cancer had low levels of transferase, an enzyme involved in the metabolism of daily foods. The enzyme breaks down galactose, a component of the milk sugar lactose. Women with low levels of this enzyme who had a high intake of daily products had an increased incidence of ovarian cancer (*The Lancet,* July 8, 1989).

Think twice about using infertility drugs, especially if you have a family history of ovarian cancer. A two- to three-times' higher rate of ovarian cancer has been found among women who took Clomid, a drug which induces ovulation (*The New England Journal of Medicine,* September 22, 1994). This finding comes from a study of 3,837 women who underwent infertility treatment between 1974 and 1985 in Seattle. Many questions remain unanswered about the safety of the ovarian hyperstimulation drugs, which are central to the treatment of infertility; more long-term information is needed. The Seattle study followed most of the women until their early forties, whereas ovarian cancer is primarily a disease of older women. Additionally, not enough women in this study were taking the newer ovarian hyperstimulation drugs like Pergonal and Lupron. So we know nothing about the long-term effects of these drugs, which are more powerful.

IF MY MOTHER HAD OVARIAN CANCER, WILL I GET IT, TOO?

Family history is the most important risk factor in ovarian cancer: an estimated 5 percent of cases of ovarian cancer are familial, and they often occur at an earlier age than others.

If one first-degree relative (mother or sister) has the disease, your risk is 4.5 percent, roughly three times that of the general population. If two first-degree relatives had the disease, your risk rises to 7 percent; a tiny subgroup in this category carry a defective gene and are thus at very high risk of developing ovarian cancer.

Having a second-degree relative (like an aunt) with ovarian cancer also increases your risk, but far less (about double the normal).

SHOULD I BE SCREENED FOR OVARIAN CANCER?

No. Testing healthy women for early-stage ovarian cancer may harm more women than it helps. This is the conclusion of the 1994 Consensus Development Conference panel on "Ovarian Cancer: Screening, Treatment, and Followup," sponsored by the National Institutes of Health.

The two screening procedures—CA-125 (a blood test for a tumor marker) and transvaginal ultrasound imaging—advocated by some doctors in order to detect ovarian cancer in its early stages have high false-positive results (erroneous evidence of cancer), which can result in anxiety and unnecessary surgery. The panel of experts did not find evidence to suggest that women with a family history of ovarian cancer could benefit from screening. If such women insist upon screening, the panel advises that it be done only within the context of a clinical trial. (The National Cancer Institute is sponsoring such a trial.)

The CA-125 test, which measures a protein that rises in the blood of women with ovarian cancer, is extremely sensitive—when the cancer is advanced. But in the early stages (which screening is intended to detect), CA-125 is positive just one third of the time, according to a review in *Contemporary OB-GYN* (February 1993).

What's more, CA-125 can be elevated for any number of other reasons, resulting in false positives. It was suggested in an editorial in *Annals of Internal Medicine* (June 1, 1993) that if all forty-year-old women were screened with this test alone, there would be 340 false positives for each true cancer detected.

If the other test, transvaginal ultrasound imaging, is added to CA-125, screening becomes considerably more accurate: there would be only eight false positives for each cancer. But the next step to distinguish the true from the false, unfortunately, is abdominal surgery (laparotomy), which carries the usual risks of infection and death associated with all major operations and general anesthesia.

UNDER WHAT CIRCUMSTANCES SHOULD OVARY REMOVAL BE CONSIDERED?

Prophylactic oophorectomy (removal of healthy ovaries) as a means of preventing ovarian cancer is a drastic choice that is usually reserved for women with a strong family history of ovarian cancer. Unfortunately, even this is no guarantee. In an eleven-year follow-up study of 324 women with a family history of ovarian cancer who opted for this operation, six developed cancer of the peritoneum (lining of the abdominal cavity), which was indistinguishable from ovarian cancer.

Oophorectomy has its costs in terms of quality of life. Even after menopause, the ovaries continue to produce a small amount of hormones, and their loss may be felt (see Hysterectomy). The effects would be more drastic in a women still in her reproductive years (see Menopause).

Women frequently develop small, benign, cystic structures on their ovaries, which have been mistaken as an early sign of ovarian cancer. For the last twenty years, for example, it has been common practice to perform a hysterectomy/oophorectomy on any postmenopausal woman with ovaries enlarged enough to be felt manually. Increasingly, however, research has cast doubt on this custom. One study found that palpable ovaries in ten of eleven postmenopausal women represented benign conditions.

If you have an ovarian mass that requires testing, it's best to discuss the possible findings and their consequences thoroughly with your surgeon. To have the biopsy (through a laparoscope) and surgery, if any, as two separate procedures will minimize the risk of unnecessary ovary removal.

DOES ALL OVARIAN CANCER REQUIRE HYSTERECTOMY?

When we hear "ovarian cancer," we generally think of the ovarian tumors that are aggressive and often fatal. But there are also other kinds of cancer, including "borderline" tumors of low malignant potential.

These tumors have a far better prognosis. Nearly 75 percent are detected when confined to the ovary, and even if they've spread, 92 percent of women survive seven years after diagnosis. According to the National Cancer Institute, twenty years after the average low malignant potential tumor has been diagnosed, 89 percent of women are still alive.

For a borderline tumor in its early stages, hysterectomy isn't absolutely necessary; the National Cancer Institute calls removal of the affected ovary alone "adequate therapy" for women who want to retain the ability to have children; when tumors are on both ovaries, it may be possible to remove the growths (cystectomy), and leave fertility unimpaired, although the chance of recurrence is higher.

Even certain more malignant tumors, if still entirely confined to the ovary, may be treated in a way that leaves the opposite ovary, and fertility, intact. This is only an option for certain types of tumor, in the absence of any evidence of spread.

HOW WILL MY CANCER BE TREATED?

Surgery is the first step, both to diagnose ovarian cancer and determine its extent, and for treatment. With few exceptions, total hysterectomy and removal of both ovaries is the rule.

For certain cancers confined to the ovary, no further treatment is required. Other tumors that are confined to the ovary or that have spread to other pelvic organs may be treated with radiation or chemotherapy. Chemotherapy after surgery is usually offered to women with cancer that has spread, at least microscopically, beyond the pelvis. The choice of drugs differs according to the stage at which ovarian cancer is diagnosed.

Ask for the clinical trial results showing the proportion of women whose lives are extended due to the chemotherapy regimen recommended by your physician. Check the chemotherapy recommendation with the information from CancerFax (see Resources). Ask what is known about the quality of life for these long-term survivors.

WILL TAXOL HELP ME?

Taxol, a drug derived from the Pacific yew tree, aroused intense excitement several years ago as a breakthrough in treating ovarian cancers that had resisted other drugs. The drug was approved by the FDA in late 1992, for women in whom all other treatments had failed to halt the disease, but it is used more widely now.

Recent research has brought a more sober reappraisal of Taxol. The 1994 Consensus Development Conference acknowledged that most oncologists in the United States are combining Taxol with platinum as the optimal first-line chemotherapy for ovarian cancer following surgery. But the consensus conference panel "declined to lend unqualified endorsement to this approach until longer term data are available."

WILL FURTHER SURGERY SERVE ANY USEFUL PURPOSE?

Most women with advanced ovarian cancer respond fully to surgery and chemotherapy, with a normal physical examination, radiology, and CA-125 tests results. In only half, however, is all microscopic evidence of disease gone. The best way to determine how complete the response was is "second-look laparotomy," a surgical procedure to take further biopsies.

Second-look laparotomy used to be done regularly, but no longer. There is simply no curative treatment when the cancer persists, and even when the second-look biopsies seem perfectly normal, the disease recurs half the time. Second-look laparotomy is no longer performed routinely. The consensus conference panel said the operation should be reserved for participants in clinical trials and for those in whom it will affect treatment decision-making.

Resources

For a free copy of the 1994 Consensus Statement on Ovarian Cancer Screening, Treatment, and Follow-up: (800) 644-6627.

Call the National Cancer Institute's hotline to learn the latest information on cancer treatments: (800) 4-CANCER (422-6237). Or, use its CancerFax service, which also draws from the computerized data base of the National Cancer Institute. The data base can be accessed directly, if you have a fax machine with a touch-tone phone. A directory of codes for each type of cancer will be faxed to you first; request the version for health care professionals because it is more substantive, particularly where it concerns the adverse effects of treatment. To use CancerFax, dial (301) 402-5874.

The hotline at The Gilda Radner Familial Ovarian Cancer Registry will answer questions and send information: (800) OVARIAN (682-7426).

A source of information on alternative cancer therapies is:

People Against Cancer
RR #1, P.O. Box 10
Otho, IA 50569
(515) 972-4444

◆ PARKINSON'S DISEASE

An estimated half million to a million and a half Americans suffer from Parkinson's disease. Most often, symptoms first appear in the years between fifty and sixty-five, but it may begin in the forties or even the thirties.

The cause is progressive destruction of neurons in a specific part of the brain (the substantia nigra) that regulates movement. The symptoms are movement abnormalities: most commonly, trembling (of hands, most often), slowness, muscle rigidity, unstable posture, and abnormal gait. In its earliest stages, symptoms are often a vague slowness, weakness, and fatigue that are mistakenly attributed to aging.

What causes the neuron destruction isn't known. Heredity is probably not a factor, except perhaps in very rare cases (several families have been reported where the disorder runs rampant). The possible role of environmental toxins is controversial. Unusually high rates of Parkinson's have been observed in some communities that share possibly contaminated well water, and in areas where certain herbicides are intensively used. Occupational exposures to manganese, mercury, or carbon disulfide can cause Parkinson-like symptoms.

HOW IS PARKINSON'S DISEASE DIAGNOSED?

A definitive diagnosis can be made only by analysis of brain tissue after death, and the accuracy of diagnosis through physical examination and tests is far from perfect. According to an editorial in *The Lancet* (May 23, 1992), what had been diagnosed as Parkinson's in one series of a hundred people was actually something else in one fourth of the cases.

Early in the disease, especially, only one or two of the basic symptoms may appear, and even the most distinctive symptoms aren't surefire indicators. About 15 to 25 percent of people with Parkinson's have no tremor, for example, and about half of people with tremor don't have Parkinson's.

Other conditions that may be confused with early Parkinson's include depression and hypothyroidism (which cause slowness), and stroke (most

Parkinson's symptoms, like the aftermath of stroke, occur first on one side of the body). About 15 to 20 percent of people with Parkinson's suffer memory loss and other mental problems, which can lead to a misdiagnosis of Alzheimer's disease.

Brain tumors or a blood clot in the brain may produce many of the same symptoms as Parkinson's disease, as can head injury. Some tests like CAT scans or electroencephalogram may assist the diagnosis of Parkinson's, chiefly by ruling out other brain disorders.

Overall, about 85 percent of people with the major symptoms of Parkinson's actually have the disease.

AM I TAKING DRUGS THAT MAY BE RESPONSIBLE?

Parkinsonism (the symptoms of Parkinson's disease) may be a side effect of many medications, including certain blood pressure drugs, the antiemetic prochlorperazine (Compazine), and metoclopramide (Reglan), a drug used for gastrointestinal disorders.

Neuroleptics, principally used for schizophrenia, very often cause Parkinsonian symptoms, which typically disappear when the drug is discontinued or the dose is lowered.

WHAT MEDICATIONS DO YOU PRESCRIBE FOR PARKINSON'S—AND WHEN?

The neurons that dwindle in number from Parkinson's are chiefly those that operate with a particular brain chemical, dopamine. So the most effective treatment used by most doctors is a drug that the body turns into dopamine: levodopa (generally combined with another chemical, carbidopa or benserazide, that allows more levodopa to reach the brain).

Levodopa (L-dopa) usually reduces most Parkinson's symptoms markedly when first used, but it has its limitations. The drug doesn't slow the progression of the disease: with time, the therapeutic response gradually wanes, while side effects (such as nausea, vomiting, heart rhythm abnormalities, and uncontrolled movements) become more of a problem.

L-dopa typically works at maximum effectiveness for three to five years of therapy. The response to the drug is no longer adequate, or adverse effects have become intolerable, for about four patients out of five after ten years. Some believe the drug may actually hasten the destruction of neurons.

For this reason, many doctors don't use any drugs at all until symptoms significantly interfere with social or working life, or begin with a dopamine agonist, such as bromocriptine or pergolide, that increases the activity of the neurotransmitter. These drugs are more expensive and less effective than L-dopa. According to a review article in *The New England Journal of Medicine* (September 30, 1993), on the basis of current information, "no compelling argument can be made for choosing any one of [these] approaches."

Some neurologists combine L-dopa with a dopamine agonist, which makes it possible to use a smaller dose of each. "For most of the duration of the illness . . . relatively low doses of two drugs are better than high doses of one drug," the *Journal* article concludes.

Another group of drugs that can sometimes relieve early Parkinson's symptoms are anticholinergics, which reduce the activity of acetylcholine, another neurotransmitter, correcting its balance with dopamine. Among these are benztropine, trihexyphenidyl, and some of the same antihistamines used for allergy symptoms, and certain antidepressants.

HOW CAN I REDUCE L-DOPA SIDE EFFECTS?

What frequently happens after several years of levodopa is the "wearing-off phenomenon"—symptoms break through or worsen as the time approaches for the next dose. Or there's the "off-on phenomenon," abrupt alternations between uncontrolled movement and immobility. If the dose is raised to overcome these fluctuations, other side effects may become intolerable.

A controlled-release preparation of levodopa-carbidopa maintains a steadier level of the drugs, and keeps the response less erratic. It may be used in combination with the standard form. It has been suggested that sustained-release levodopa spares the brain damage by avoiding repeated swings between high and low serum concentrations of the drug. "Further studies are needed to confirm or refute this association," according to *The New England Journal of Medicine* review article.

In about 20 percent of people, the response to levodopa is influenced by diet. Taking the drug before meals and avoiding high-protein foods before evening may moderate fluctuations. Solid food, especially protein-containing foods, delay the absorption of levodopa.

WHEN ARE DEPRENYL OR VITAMIN E PRESCRIBED?

In recent years, considerable interest has surrounded the possible use of deprenyl (also called selegiline) and tocopherol (vitamin E) in so-called neuroprotective therapy. In different ways, both compounds aim to prevent damage to nerve cells by oxidation caused by free radicals, such as peroxides and superoxides, which are implicated in Parkinson's and other degenerative diseases. In theory at least, both compounds could slow the progression of early Parkinson's disease.

In a large multicenter, controlled clinical trial of these approaches (the DATATOP study), eight hundred people with early Parkinson's were randomly assigned to groups that received deprenyl, tocopherol, both drugs, or placebo.

After follow-up that averaged fourteen months, deprenyl significantly delayed the onset of disability requiring L-dopa therapy, compared with placebo. Tocopherol, on the other hand, had no apparent effect, either alone or combined with deprenyl (*The New England Journal of Medicine,* January 21, 1993). Side effects with both drugs were neither frequent nor serious.

Just how deprenyl delays disability, and whether it actually protects neurons from damage is unclear, the authors said. Whether the drug, which is expensive, should be routinely prescribed early in the course of Parkinson's disease is a matter of some dispute.

DO YOU CONSIDER SURGERY AN OPTION?

Thalamotomy, surgery to destroy a small part of the brain, can reduce tremor on one side of the body, but it has no effect on slowness, rigidity, or other symptoms, and may worsen speech. Among potential adverse effects are weakness, numbness, uncontrolled movements or memory loss. The procedure is used, if at all, for some younger patients who are seriously disabled by a tremor that resists all medical therapy.

The possibility of transplanting fetal brain cells to replace those destroyed by Parkinson's disease, or cells that produce dopamine from one's own adrenal gland, has understandably fired the imagination in recent years.

Both approaches have brought about some benefits in experimental settings. According to a review article in the *Mayo Clinic Proceedings* (June 1993), among persons treated by fetal transplantation, eight had no or mild improvement; eleven had moderate improvement; and fourteen showed marked improvement, which was maintained for up to four years. A third surgical approach, adrenal to brain transplant, has been poorer, largely due to graft failure.

Transplant must be regarded as highly experimental. "Cerebral transplantation has considerable promise as a treatment strategy," the Mayo Clinic review said. "The experience in human and animal studies, however, suggests that many unanswered questions need to be addressed. Therefore, this exciting therapeutic adventure is only in the earliest stages."

ARE THERE NONDRUG WAYS TO MAKE LIFE EASIER?

The benefits of physical therapy haven't been confirmed by many controlled studies, but most people think that regular exercise is important to prevent weakness and muscle wasting from worsening the actual symptoms of Parkinson's. It's necessary to tailor your exercise to your capacities and disabilities: walking and swimming are ideal for some, but balance or stiffness problems can make them hazardous without supervision.

A physical or occupational therapist can provide useful instruction and advice about getting around safely despite disability, and adaptive equipment (such as railings, dressing aids, and specially designed eating utensils and kitchenware) can help you maintain an independent life.

Resources

You can get information about Parkinson's disease, support groups, and sources of special equipment from:

National Parkinson Foundation, Inc.
(800) 327-4545
In Florida, (800) 433-7022

American Parkinson Disease Association
(800) 223-APDA (2732)
In New York, (718) 981-8001

• PELVIC INFLAMMATORY DISEASE

Pelvic inflammatory disease (PID) is not the kind of illness people like to talk about; three times out of four, it is sexually transmitted, often by the organism that causes gonorrhea. Yet because it's common, potentially serious, and largely preventable, PID isn't something to ignore.

About a million women yearly have episodes of PID, sometimes with mild symptoms. No matter how mild or severe their attack, one woman in four who has PID will suffer severe consequences: they are seven times more likely than other women to have an ectopic pregnancy, and one in eight will be infertile. Repeat infections, which multiply the risk of complications, are more likely.

PID is an infection of the female reproductive organs—the fallopian tubes, ovaries, and lining of the uterus—caused by a variety of organisms. Three quarters of the time these include chlamydia and gonococcus, which are sexually transmitted.

When the fallopian tubes are involved, they may become scarred, which can block the descent of the egg necessary for normal conception. Fertilized eggs are more likely to be implanted in infection-scarred tubes— which means ectopic pregnancy, with its risk of life-threatening rupture and hemorrhage.

HOW DO YOU KNOW IT'S PID?

The only accurate way to diagnose PID is by laparoscopy—a tubular fiberoptic instrument allows the doctor to visually inspect the pelvic organs for evidence of infection. But this is an invasive surgical procedure, and it's generally used only when treatment runs into trouble.

For the most part, doctors conclude PID by inference. The classic symptoms are severe pain on both sides of the lower abdomen, tenderness on examination, and fever as high as 104. But symptoms can be more subtle, with milder pain and low fever, particularly when caused by chlamydia. A white blood cell count and other lab tests can help establish the diagnosis.

A sensitive pregnancy test will rule out ectopic pregnancy, which can cause similar symptoms.

Another factor in diagnosing PID is you. "Ranking in importance only after the signs and symptoms of the current episode is a patient's sexual history," according to an article in *Contemporary OB-GYN* (November 1992).

Basically, the risk factors are the same as for gonorrhea and chlamydia. Women younger than thirty and those who began sexual activity early in life are more likely to have PID. The risk rises with the number of past sexual partners, according to an article in the *Journal of the American Medical Association* (November 13, 1991).

Douching can also increase the risk. A study of nearly a thousand women found that those who douched three or more times a month had 3.6 times as much PID as those who douched less than once a month or not at all. The more they douched, the higher their risk (*Journal of the American Medical Association*, April 11, 1990).

It's possible that douching kills harmless bacteria that normally live in the vagina and keep pathogens in check. Or douching could flush microbes up from the vagina and cervix into the uterus, where they can establish an infection. The study found the risk of PID higher for women who used commercial preparations (which might kill harmless bacteria more effectively) than homemade solutions like vinegar and water.

SHOULD I BE IN THE HOSPITAL?

PID should be treated quickly and aggressively, to prevent the formation of abscesses that might require surgery, and to keep tubal damage that could impair fertility to a minimum.

This means substantial doses of antibiotics. Most experts recommend drug combinations, because the infection is likely to involve more than one organism. Once gonococcus or chlamydia initiate the infection, the pelvis becomes vulnerable to other microbes that are best treated with different drugs.

According to the 1991 *Journal of the American Medical Association* article, many experts believe that any woman with PID should be treated in the hospital, so that she can receive intravenous antibiotics and have her condition closely observed. This is particularly important for women who want to protect their ability to have children. Especially with today's heightened consciousness of medical costs, however, many women with milder PID are treated as outpatients.

The Centers for Disease Control advocate hospitalization under certain conditions. Among them: when the diagnosis is unclear, particularly if appendicitis or ectopic pregnancy can't be ruled out; if there's the possibility of pelvic abscess; or when the woman is pregnant or an adolescent.

HOW CAN I PROTECT MY FERTILITY?

Prompt diagnosis and treatment will eliminate the infection, "but apparently only have a marginal impact on PID sequelae such as infertility, particularly if tubal damage already exists when treatment is started," according to the paper in the *Journal of the American Medical Association*. Tubal scarring can be caused by quite modest attacks of PID, even those so mild that they escape notice. Up to half of women with tubal damage do not recall ever having had PID.

One way to keep PID from developing is by treating infections in the cervix and vagina before they can ascend to the upper reproductive organs. Women with symptoms suggesting gonorrhea or chlamydia who are treated quickly and adequately are at reduced risk for subsequent PID, according to the *Journal* paper.

Early sexual activity apparently increases the risk for PID, not only because of increased exposure, but also because very young women probably have fewer protective antibodies, and their cervical mucus is more easily penetrated by the pathogens. This is an age when the potential consequences for fertility are particularly severe.

At any age, limiting the number of sex partners and choosing them on the basis of sexual history will reduce the chance of becoming infected with a sexually transmitted disease (STD) that can lead to PID.

If you've ever had PID, your chances of another episode are heightened. Precautions valuable for others are essential for you.

WHAT'S THE BEST CONTRACEPTIVE FOR ME?

Sexual intercourse is the most common way to be infected with PID, not only because it introduces the responsible microbes but also because it effectively gets them to the pelvic organs. "Many organisms that alone do not seem to be sufficiently mobile may ascend the genital tract on the back of spermatozoa" is how a paper in the *British Medical Journal* (April 28, 1990) put it.

For this reason, a barrier contraceptive—condom, cervical cap, or diaphragm—is a good choice for prevention. Condoms appear to be very effective in blocking the bacteria responsible for PID, and the diaphragm and cervical cap also seem to decrease the risk of disease. Adding a spermicide to a barrier contraceptive may further increase its effectiveness.

Oral contraceptives appear to reduce the risk of PID caused by chlamydia, but not by gonococcus or other organisms.

Considerable attention in recent years has surrounded the association between PID and intrauterine devices (IUDs). Data collected during the 1980s suggested that this means of contraception doubled the risk of PID. Today, the consensus is that IUDs increase the disease just slightly, if at all, at least in women who are at low risk of STDs. Modern devices that are medicated with copper or hormones apparently carry less risk than older ones (*The Lancet,* March 28, 1992).

The incidence of PID rises temporarily after the IUD is inserted (for a time that is estimated as twenty days to four months), which is a good argument for using a device that can be left in place for as long as possible.

Whether or not IUDs actually increase the risk of PID, they don't offer the protective benefits of barrier contraceptives.

Resources

Call the National STD Hotline, sponsored by the American Social Health Association (North Carolina), (800) 227-8922.

◆ PREMENSTRUAL SYNDROME (PMS)

Many women experience some physical discomfort and/or emotional distress as their menstrual periods approach. For an estimated 5 percent, it's severe enough to disrupt normal life, and merits the term premenstrual syndrome (PMS).

PMS is defined extremely broadly: more than a hundred and fifty different symptoms have been ascribed to it. The most common physical complaints are abdominal bloating, breast pain, headache, dizziness, and muscle aches. Frequent psychological symptoms are tension, depression, irritability, and anger.

Whether PMS is a real illness has been an ongoing controversy, fueled as much by political as medical disagreement. It has been suggested that its recognition legitimizes the "raging hormone" rationale for denying women access to positions of power; on the other hand, argue others, failure to recognize PMS denies real suffering the serious attention it deserves. The status of PMS could have legal repercussions (as a defense in criminal cases, or as a factor in child-custody disputes).

HOW DO I KNOW THAT WHAT I HAVE IS PMS?

Although PMS is, by definition, related to events of the second half of the menstrual cycle, presumably involving ovulation, no biological pathway has been mapped out. "To date, attempts to find consistent hormonal or other biochemical abnormalities in women suffering severe premenstrual symptoms have failed," said an editorial in *New Scientist* (July 31, 1993).

The condition is diagnosed more by timing than symptoms. PMS occurs during the second half of the menstrual cycle, lasts up to two weeks, and disappears, often abruptly, at the time of menstruation. If your symptoms are more constant, you don't have PMS, or you have something in addition to it.

The best way to track your symptoms is to keep a diary or chart, recording them day by day for several months. Merely thinking back and trying to reconstruct the pattern from memory leads to overdiagnosis of PMS, according to an article in *Contemporary OB/GYN* (January 1994).

COULD MY SYMPTOMS BE CAUSED BY SOMETHING ELSE?

Given the diversity of PMS symptoms, it's unsurprising that many other disorders often must be ruled out. These include thyroid disease, diabetes, endocrine disorders, and depression. An evaluation for PMS should include basic laboratory tests to investigate these and other possibilities.

DO YOU TREAT PMS AS A PSYCHIATRIC ILLNESS?

The most recent PMS controversy surrounded the inclusion of "premenstrual dysphoric disorder" in the 1994 edition of the American Psychiatric Association's *Diagnostic and Statistical Manual IV* (DSM-IV) as a kind of depression. This definition focused on the emotional symptoms that resemble those of depression (see Depression), and specified that they must be pronounced enough to severely interfere with functioning. (The diagnosis also was included in an appendix, indicating it needs further study.)

The categorization, many think, is a two-edged sword. On the one hand, it recognizes the seriousness of PMS; on the other, it can carry the stigma associated with emotional illness. How the concept affects treatment of PMS depends in large part on the extent to which you and your doctor are free from the ignorant bias that sees psychiatric disorders as shameful and blameworthy, and able to accept their reality as compassionately as you would a medical disease.

CAN MY USE OF NONDRUG APPROACHES HELP PMS?

PMS often improves substantially with changes in lifestyle, exercise, and diet, and with simple strategies to reduce stress. "Such approaches are more appropriate for many women than are hormones, surgery, and psychiatric consultation," according to a review article in the *British Medical Journal* (December 4, 1993).

The *Contemporary OB/GYN* article recommends small regular meals consisting of fresh foods, with the emphasis on whole grains, fruits, and vegetables. Fat, sugar, caffeine, and refined foods should be limited—good dietary advice that goes beyond controlling PMS. Many women have a craving for carbohydrates at this time, and this nutrient may help ease symptoms by increasing blood levels of the neurotransmitter serotonin, which may be in short supply.

Vitamins and minerals (vitamin A, B_6, calcium, and magnesium) and other dietary supplements (evening primrose oil) appear to help some women with PMS, although evidence supporting their effectiveness is mixed, according to the *British Medical Journal* article. In one double-blind study of thirty-two women, magnesium supplements improved depression and mood swings (*Obstetrics and Gynecology,* August 1991). In another, twenty-eight women who took supplements of magnesium and vitamin B_6 had significantly less severe symptoms than those who took a placebo (*Journal of the American College of Nutrition,* 1991, vol. 10, no. 5).

Vitamin B_6 and magnesium can be toxic in large doses; if you take a supplement, make sure it's at a safe level. A safe dose of vitamin B_6 is 50 milligrams per day, according to Patricia Hausman, M.S, author of *The Right Dose: How to Take Vitamins and Minerals Safely* (New York: Ballantine, 1987), but doses in the 50- to 200-milligram range are well tolerated by many people. As for a safe dose of magnesium, Hausaman found that a combined intake of 1,000 milligrams from diet and supplements should be safe for anyone without kidney impairment.

Evening primrose oil appears helpful in alleviating breast tenderness, but not significantly effective in easing other PMS symptoms.

Women who are in good aerobic condition appear to suffer less PMS than those who are less fit. This may be related to the physical effects of exercise (such as release of beta-endorphins—the body's own natural pain-killers), or to the general stress-reducing benefits of exercise.

DOES STRESS WORSEN PMS?

Like virtually all physical and emotional disorders, PMS can be worsened by stress—at home, on the job, or anywhere else. The life-disrupting symptoms of PMS, in their turn, can cause considerable stress, creating a vicious cycle.

What helps reduce stress is largely a personal matter: the smorgasbord of remedies runs the gamut from meditation to psychotherapy to hot baths to joining support groups. Whatever works for you is worth the time and effort; it will help your ability to cope with PMS and perhaps reduce the symptoms themselves. If your doctor can't help you work out a stress-reduction program, ask him or her to refer you to someone who can.

ARE DRUGS USED FOR PMS?

Many medications have been tried, but none has been proven useful for all the symptoms of PMS. Certain drugs, however, can help some women with some aspects of the disorder. Certain diuretics (usually spironolactone) may relieve abdominal bloating and breast tenderness—but only if there is actual water retention, as evidenced by periodic weight gain, according to the *British Medical Journal* article. Among the possible risks of spironolactone are masculinization effects in women, such as deepening of the voice and excessive hair growth.

Some doctors prescribe bromocriptine (Parlodel) to reduce breast tenderness, but this is a drug approved for relief of symptoms of Parkinson's disease and several endocrine disorders. Its safety and efficacy is not proven for breast tenderness. To use it for this purpose would be like killing a flea with a sledge hammer. The side effects of spironolactone and bromocriptine could be worse than the symptoms of PMS.

Considerable interest has surrounded the use of the newer antidepressants, such as fluoxetine (Prozac), which seem particularly helpful for the psychological suffering of PMS. These drugs specifically increase activity of serotonin, which appears diminished by the disorder.

In one double-blind, placebo-controlled trial, sixteen women with severe PMS were given fluoxetine for three months, then placebo (or vice versa). Fifteen had a "good" or "very good" response to fluoxetine, compared with three to placebo. Psychological, behavioral, and physical symptoms all improved, to the point where on average, they were scarcely worse than in a control group that didn't have PMS (*British Medical Journal*, August 8, 1992). Given the short duration of this trial, the use of fluoxetine for PMS must be considered experimental.

WHAT ABOUT HORMONES?

The association of PMS symptoms with the menstrual cycle leads naturally to the assumption that sex hormones are to blame. But repeated studies have never found consistent differences in hormone levels between women with and without PMS. It seems that a disturbed response to hormones, rather than abnormalities in the hormones themselves, is more likely responsible for PMS (*Journal of the American Medical Association,* October 14, 1992).

The hormone progesterone, particularly in the form of a vaginal suppository, is the most widely used treatment for PMS, despite its ineffectiveness. This was proven at the University of Pennsylvania in a well-designed clinical trial of 168 women who received progesterone in 400 milligrams, 800 milligrams, or placebo (*Journal of the American Medical Association,* July 18, 1990).

WHAT CAN BE DONE FOR VERY SEVERE PMS?

Gonadotropin-releasing agonist drugs and Depo-Provera, two treatments prescribed for intractable, life-disrupting PMS, have not been proven safe or effective for this purpose. These drugs are approved by the FDA for other purposes, such as palliative treatment of certain forms of advanced cancer. When prescribed for severe PMS, this is what is called an "off-label" usage. It is unethical for a doctor to prescribe these drugs for PMS without informing you of the complete lack of information about their safety and efficacy for this condition.

Gonadotropin-releasing agonist drugs will inhibit ovarian activity altogether and produce a "medical hysterectomy" which is similar to, but perhaps more extreme than, those of menopause (see Menopause and Hysterectomy). Neither these drugs nor Lupron are suitable for long-term use, and symptoms generally return quickly when they're stopped.

Surgical removal of the ovaries and uterus is a drastic step and is rarely, if ever, an option, except for women who are considering the surgery for other reasons (see Hysterectomy). Along with menstruation, PMS ends naturally at menopause.

◆ PROSTATE CANCER

Cancer of the prostate is something of an enigma. In recent years, a blood test to detect it early has become widely available—yet many experts have serious doubts about the wisdom of screening. The incidence of prostate cancer appears to have risen enormously, but it may actually be little if at all more common than before.

Despite a great increase in surgical and radiation treatments for the condition, mortality rates have not fallen. And a convincing argument can be made that many men will do as well or better with no treatment at all.

What is clear, however, is the magnitude of the problem. An estimated 165,000 men were diagnosed with prostate cancer in a recent year, and 35,000 died of the disease—making it second only to lung cancer as a cause of cancer deaths among men. The average age of diagnosis is seventy.

AM I AT RISK?

An estimated 13 percent of men will be diagnosed with prostate cancer at some point in their lives, and 3 percent will die of it. The risk rises steeply with age: according to the National Cancer Institute, the annual rate is 22.7 per 100,000 men under age sixty-five, and 884.1 cases per 100,000 older men.

Race is a significant factor. African Americans are about a third more likely to get prostate cancer than whites (in fact, their rate may be the highest in the world), and if they develop the disease, they are more likely to die of it. Asian Americans are at considerably lower risk.

Genetics apparently plays a role. If your father or a brother has had prostate cancer, your chances of getting it are significantly increased.

HOW CAN I PROTECT MYSELF?

The impact of lifestyle and environment on prostate cancer risk is less clear. Epidemiological research generally finds higher rates of prostate cancer in groups that consume more fat, particularly animal fat, but other studies are inconsistent. One recent study of over fifty thousand men that appeared in the *Journal of the National Cancer Institute* (October 6, 1993) linked fat consumption to advanced prostate cancer; red meat, in particular, was associated with more than double the incidence. It may be that some fats don't initiate cancer, but do promote its progression.

Another study, of fourteen thousand Seventh Day Adventists, associated certain vegetables—beans, lentils, peas, tomatoes, raisins, dates, and other dried fruits—with significantly *reduced* prostate cancer risk (*Cancer,* August 1, 1989).

WILL VASECTOMY INCREASE MY RISK?

A number of studies have suggested that it will, but the magnitude of the increase is by no means clear. In a study that followed nearly fifty thousand men for four years, those who had had a vasectomy were about 50 percent more likely than others to develop prostate cancer; among those who had undergone the procedure at least twenty-two years previously, the risk was higher (*Journal of the American Medical Association,* February 17, 1993).

A large multiethnic study conducted in the U.S. and Canada contradicted this finding. It found no increased incidence of prostate cancer among men who had undergone a vasectomy (*Journal of the National Cancer Institute,* May 3, 1995).

HOW IS THE PSA TEST USED FOR SCREENING?

For years, the National Cancer Institute and American Cancer Society have recommended yearly digital rectal examination for men over forty: the doctor inserts his finger into the rectum and feels the prostate for lumps and texture changes that indicate a possible tumor. Several years ago, a blood test, prostate specific antigen (PSA), became widely available.

Prostate specific antigen is a protein secreted by the gland. Cancer leads to significantly greater blood levels of this antigen. But so, for that matter, do some far more common conditions like infection and prostate enlargement (benign prostatic hyperplasia). Because there are so many false positives with PSA, it is at best a screening test that suggests the need for further investigation such as ultrasound and biopsy.

When are more tests indicated? Normal PSA is below 4 nanograms/milliliter (ng/ml). According to Fred Lee, M.D., clinical professor of radiology and urology at Wayne State University in Detroit, readings above 10 ng/ml indicate a high likelihood of cancer and warrant a biopsy. But between 4 and 10 ng/ml is a gray area. Dr. Lee strongly questions the common practice of many urologists to follow up such findings with an immediate ultrasound and biopsy.

PSA is simply not very accurate. In addition to yielding false-positive results, it remains normal in 40 percent of men who do have cancer. Even among health organizations, there is disagreement about the value of screening: the American Cancer Society and the American Urological Association advise yearly PSA tests for all men over fifty; the National Cancer Institute and the U.S. Preventive Services Task Force do not. (The NCI has initiated a randomized prospective study on the effect of screening on prostate cancer mortality.)

After reviewing all relevant articles on screening, a paper in *Annals of Internal Medicine* (November 1, 1993) concluded that "the net benefit from widespread screening is unclear . . . Although screening for prostate cancer has the potential to save lives, because of possible overdiagnosis, screening and subsequent therapy could actually have a net *unfavorable* effect on mortality or quality of life or both."

WHEN IS A BIOPSY INDICATED?

When PSA levels are elevated, the usual next step is an ultrasound examination and, if indicated, a biopsy of prostate tissue. The trouble is, many urologists do their own ultrasound without much expertise in interpreting the findings, and then rush to biopsy. Dr. Lee says: "What you've got is all these urologists out there who have ultrasound equipment, and they've got this [elevated] PSA, and they don't know what the hell to do with it, so they're bringing all these poor souls in and biopsying them."

Unnecessary biopsy isn't just a waste of time: the procedure carries some definite risks. To obtain a prostate tissue specimen, a needle is inserted via the rectum, which is loaded with bacteria, so infection of the prostate is very likely. Prophylactic antibiotics, commonly given, aren't very effective because the prostate concentrates drugs poorly. A low-grade infection may linger, raising PSA levels still higher, which leads to a second biopsy.

"So they're in a cycle," Dr. Lee says. One third of the men he sees are referred to him after just such a cycle.

Used appropriately, ultrasound can eliminate many unnecessary biopsies. In a study that appeared in *Cancer* (March 1, 1992), Dr. Lee described an approach that correlates PSA with prostate size. A skilled interpreter can determine the volume of the gland by ultrasound, and thus identify the many elevated PSA readings that are caused by prostate enlargement and don't require biopsy.

It's important to remember, too, that prostate cancer is typically slow-growing, so biopsy isn't an urgent matter. "You can have a repeat PSA in four to six months," Dr. Lee advises. "Don't let anyone biopsy you just because your PSA is elevated. The next step should be an ultrasound to have the volume of your gland measured."

There are doubts, for that matter, about the need and effectiveness of treatment that raise questions about the value of the whole early-detection enterprise.

IF I HAVE EARLY PROSTATE CANCER, WHAT WILL I GAIN FROM TREATMENT?

Early cancer of the prostate usually has no symptoms. Nearly one third of men over fifty have some cancer cells in that organ, detectable by microscopic examination. This rises to half of men over seventy, and 90 percent over ninety. But it is often an extremely slow-growing cancer: so slow that the vast majority of men who have latent cancer eventually die of other causes, often without ever having had symptoms. It is estimated that only one in three hundred and eighty men with such evidence of prostate cancer actually dies of the disease.

A minority of prostate cancers, however, are aggressive; they spread to other organs and cause death. Right now, there is no way to distinguish the accuracy of one type from the other, in the early stages. Most important, there is no evidence that early intervention is effective even for the fast-growing prostate cancer.

Prostate cancer incidence has increased continually, by an average of 3.3 percent per year since 1975, and took a quantum leap of 16 percent in the single year from 1989 to 1990. To a great extent, this reflected increased detection, first from tissue specimens obtained as transurethral resection of the prostate became more widely used for enlarged prostate, and then as a result of increased PSA testing, according to the *Journal of the National Cancer Institute* (June 16, 1993).

Many of these cancers were symptomless. Did early detection save lives? According to the National Cancer Institute, five-year survival of men diagnosed with prostate cancer rose from 66.7 percent in 1974–76 to 77.6 percent in 1983–89. But it is impossible to say how much of the apparent improvement was due to treatment, and how much due to the fact that detection at an early stage simply increases the time between diagnosis and death (what investigators call "lead-time bias").

Actually, the mortality rate from prostate cancer (deaths per hundred thousand men) has increased steadily from 1973 to the present, by about 1 percent per year. Since 1986, the rise has been 2.6 percent per year. Some of this is probably due to increasing numbers of men surviving to the years when prostate cancer is most common, and also to the fact that, with increasing detection, more deaths are attributed to cancer that may actually be due to other causes. It is also possible that more men are dying of the treatment for prostatic cancer. Death rates from this cancer have not dropped in states with the highest rates of PSA screening and radical prostatectomy (*Journal of the National Cancer Institute,* September 21, 1994).

DOES TREATMENT OF EARLY PROSTATE CANCER MAKE A DIFFERENCE?

This is a question that challenges some of our most cherished beliefs about the value of medical care.

But it is unavoidable. The standard treatment for cancer confined to the prostate (about 60 percent of tumors) is radical prostatectomy—removal of the entire prostate—or radiation therapy.

Neither treatment method is without serious drawbacks. According to a report in the *Journal of the American Medical Association* (May 26, 1993), 8 percent of men ages sixty to seventy-five suffer cardiovascular complications within thirty days after surgery, and 2 percent die. Impotence was almost inevitable with the older prostatectomy procedure, and incontinence was common, but with newer "nerve-sparing" techniques 50 to 80 percent of men recover sexual capacity within a year, and incontinence is also significantly less common. Radiation can damage tissue around the prostate and carries a similar risk of impotence.

The procedures are comparably effective. A literature review in *The New England Journal of Medicine* (January 24, 1991) found that 90 percent of men survived at follow-up fifteen years later.

This sounds convincing, until you realize that men with the same early stage of prostate cancer apparently do just as well with *no* treatment. In a classic Swedish study of 223 men who received no treatment at all for cancer confined to the prostate, 8.5 percent had died of the disease ten years after diagnosis.

According to the *Journal of the American Medical Association* article, "watchful waiting" (doing nothing unless there is sign of cancer spread, at which time hormonal therapy is indicated) is a reasonable alternative. "In reviewing the medical literature, we could find no definitive evidence that either radiation therapy or radical prostatectomy is superior to watchful waiting (with delayed hormonal therapy) for patients with clinical stage A or B prostatic carcinoma," the authors said.

In deciding what course to follow, age is a factor. According to the authors' analyses, men over seventy gained, on average, less than six months of additional life by aggressive treatment, and this benefit was overshadowed by the potential for complications. "One finding is very clear," they said. "Men aged seventy-five years and older are not likely to benefit from either radiation therapy or radical prostatectomy when compared with watchful waiting."

Men under seventy gained an average of a year of life. Even for them, the authors said, watchful waiting should be considered a reasonable alternative. Men in their fifties and sixties are less likely to die or become impotent as a result of the surgery, and it seems logical that they have more to gain. But there simply is not enough information to prove that surgery does more good than watchful waiting.

In view of these conclusions, the dramatic increase in radical prostatectomy in recent years (partly a result of improvements in technique) is questionable. A study in the same *Journal* issue found that the rate of prostatectomies increased almost sixfold from 1984 to 1990. The increase among men over seventy-five was particularly striking.

CAN ANYTHING HELP MORE ADVANCED CANCER?

When cancer has spread beyond the prostate, surgery is no longer an option. There is no curative treatment; the aim is to slow the progress of the cancer and relieve its symptoms.

The standard approaches are radiation (if the cancer is still restricted to nearby tissues); hormonal therapy; surgical removal of the testicles; or administering female hormones, or antiandrogen drugs. Since the growth of cancer derived from the prostate is fueled by male hormones, no matter where it has spread, these strategies can often slow or reverse the cancer's progression.

Survival with these more advanced stages of cancer depends largely on how far the disease has spread. If it is still "regional," involving lymph nodes in the area, 80 percent of men are still living five years later; if it has gone further by the time it is diagnosed, 30 percent have survived at five years.

Resources

Use CancerFax to receive a printout on prostate cancer from the computerized database of the National Cancer Institute. You will need access to a fax machine with an attached telephone. Dial (301) 402-5874 on a touch-tone phone and receive a faxed report on state-of-the-art treatments for prostate cancer. Request the physicians' version.

◆ PSORIASIS

Psoriasis is not life-threatening and is rarely severe enough to be disabling. But the discomfort and distress it can cause makes the "heartbreak" image used to hawk remedies for this skin disease seem no exaggeration. Two to eight million Americans endure the itching, scaling, and unsightly red plaques of psoriasis, which may cover a tiny bit of skin or nearly the entire body.

Heredity and environment both play a role in psoriasis. What runs in families, apparently, is the tendency to develop the disease. Depending on various other factors, that tendency may never be expressed—you might go your entire life without an outbreak of psoriasis—it may be a minor annoyance, or a lifelong struggle.

Typically, psoriasis waxes and wanes in extent and severity: change of seasons, skin injury, or stress may trigger it, or it may flare and disappear without apparent cause.

What goes awry in psoriasis is apparently an acceleration of the process that renews skin cells. Normally, the cycle that brings cells from the deep layers of the skin to the surface where they are shed takes nearly a month; in psoriasis, the time is cut to three to four days. The excessive skin cells accumulate on the skin's surface and form scaly plaques. The increased blood supply to the skin demanded by the accelerated process causes the plaques to look red.

IS PSORIASIS TREATABLE?

There is no real cure for psoriasis—once you have it, you have it—but a broad spectrum of treatments can relieve symptoms and may induce remissions.

When the lesions are localized to limited parts of the body, topical treatment with creams and lotions is often enough. The most commonly prescribed preparations are corticosteroids, which reduce inflammation and redness. However, corticosteroids are good only for short-term relief;

long-term use decreases their effectiveness and increases the risk of side effects, such as skin atrophy. For these reasons, use of corticosteroids requires expert supervision. Another helpful topical treatment is coal tar, which can relieve itching and improve the skin's appearance. Though its exact mechanism of action is unknown, coal tar is thought to work by slowing down cell reproduction.

More extensive, severe, and resistant psoriasis is often treated with systemic drugs, including some powerful ones like retinoids (chemicals related to vitamin A), methotrexate (an anticancer drug), and even cyclosporin, which was developed to assist in organ transplants. Retinoids affect psoriasis by slowing down the rate of skin cell multiplication. Methotrexate and cyclosporin work through their immunosuppressant abilities, which help reduce inflammation. One or another of these drugs can almost always effect dramatic improvement or induce remission in even the most formidable psoriasis. But all have the potential to cause serious side effects; deaths have been reported with the use of methotrexate in the treatment of psoriasis, for example.

CAN SUNLIGHT HELP?

Most people with psoriasis have discovered that exposing affected parts to sunlight can bring improvement, often quite dramatically.

The part of sunlight that actually helps—the tanning, burning rays of the ultraviolet spectrum—have become an important part of psoriasis treatment: phototherapy. UVB (the more potent wavelengths of ultraviolet) is applied alone, and UVA (the lower energy end) is frequently used in combination with psoralens, chemicals that makes the skin more light sensitive, in "PUVA" therapy.

DOES ALL THIS UV EXPOSURE RISK CANCER?

Like extensive exposure to sunlight, phototherapy does increase the danger of skin cancer. The risk is higher with PUVA than UVB therapy. A Swedish study that followed 4,799 persons who had received PUVA for psoriasis for about seven years found that the rate of squamous cell cancers of the skin increased in proportion to the total dose received. Men who had had more than two hundred treatments had over thirty times the number of such cancers as the general population (*The Lancet,* July 13, 1991).

The study also found less striking increases in pancreatic cancer in men, kidney and colon cancer in women, and respiratory cancer in both.

This doesn't mean that phototherapy, which can make a big difference in the quality of life for people with severe psoriasis, must be avoided. But it shouldn't be overused as a maintenance therapy, for example, and cumulative exposure should be tracked and limited.

CAN DIET AFFECT PSORIASIS?

People have reported improvements in the disease with such diverse eating plans as a rice-based diet, the Weight Watchers program, a diet that avoids yeast-promoting foods, and diets that emphasize or exclude dairy products. Some have suggested that food allergies, which vary from one person to another, can trigger or exacerbate psoriasis.

According to the National Psoriasis Foundation (NPF), no double-blind studies have been conducted to confirm the value of any of these dietary approaches. If you try one of them on your own, particularly if it departs drastically from eating patterns you're used to, the NPF advises consulting with a nutritionist or knowledgeable physician to make sure you stay adequately nourished.

One nutritional factor with psoriasis benefits that has stood up to scientific scrutiny is fish oil—specifically eicosapentaenoic acid (EPA), which is found abundantly in cold-water fish like salmon or mackerel.

In one British study (*The Lancet,* February 20, 1988), twenty-eight people with chronic psoriasis took either fish-oil capsules or placebo capsules for eight weeks. Those who took the fish oil had a significant improvement in itching, scaling, and redness; the placebo group did not. (To get the amount of EPA taken in the trial from your diet, you'd need about six ounces of oily fish daily.)

The apparent benefit of fish oil comes from an anti-inflammatory effect: the authors of the study suggested that EPA may shift the body's metabolism of fats to produce fewer powerful inflammatory chemicals.

SHOULD I TAKE VITAMINS?

Retinoids, which are chemically related to vitamin A, have been used for years in treating severe psoriasis. More recently, doctors have been investigating the effect of vitamin D derivatives, both taken internally and applied topically. The results have been promising—and surprisingly free from skin side effects. An editorial in the *Mayo Clinic Proceedings* (September 1993) called vitamin D compounds "a new therapeutic era for dermatology in the 21st century."

This does *not* mean that large doses of vitamin A or D will provide comparable benefits. Both vitamins are stored by the body, and are toxic when ingested in quantities exceeding normal intake. In the case of vitamin D, the transformation of the vitamin to the active compound shown to help psoriasis is tightly controlled by the body: taking more vitamin D will not increase the derivative.

Topical vitamin D_3, or calcipotriene, was approved by the FDA in 1993 for the treatment of mild to moderate psoriasis. It is a prescription drug, marketed in the United States under the brand name Dovonex. Studies show Dovonex can be safely taken for at least a year. Thus far, its only known side effect is a burning sensation in 10 to 15 percent of cases. Some improvements are noted within two to three weeks; most often, however, full benefit will take two months or longer.

DOES STRESS CAUSE PSORIASIS?

No. If you don't have the genetic predisposition, all the stress in the world won't give you psoriasis. It seems quite clear, however, that stress (among other things) can trigger or exacerbate outbreaks of psoriasis in some people who have the disease. Various studies have estimated that 40 to 80 percent of sufferers report that their skin worsens with stress.

By the same token, stress control has been shown to be effective. Hypnosis, biofeedback, relaxation exercises, psychotherapy, and group therapy are reported to improve psoriasis (in small, and generally uncontrolled, studies). These approaches, as always, require more commitment than taking medication, and vary greatly in individual response.

Whether or not stress causes psoriasis, it seems unquestionable that psoriasis causes stress. Embarrassment and stigmatization are cited by many people as the worse aspects of the disease. Before 1908, psoriasis was confused with leprosy, and subject to the same superstitious dread. While it is now known that psoriasis is entirely noncontagious and has nothing to do with personal hygiene, backward attitudes may continue to haunt sufferers.

Support groups, in particular, are useful in helping members to deal with negative attitudes of others and negative feelings of one's own.

CAN ANYTHING ELSE TRIGGER PSORIASIS?

Certain drugs (antimalarials, beta-blockers, nonsteroidal anti-inflammatories, lithium) may trigger or worsen psoriasis. So can skin injury, even the minimal trauma caused by scratching and picking at lesions.

Recent reports have focused on alcohol consumption as a factor in psoriasis, at least in men. A Finnish study of over four hundred men with psoriasis and other skin diseases found that the consumption of alcohol in the year before their illness appeared had been twice as high in the psoriasis group as in the others (*British Medical Journal*, March 24, 1990). It may be that alcohol triggers the disease in those who are genetically susceptible.

In a North American study (*Journal of the American Academy of Dermatology*, May 1993), men who drank heavily responded markedly less well to psoriasis treatment: more than half the time, they improved less than 10 percent as much as more moderate drinkers.

Resources

The National Psoriasis Foundation provides educational brochures about psoriasis and its treatment, publishes a newsletter, and can put you in touch with local chapters and support groups:

National Psoriasis Foundation
6600 S.W. 92nd Avenue, Suite 300
Portland, OR 97223
(800) 248-0886 or (800) 723-9166

◆ RHEUMATOID ARTHRITIS

Rheumatoid arthritis (RA) is an autoimmune disease; i.e. the immune system that normally protects the body attacks it instead. The primary target of attack in RA is the synovial membrane that lines the joints, although other parts of the body may be affected as well.

The immune attack produces inflammation, causing pain, swelling, and eventual joint destruction. Disability is a real threat in RA: ten years after the disease begins, less than half of sufferers are still working.

RA is not rare: it affects an estimated 1 percent of the American population—about two and a half million people—three times as many women as men. Genetics plays a role (it's more common in close relatives of those with the disease), but exactly *what* role is unclear. Most likely, what you inherit is a vulnerability to the disorder, which may or may not develop, depending on environmental factors. One strong possibility is that infection by a virus or bacteria triggers the immune system to produce antibodies that then attack the joints.

RA varies considerably in course and severity. About 70 percent of people have progressive, chronic disease; one quarter have brief attacks and long remissions, and the rest have extremely severe disease that affects the entire body, particularly blood vessels. Quite possibly, severity, as well as vulnerability, is inherited.

HOW SHOULD I DECIDE WHICH DRUGS TO USE FOR RA?

Only in recent years has the seriousness of RA been fully appreciated. It's not just a potentially crippling disease, but a life-threatening one as well. People with RA die ten to fifteen years earlier than others matched for age and sex, and a twenty-five-year British study found that one third of such deaths were due to RA itself. Among individuals with extremely severe disease that involves many joints and other parts of the body, five-year survival is less than 50 percent—comparable to advanced Hodgkin's disease and extensive coronary heart disease.

In addition, it's become clear that much irreversible damage in RA, namely, the joint erosion that eventually leads to disability, takes place in the early stages of the disease—within a year or two after it is diagnosed.

The therapeutic strategy has changed accordingly. A decade ago, doctors followed a "treatment pyramid" plan, starting with relatively mild drugs and waiting as long as possible before graduating to more potent, potentially toxic, agents. Nowadays, it's typical to bring in the heavy artillery if anti-inflammatories do not halt the disease within a month or two.

The first-line drugs are still nonsteroidal anti-inflammatory drugs (NSAIDs). It is still not completely understood how these drugs work, but they appear to reduce the concentration of prostaglandins and related compounds. NSAIDs are often supplanted quickly by potent medications that suppress the immune system or put a damper on cell activity, such as methotrexate (which was first used in cancer chemotherapy), sulfasalazine, corticosteroids, azathioprine, gold or cyclosporin. These drugs are called DMARDs (disease-modifying antirheumatic drugs). The goal is not just to relieve symptoms, but to stop the disease process and induce remission.

HOW WELL DO THESE DRUGS WORK?

Practicing rheumatologists seem to have little doubt about the efficacy of DMARDs. In a survey several years ago, specialists cited methotrexate (along with hip replacement surgery) as the principal milestones in the treatment of RA since the mid-1960s.

But as with so much else in medicine, what everyone knows hasn't yet been proven. "These drugs alter disease outcome in rheumatoid arthritis, although the extent to which they do so is unclear," according to a review article in The Lancet (January 30, 1993). "There is no doubt that the rate of functional deterioration is reduced by these drugs," the author went on to say, but long-term studies must still be done to determine exactly the impact of early treatment with such strong drugs.

ARE RA DRUGS SAFE?

All the drugs used for RA can have adverse effects, some serious. NSAIDs frequently cause gastrointestinal problems, including bleeding and ulcer. Methotrexate can lead to liver damage and reduced white cell counts. Other disease-modifying agents may produce these or other problems, including kidney damage, hypertension, infection, and cancer. All can interact with other drugs and may be contraindicated if you have other medical conditions.

For this reason, it is essential that drug therapy be done carefully and monitored appropriately, with regular blood tests and tests of kidney or liver function. This is something to be discussed fully with your doctor. Make sure you know what risks are involved and what steps are being taken to protect your health.

DO ANTIBIOTICS HAVE A ROLE IN THE TREATMENT OF RA?

This is a controversial suggestion that recently received validation for some cases of rheumatoid arthritis. Research dating back to the 1950s indicates that a persistent Mycoplasma infection may cause rheumatoid arthritis, and long-term antibiotics could provide successful treatment. Since then, studies have produced contradictory results. In 1995, however, a well-designed study showed that the antibiotic minocycline is safe and effective for people with mild to moderate rheumatoid arthritis. The study involved over two hundred people who received either minocycline or a placebo for forty-eight months (*Annals of Internal Medicine,* January 15, 1995).

IF I CAN STAND THE PAIN, MUST I TAKE DRUGS?

Stoicism is out of place in RA. For one thing, RA is a systemic condition, affecting more than just the joints, and drugs reduce the inflammation and other aspects of the disease process that apparently hasten permanent damage.

What's more, some research suggests that pain itself can feed the disease process. Substance P, a chemical produced when you have pain, appears to increase inflammation.

But drugs shouldn't be your only defense against pain. As with any kind of arthritis, it can be extremely helpful to learn techniques that reduce the muscle tension that can increase pain, like relaxation, biofeedback, or hypnosis. Applications of heat and cold, either as compresses or lotions, are basic weapons to relieve pain and joint stiffness. Massage can be soothing, relaxing, and pain relieving.

You can educate yourself about nondrug approaches to pain, but you also can get a lot of help from a physical therapist. Question your rheumatologist and the physical therapist about the latter's experience in treating people with RA. Massage should be given only by someone with expertise, to minimize the risk of damaging weakened joints and muscles.

HOW ELSE CAN I HELP MYSELF?

Drug treatment is only one part of RA management; the rest is largely up to you. Exercise is vital. The proper program will reduce joint stiffness and prevent the muscles that support the joint from wasting away, minimizing disability.

Specific exercises are targeted to the particular joints that are affected: gentle stretching is essential to maintain range of motion; strengthening exercises will keep them functioning well. Here again, a physical therapist is invaluable as a "coach" to teach you how to exercise safely and effectively. RA can flare and subside, even from day to day. You should adjust your exercise regimen to how you feel, although it is important to do *some* exercise every day, even if it's just minimal stretching, to prevent stiffness from getting worse.

You should also learn ways to make exercise easier and more effective—applying heat, for example, to relax muscles and loosen joints before you start exercise. Many people find they can do stretching work in the morning, when joints are stiffest, in or just after a hot shower.

The other side of exercise is rest. Fatigue is a significant problem for people with arthritis, both a consequence of trying to stay active despite pain, and of the disease itself. A full eight hours of sleep—or rest in bed, if you can't sleep—should be a goal.

CAN EXERCISE INJURE ARTHRITIC JOINTS?

Arthritic joints do become fragile, and trauma can compound the damage of the disease. If exercises are done carefully, however, with guidance from a good physical therapist or doctor, there's little risk of joint injury.

In addition, lifestyle modifications can protect joints and enable you to keep active. How you stand, sit, and work makes a real difference. There are a host of joint-sparing devices, such as tools and utensils with thickened or lengthened handles, that keep strain to a minimum. Which are best for you depends on the location and severity of your disease. The guidance of a physical or occupational therapist is invaluable here.

DOES DIET MAKE A DIFFERENCE?

Over the years, many special diets have been advocated for arthritis (such as eliminating vegetables of the nightshade family, which includes tomatoes, potatoes, and peppers), but for the most part, they haven't been subjected to scientific scrutiny. In recent years, however, several nutritional approaches have shown promise.

Three studies over the last fifteen years found that fasting reduces pain, stiffness, tenderness, and swelling in arthritic joints. But this, for obvious reasons, can't be a long-term therapy. A Finnish trial suggested that a vegetarian diet can maintain the gains of a brief period of fasting (*The Lancet,* October 12, 1991).

In this trial, twenty-seven people with RA spent a week to ten days on a partial fast (nothing but vegetable extract), then three to five months on a gluten-free vegan diet (no meat, dairy, refined sugar, citrus fruits, or wheat products), and then a lactovegetarian diet consisting of vegetables, fruits, grains, and dairy products. At the end of a year, they had significant improvements in arthritis symptoms. (In a control group of those who ate an ordinary diet, pain was improved after a year, but nothing else.)

There is also reason to believe that a small but real minority of people have RA symptoms worsened by food allergies. Perhaps 5 percent of people with RA, small studies suggest, may benefit from eliminating foods like milk, shrimp, or nitrate-containing foods.

Will these approaches work for you? There's no harm in trying (a vegetarian diet can be healthful for any number of reasons), as long as you maintain good nutrition. As with any chronic disease, an adequate supply of essential nutrients is necessary. If you plan any major modification from your customary diet, it's wise to consult with a qualified nutritionist.

WHAT ABOUT SUPPLEMENTS?

Some very interesting recent research suggests that supplements of fish oil can reduce the inflammation of RA. In one study, twenty-one people took a sizable dose of this supplement daily for fourteen weeks: fatigue and number of tender joints decreased significantly, compared with nineteen others who were given a placebo (*Annals of Internal Medicine,* April 1987).

In theory, adding these specific fatty acids to the diet alters the function of the immune system, and laboratory tests in fact indicated that the production of some inflammatory chemicals was reduced.

The anti-inflammatory effect of fish oil appears real, but may be quite limited. Whether or not it can influence the progression of RA is unknown. There's no evidence to suggest it can replace conventional arthritis therapy, but it may well be a helpful adjunct.

A small, preliminary study reported in *Science* (September 24, 1993) suggests that another supplement, derived from chicken cartilage, may be promising. The preparation contains Type II collagen, a possible target of immune attack in RA; the idea is to induce "toleration" of this substance, in a process that may involve T-cell lymphocytes.

Three months after sixty people with RA stopped other arthritis drugs and took either the collagen extract or a placebo, joint swelling and pain was reduced 25 to 30 percent for those in the collagen group, while the others had slightly worsened symptoms.

Most other experts are reserving judgment until larger studies are done. Collagen supplements are available at health food stores, but since dosage and collagen type appear crucial, it's unlikely that this route will bring much benefit, the researchers say.

DO EMOTIONS AFFECT ARTHRITIS?

No one seriously believes, nowadays, that RA is caused by stress or emotional conflict (a respectable theory fifty years ago), and there's no indication that any personality type is particularly prone to it. Perhaps surprisingly, however, attitude and state of mind appear to have a significant effect on its course.

In particular, it seems that confidence in your ability to deal with arthritis materially influences severity and disability. Self-efficacy—the belief that you can cope with the problems of the disease—has been significantly related to ability to function. Conversely, people who feel helpless suffer more impairment and disability.

Most surprisingly, perhaps, an individual's own subjective rating of how well he or she can function can predict how likely he or she is to become disabled in the years to come (and even how long he or she will live) more accurately than objective measures of disease severity like X rays or blood tests.

From such studies, it's impossible to say whether subjective feelings simply reflect the seriousness of RA more precisely than science can, or if a more positive attitude can itself slow progression. Still, it's unquestionable that confidence and coping make RA easier to live with, and taking steps to increase your confident control of RA should be a central part of your efforts.

To this end, learning ways to minimize pain and stay active, participating actively in RA management, even seeking psychotherapy to fight the depression and discouragement that serious illness can bring, are worth considering. Support groups can be extremely helpful.

A six-week course, developed at Stanford University, was shown to reduce pain in all kinds of arthritis by 15 to 20 percent, lessen depression, and reduce the number of doctor visits—benefits that were maintained even four years later. Although the self-help measures taught by the course (nutrition, exercise, coping, and pain control) no doubt played a role, the single factor most closely related to improvement was an increase in feelings of self-efficacy.

The Arthritis Self-Help Course, modeled on the Stanford research, is now available throughout the country through local chapters of the Arthritis Foundation.

Resources

The Arthritis Foundation is a good source of information and guidance, offering educational brochures on RA and a booklet, "Coping with Pain," that will help you design your own pain management program.

Arthritis Foundation
P.O. Box 19000
Atlanta, GA 30326
(800) 283-7800

The organization also publishes the *Guide to Independent Living for People with Arthritis*, which includes descriptions, pictures, and ordering information for over six hundred joint-sparing devices and other helpful items: $9.95 plus $2.00 for shipping and handling.

If you're interested in the Arthritis Self-Help Course, the above toll-free number can put you in touch with local chapters that sponsor it.

◆ SHINGLES

The most significant thing about shingles (herpes zoster) is pain. Although some people get away with itching and aching (and a few have no pain at all), the sharp, burning, shooting pains of shingles can be agonizing. What's worse, a significant proportion of people suffer neuralgia that lingers after the disease itself is gone—sometimes for months or years.

Strangely, behind all this suffering is the same virus that causes what is usually an innocuous childhood malady: chicken pox. The varicella-zoster virus doesn't disappear when the rash fades into memory, but settles, dormantly but permanently, in bundles of nerve cells (ganglia) near the spine. If a time comes when the immune system can't keep them in check, the virus migrates up one or more nerves to the skin.

First comes the pain—typically, sharp or burning pains on one side of the trunk (*zoster* is a Greek word meaning *belt* or *girdle;* the Latin *cingula*, from which we get *shingles,* means the same thing), head or face. The red, blistering rash appears several days later; crusts form, harden and fall off, and within three to five weeks it's over. But sometimes it's not *all* over.

WHY DO OLDER PEOPLE GET SHINGLES?

A decline in immune system function is one of the normal, predictable consequences of aging. As the body's self-defense weakens, the varicella-zoster virus can proliferate and travel. While it's possible to develop the disease at virtually any age, the risk increases markedly with advancing years: by the age of eighty-five, about half of this age group will have had shingles.

The incidence of shingles has risen noticeably over the decades (about three hundred thousand Americans a year now have episodes), and this is due largely to increasing numbers of older people.

WHEN IS SHINGLES TREATED AS LIFE-THREATENING?

Another group of people at risk for the disease are those whose immune system has been severely depressed by other illness. About 10 percent of those with leukemia and one third of those with Hodgkin's disease develop shingles. People with AIDS are another high-risk group.

In immunity-impaired people, there's the danger of *disseminated* shingles, which spreads over the skin and infects internal organs as well. If the brain or lungs are affected, it can be fatal. The same thing can happen to people who develop shingles while taking immunosuppressive drugs, such as those used after organ transplants.

While otherwise healthy older people are not prone to such complications, they are far more likely than younger ones to develop postherpetic neuralgia, the lingering agony of which is the leading cause of suicide among chronic pain sufferers over age seventy.

IS THERE PROTECTION AGAINST EYE DAMAGE CAUSED BY SHINGLES?

Shingles that has invaded the trigeminal cranial nerve (large nerve on each side of the face that splits into three branches, which among other things, supply sensations to the face, scalp, nose, teeth, lining of the upper eyelid, sinuses, and front two thirds of the tongue) may affect the eye: the warning sign is a rash on the tip and side of the nose. The incidence may be as high as 15 percent, predominantly in older persons.

Ocular herpes zoster can cause severe inflammation in various parts of the eye and can lead to cataract, glaucoma, and even loss of sight. It should be treated by an ophthalmologist. Steroids and acyclovir, applied directly to the eye, have both been used, but their relative effectiveness hasn't been subjected to controlled studies.

IS SHINGLES CONTAGIOUS?

You can't catch shingles itself from anyone. But the virus that causes both it and chicken pox is one of the most contagious known. Someone who has never had chicken pox—usually a small child—is very likely to develop it after exposure to a person with shingles.

WHAT DRUGS ARE PRESCRIBED FOR SHINGLES?

Like most viral diseases, herpes zoster must run its course with or without medication. In uncomplicated cases, treatment aims to reduce pain and itching until it goes away. Aspirin, sedatives, and cool compresses are often sufficient; certain antidepressants can relieve the pain as well.

The antiviral drug acyclovir, widely used for genital herpes (caused by a related virus) apparently can shorten the course of shingles, but only in extremely high doses. It is often given intravenously to immunocompromised patients who are at risk of dissemination (this treatment requires hospitalization).

CAN POSTHERPETIC NEURALGIA BE PREVENTED?

Unfortunately, postherpetic neuralgia, the disabling pain that can persist long after the acute phase of shingles is over, is notoriously resistant to prevention.

In a preliminary study of elderly British people with shingles, high-dose oral acyclovir (800 milligrams five times a day for seven days) lowered the rate of postherpetic neuralgia by 30 percent (*British Medical Journal,* October 29, 1994). The study also showed that oral acyclovir alone, without topical acyclovir, provides ocular protection in people with the shingles rash near the eye. This is the first long-term follow-up study (five years) of people with shingles given either high-dose acyclovir or a placebo.

"Shingles should be treated as a pain emergency," said Daniel B. Carr, M.D., at a 1994 press briefing on pain treatment, sponsored by the American Medical Association. "Now there's fairly good evidence that if you intervene early, you can abort the attack," explained Dr. Carr, who is the Saltonstall Professor of Pain Research at New England Medical Center in Boston. The intervention is a combination of an oral antiviral drug, such as acyclovir, and a nerve block. The latter involves an outpatient hospital treatment in which a local anesthetic is injected into an area of the body that corresponds to the site of the shingles rash. Reports in the medical literature indicate that the nerve block, which deadens pain and decreases inflammation surround affected nerve roots, must be applied within days to a few weeks after onset of the rash. (See Resources to find a pain specialist who can administer a nerve block.)

WHAT CAN I DO FOR POSTHERPETIC NEURALGIA?

Several nonmedical therapies are used in the treatment of postherpetic neuralgia, but there is little or no scientific evidence to demonstrate efficacy. They include topically applied vitamin E oil, vitamin C supplements, and lysine (an amino acid) supplements, all of which can be purchased in health food stores.

A relatively new, and apparently quite helpful, treatment comes from an unexpected source: capsaicin, an active component of red pepper. Half or more of people treated with a topical capsaicin cream on painful areas have experienced substantial relief, in various studies. One side effect, an intermittent burning sensation that can range from uncomfortable to intolerable, usually subsides if treatment is continued.

Apparently, capsaicin depletes affected nerves of substance P, a natural chemical essential for the transmission of pain impulses to the brain. The cream, available over the counter as Zostrix, Capsaicin, and ToppSation, should never be used before the actual rash of shingles has cleared completely. The manufacturer is currently testing a more potent version, in clinical trials. Those results should be available in 1995 or 1996.

Another promising, research-backed treatment involves aspirin dissolved in chloroform and applied directly to the painful area. Two published studies show that this treatment relieves the pain of both shingles and postherpetic neuralgia (*Pain,* March 1992, and *Archives of Neurology,* October 1993). Each study involved about forty-five participants.

The 1992 study, which was conducted in Milan, Italy, reported: "A striking reduction in the percentage of [shingles] patients developing postherpetic neuralgia was observed in the treated group, as compared with [untreated cases] reported in the medical literature (4 percent vs. 50 to 70 percent)." The 1993 study, which was conducted at the State University of New York Health Science Center, Syracuse, New York, showed that the aspirin/chloroform treatment helped people in the acute phase of shingles and those suffering postherpetic neuralgia. "All participants reported substantially decreased pain promptly after treatment, with maximum relief at twenty to thirty minutes and lasting two to four hours.''

The chloroform removes the skin oils and dead cells, thus allowing deeper penetration of the aspirin. Since chloroform is not readily accessible to most people, some doctors advise using an over-the-counter skin lotion like Vaseline Intensive Care Lotion, though it is not as effective as chloroform.

IS THERE A VACCINE AGAINST SHINGLES?

A vaccine has been developed to prevent chicken pox, which is caused by the same virus. In theory, a person who never gets chicken pox won't have to worry about shingles. But because the vaccine uses weakened, but not killed, varicella-zoster virus, this is not certain, and in fact, some worry whether shingles may occur years after vaccination, the same way it does after chicken pox.

On the other hand, it's possible that the same vaccine, given to older persons who have already had chicken pox, can prevent the virus from coming back as shingles. A small study of people ages fifty-five to eighty-seven found that in the majority of cases, the vaccine boosted immune response to varicella-zoster virus up to the level of much younger people. A large clinical trial is now under way, to see whether vaccination will actually reduce incidence of the disease.

Resources

American Society of Regional Anesthesia, 1910 Byrd Ave. #100, P.O. Box 10086, Richmond, VA 23230-1086, (804) 282-0010. Call weekdays, 7:00 A.M. to 4:00 P.M. eastern time, for the name of one of 53 pain programs in the U.S. which are accredited by the American Council of Continuing Medical Education.

National Chronic Pain Outreach Association, 7979 Old Georgetown Road, Suite 100, Bethesda, MD 20814-2429. The NCPOA maintains a registry of chronic pain support groups in the U.S. and Canada; provides referrals to NCPOA member health care professionals and medical facilities nationwide; operates as an information clearinghouse for pain sufferers and health care providers; and publishes a monthly newsletter on such topics as pain management methods and coping techniques.

◆ SINUSITIS

If you suffer from sinusitis, your misery has lots of company. Affecting over thirty-one million Americans, it is our number-one chronic illness. Millions more have episodes of acute sinusitis that cause a few days or weeks of discomfort and then disappear spontaneously.

The sinuses are four pairs of air-filled spaces lined by mucus membrane located in the bones of the skull surrounding the nose. Normally, natural secretions empty from the sinus into the nose, but when the opening is blocked, secretions trapped in the sinus provide a perfect medium for bacteria to thrive. Infection and inflammation follow, causing pain (often a headache or toothache that worsens when you lie down), nasal congestion, or discharge (typically yellow or green in color), and postnasal drip.

Among those especially susceptible to sinusitis are people with allergies, cigarette smokers, and people with anatomic abnormalities of the nose, such as deviated septum, that interfere with drainage.

HOW CAN A DOCTOR TELL IF I HAVE SINUSITIS?

It's not always easy. The symptoms of sinusitis aren't terribly different from those of other respiratory disorders such as colds and viral infections. Allergic rhinitis—inflammation of the nose caused by reactions to pollen ("hay fever"), molds, or dust mites—can cause very similar miseries. So can some licit drugs, such as certain antihypertensives, illicit drugs like cocaine, or overuse of nose drops.

Acute sinusitis may in fact develop as a consequence of one of these other conditions: for example, when a cold or allergy blocks the sinus openings, trapping secretions that become and remain infected after the original illness is history. Doctors generally diagnose sinusitis by asking questions and doing a physical examination. But it's no precise science, as studies in two major journals, *British Medical Journal* and *Annals of Internal Medicine,* showed.

In the *British Medical Journal* study (September 19, 1992), Dutch physicians reviewed 441 cases of sinusitis. The diagnostic strategy that worked best focused on five clues: symptoms beginning with a cold; yellow-green nasal discharge; pain at bending; pain on one side of the upper jaw; and pain in teeth. Doctors who used this strategy made the diagnosis correctly (as confirmed by ultrasound) in 243 cases. But the strategy missed 44 cases, gave a false-positive diagnosis in 44 others and left 110 cases uncertain.

The American study, reported in *Annals of Internal Medicine* (November 1, 1992), found that a different group of symptoms (toothache, poor response to nasal decongestants or antihistamines, a history of yellow-green discharge or yellow-green discharge seen by examiner placing a light source either externally or within the mouth) best identified sinusitis.

These two studies are among the few systematic attempts to standardize the diagnosis of sinusitis. They demonstrate the need for more research.

For a more definite diagnosis, a doctor may use X rays, CAT scans, or ultrasound to see what's happening inside the sinuses. Even these are not as accurate, however, as a bacterial culture made from fluid drawn out by needle from the sinus (an invasive test that is not used routinely).

CAN I TREAT SINUSITIS ON MY OWN?

If you have symptoms that appear to be sinusitis, there's no reason not to try home treatment before seeing a doctor. *The CareWise Handbook,* published by the nonprofit HealthWise organization, suggests this approach (adapted with permission of HealthWise):

- Lie on your back and apply hot and cold compresses to forehead and cheeks, one minute each, for ten minutes. Repeat, if necessary, four times a day, ending at bedtime. This should stimulate the release of mucus.
- Apply decongestant nose drops or nasal spray (containing phenylephrine) while lying down. *Important:* Follow product directions and don't use them for more than three days, or you're likely to make congestion worse.
- Repeat the letter *K* for thirty seconds, to open the sinuses.
- If you're troubled by postnasal drip, gargle with warm water to clear the throat of mucus draining from the sinuses.

- Increase humidity in your home (this is especially important in the winter, in your bedroom).
- Drink lots of liquids (eight ounces of water or juice every hour) to keep mucus thin and less likely to accumulate.
- Treat headache, face, or tooth pain with aspirin or acetaminophen (children under fifteen should avoid aspirin because of the danger of Reye's syndrome).

Some other self-help hints: Avoid respiratory irritants like tobacco smoke and exposure to cold air while your symptoms are troublesome. Some people get relief by inhaling steam from a kettle or pan, which thins mucus secretions so they will drain more easily.

WHEN SHOULD I SEE A DOCTOR?

If untreated and recurrent, acute sinusitis can become chronic. There is also the risk, although small, of serious complications, such as osteomyelitis (an infection of the bone) or meningitis.

You should seek medical assistance if your symptoms haven't improved after two days of home treatment, if your sinusitis symptoms are associated with a fever over 101 degrees, or if you notice facial swelling, blurring, or other changes in vision, bleeding from the nose, or increased yellow-green nasal discharge.

An infection in the ethmoid sinus (next to the nose and just below the eye) poses particular risk of severe complications. Pain along the ridge between nose and lower eyelid deserves a prompt doctor visit.

WHY ARE ANTIBIOTICS PRESCRIBED FOR SINUSITIS?

Because sinusitis is generally caused by a bacterial infection, antibiotics are the first line of defense. They usually work quite well, but not always right away. The infection may be caused by a combination of bacteria, including anaerobic species, which don't respond to the penicillinlike antibiotics most commonly used. And because the sinuses are closed spaces without a rich blood supply, infections hold on longer there than elsewhere.

Acute sinusitis should respond to antibiotic treatment within two to three weeks. If it doesn't, it's now considered chronic sinusitis and merits a visit to a specialist. "Acute sinusitis is usually taken care of very well by the general practitioner, but chronic sinusitis is tough," says James Shenkiewicz, M.D., professor and vice chairman of the department of otolaryngology and head/neck surgery at Loyola University Medical Center, Chicago.

There are studies in the medical literature to guide doctors in choosing drugs for acute sinusitis, but none for chronic sinusitis. The superior experience and expertise of an otolaryngologist (ear, nose, and throat specialist) puts him or her in a better position to plan an antibiotic strategy likely to work in resistant cases, Dr. Shenkiewicz says. A specialist may culture a sample of mucus directly from the sinus to identify the bacteria responsible and find antibiotics that work best against them.

Even when the right antibiotics have been chosen, it may take four to six weeks for chronic sinusitis to be eradicated completely.

WILL I NEED SURGERY?

If antibiotics don't work, the next step may be washing out the sinuses. A needle is inserted into the sinus, some of the mucus is drawn out, and salt water is injected to flush out secretions.

This won't be effective, however, if the lining of the sinus has been permanently damaged by lengthy inflammation or if an anatomical abnormality interferes with normal drainage. Then surgery may be performed to make a permanent opening in the wall between nose and sinus.

Such surgery appears to have been far more common in recent years (although formal statistics are not kept for outpatient procedures), largely because of improvements in technique. What used to be an extensive operation requiring hospitalization and often causing more pain than the condition it was intended to alleviate has become an outpatient procedure that takes sixty to ninety minutes and may even be performed under local anesthesia.

What has made the difference is the endoscope, a thin tube that makes it possible for a surgeon to see the sinus and widen its opening so that secretions can drain more readily. The idea is to drain the sinus cavities, allow them to heal, and thus end the cycle of recurring infections. No external incision is necessary.

Like many surgical procedures, endoscopic sinus surgery was widely accepted before it was fully evaluated for safety and effectiveness. One of the few studies (*Ear, Nose and Throat,* May 1993) involved a review of eighty people who had the surgery, with follow-up averaging twenty-two months. Overall, the operation was largely successful in 93.5 percent of cases in dealing with chronic headache and infection. Thirty people experienced complications ranging from taste disturbance to acute facial pain five days after surgery.

Although modern sinus surgery appears reasonably safe and effective, like any outpatient procedure for a common problem, it is likely to be overdone. You may have seen ads inviting you to call an 800 number for a free consultation about nasal obstruction, sinus pain, or other similar complaints.

"Ignore these ads," advises Dr. Shenkiewicz. "Most intend to get people directly to the operating table before they have been given the maximum chance at drug therapy." The procedure, at two thousand to ten thousand dollars, is lucrative, and the competition is fierce. "I couldn't denounce them [doctors who advertise nasal surgery to the public] more strongly," Dr. Shenkiewicz says.

◆ SKIN CANCER (NONMELANOMA)

Nonmelanoma skin cancers are the most common malignancies in the United States, with about six hundred thousand new cases yearly (some say this is a conservative estimate). The rate has been increasing dramatically—by perhaps 65 percent during the decade of the 1980s, according to some limited studies.

Although these cancers are rarely fatal, they are far from trivial: they cause an estimated two thousand deaths each year (about one third as many deaths as from melanoma). The lesions are often deeper and wider than they look, and their removal can entail functional impairment and, insofar as 80 percent are found on the head and neck, considerable disfigurement.

The most common kind of skin cancer, basal cell carcinoma, accounts for some half-million cases yearly. Squamous cell carcinoma is less common (about a hundred thousand cases) but more dangerous: they cause almost all the deaths due to nonmelanoma skin cancer.

WHY BOTHER TREATING SKIN CANCERS EARLY?

Although there is little to be gained in reduced mortality, a strong argument can be made for early treatment: small lesions can be removed more cheaply and easily, require less extensive procedures, and cause less scarring and disfigurement.

IF I HAVE A SKIN CANCER, WHAT IS THE BEST TREATMENT?

There are a number of treatments for skin cancer: various kinds of surgery to cut it out, cryosurgery to freeze it off, electrodesiccation and curettage to burn and scrape it away, topical chemotherapy and radiation. Randomized trials comparing the risks and benefits of these methods haven't been done. "In most cases," a review article in *The New England Journal of*

Medicine (December 3, 1992) says, "there is no single treatment that is superior with respect to effectiveness, associated morbidity, cost, and cosmetic outcome."

Particularly in view of the fact that these cancers are rarely life-threatening, the choice among different treatments should be yours, although not every doctor will go to great lengths to make sure you know this.

Each approach has its advantages and drawbacks, which your doctor should explain to you. The best choice may depend on the type of tumor, where it is located, your age and, for that matter, the coverage offered by your health insurance for the various treatments.

According to the *Journal* review, an advantage of surgery is the ability to examine the area around the lesion; if all malignant cells aren't excised, the chance of cancer recurrence is 16 to 48 percent. Mohs' surgery, which involves removal of the area around the malignancy in stages and microscopic examination of each, is designed to get all the tumor out while keeping the extent of the procedure to a minimum. Because it is considerably more expensive than conventional surgery and takes longer, the technique is often reserved for tumors likely to recur, and where it is important to preserve normal tissue.

Cryosurgery and electrodesiccation and curettage are usually used for smaller, less aggressive tumors, especially on less visible parts of the body. Radiation, which is expensive, is most often a choice for older people and those at risk of surgical complications. "Longer-term difficulties, including carcinogenesis and radiation dermatitis, argue against its use in patients under fifty years of age," the *Journal* review says.

Topical chemotherapy, in which a cream or solution is applied directly to the skin for four to six weeks, is best used only for superficial tumors, and may leave a greater risk of recurrence. Laser can be used in the same way as electrodesiccation and curettage, but no comparative studies show it to be any better than these procedures.

SHOULD I HAVE PRECANCEROUS LESIONS TREATED?

Actinic (or solar) keratosis is a roughened patch of skin that has an estimated 25 percent chance of developing into skin cancer over a ten-year period.

Some disappear on their own, but they can be removed by freezing or by the application of 5-fluorouracil, a chemotherapy agent. A skin peel can get rid of them, but they may grow back.

Tretinoin (Retin-A), a topical drug that repairs sun damage, has been used to reduce the risk of skin cancer from such lesions, but its effectiveness isn't clear. In some animal studies, topical retinoids actually enhanced tumor growth.

An Australian study of 588 people found that regular sunscreen use reduced the number of actinic keratoses in the course of a single summer, while they increased in a control group. Those who used more sunscreen had fewer new keratoses and more remissions of existing ones.

Actinic keratoses that aren't removed should be watched closely for signs of malignancy; have a total body examination yearly to detect cancers elsewhere.

CAN I GUARD AGAINST RECURRENCES?

Between 1 and 39 percent of basal cell carcinomas recur, according to various studies: two thirds recur within three years after treatment. Tumors around the nose, eyes, ear, scalp, and forehead are especially likely to recur, while those on the neck, body, or legs are least likely to do so. One recurrence increases the chance of a second.

An estimated 1 to 20 percent of squamous cell carcinomas recur; the risk is highest for those on the legs or those associated with scars.

If you've had one skin cancer, the chances are good you'll have another one later. A study of a thousand people who had had one basal cell carcinoma found that more than one third developed a second within five years (Cancer, 1987, no. 60). About half of those who have had two or more skin cancers will have another in that period. Men, and people who burn easily or who have been exposed to a lot of sun are at increased risk.

HOW CAN I REDUCE MY RISK OF SKIN CANCER?

Sun exposure is the primary risk factor for basal cell and squamous cell carcinoma. Tucson, Arizona, has more than double the skin cancer rate of Rochester, Minnesota; in subtropical latitudes of Australia, nearly one person in a hundred is diagnosed with skin cancer each year.

Lifetime protection against the sun, inconvenient as it may be, is the most important strategy for prevention: avoid exposure in the hours when the sun is strongest, use sunscreens (even for brief, casual outdoor activities), and wear protective clothing. It has been estimated that using an SPF-15 sunscreen up to age eighteen would reduce skin cancer risk by 78 percent.

Modern tanning equipment emits UVA light, which its marketers claim carries less risk. But animal studies show that the dose required for an equivalent tan is as carcinogenic as UVB, the primary burning rays of sunlight.

Sun protection is especially important for light-skinned, blue-eyed people who burn easily, and who are at higher than average risk of skin cancer.

Resources

Use CancerFax to receive a printout on skin cancer from the computerized data base of the National Cancer Institute. You will need access to a fax machine with an attached telephone. Dial (301) 402-5874 on a touch-tone phone and receive a faxed report on state-of-the-art treatments for skin cancer. Request the physicians' version.

✦ STREP THROAT

Sore throat (also known as pharyngitis) brings adult Americans to their doctors for more than forty million visits each year. The disease is far more common in children: in the first three years of life, the average infant has about four upper respiratory illnesses (which also include colds, earaches, and sinusitis) per year; those in day care have six or seven.

A sore throat can be caused by any number of organisms, both viral and bacterial, and for the most part, it simply inflicts a few days of discomfort and then goes away, with or without medical help. Drugs, whether over the counter or prescribed, have little if any effect.

The exception is sore throat caused by the group A β-hemolytic streptococcus bacterium—familiar to all as "strep throat." Although a strep throat is likely to make you a lot more miserable than a run-of-the-mill sore throat, it too will almost always run its course in less than a week. But there's the danger that it won't—and that it will lead to complications like ear infections or even heart or kidney disease. That's why it's important to seek prompt diagnosis and treatment.

Strep throat is most frequent in children ages five to ten. Some surveys find the organism in 40 percent of sore throats in this age group.

HOW DO I KNOW IF IT'S STREP THROAT?

Strep throat often, but not always, causes particularly severe throat pain, which can make swallowing difficult. However, symptoms, such as fever and pain, and physical examination cannot differentiate infallibly between strep throat and less severe ailments.

In estimating the likelihood that strep is involved, the doctor will probably take several other factors into account. A discharge on the tonsils (clumps of lymph tissue in back of the throat), fever, swollen lymph nodes in the front of the neck, and the absence of a cough and hoarseness are warning signs: if an adult has all four of these symptoms, the odds are fifty–fifty that his or her sore throat is caused by strep, according to an article in *Patient Care* (May 30, 1991).

There are two basic lab tests for diagnosing strep throat. The definitive one is a bacterial culture of material swabbed from the back of the throat. It gives a clear yes or no answer, but it takes several days to get results. More recently, several ten-minute office tests have become available. They vary in accuracy, but for the most part, they are fairly sensitive (about 80 percent) and extremely selective. That is, a positive finding almost always means strep, while you can have strep despite a negative result.

CAN ANTIBIOTICS HELP?

Doctors differ widely in their eagerness to use antibiotics for sore throat. According to a review article in the *Medical Journal of Australia* (May 4, 1992), Australian doctors seem very likely to prescribe these drugs, British doctors considerably less so, while American doctors fall between. In this country, family physicians give more antibiotics for sore throats than pediatricians. At least some antibiotics prescribed by doctors would seem to be unnecessary.

Since most sore throats get better spontaneously, and since viruses won't respond to antibiotics in any case, the general feeling is that antibiotics are justified only when sore throat is caused by strep. It will probably make you feel better faster—shortening the illness episode from four days to three, for example—and lessen the chance that the infection will spread to the ear or sinuses.

The most important reason to give antibiotics is to prevent more serious complications. Glomerulonephritis, a kidney disease, and rheumatic fever, which can cause permanent heart damage, can result from an immune reaction, triggered by the strep bacteria, against the body's own tissues.

Treating strep promptly can lessen the risk of glomerulonephritis and can largely prevent rheumatic fever. (Rheumatic fever has declined considerably since the 1940s, but there have been renewed outbreaks in recent years, in a number of states; the disease is far from extinct.) On the other hand, there's no reason to add the adverse effects of antibiotics, which can include diarrhea, rash, and yeast infections, to your sore throat experience unless it's likely to do some good.

What many doctors do is give the office strep test to people with sore throats. If it's positive, they put them on antibiotics; if negative—but there's still some doubt—the next step might be a throat culture, with antibiotics at least until the results are in. How common strep throat is in your area may help the doctor decide how readily to give antibiotics.

Some research suggests that many antibiotic prescriptions are written not on medical, but on marketing, grounds by doctors who assume that those who come to see them expect a prescription or will feel better if they walk out with one in hand. However, a study cited in the *Medical Journal of Australia* paper found that "patient satisfaction is not altered by the provision of a prescription" and "patients are happy not to be provided with antibiotics."

Would ten days of antibiotics, whether you need them or not, make you feel you got your money's worth out of your appointment? Let your doctor know.

WILL ANTIBIOTICS BE STARTED RIGHT AWAY?

For a number of years, some researchers have been saying that antibiotic therapy for strep throat should be delayed for several days, to allow the body to build a stronger immune response that will prevent future attacks. It has been shown, in fact, that such a delay results in higher levels of certain antistreptococcus antibodies.

What has *not* been shown, according to an article in *The Pediatric Infectious Disease Journal* (October 1991), is a rise in other antibodies that may be more important and—bottom line—whether the difference, whatever it is, actually makes recurrence less likely. The author of that article didn't think it made sense to wait.

On the other hand, there doesn't seem to be much harm in waiting; glomerulonephritis and rheumatic fever are no more likely if antibiotics are held back for a day or two. Starting antibiotics right away will probably make you feel better sooner, however, and less likely to spread the illness to your family and beyond. There is evidence that the strep organism becomes more virulent, and more likely to cause rheumatic fever when it is transmitted to the next person.

WHAT CAN I DO FOR RECURRENT STREP THROATS?

A child who has three or more bouts of sore throat in a single year probably needs further tests, which could mean a workup by a otolaryngologist.

One option the otolaryngologist may suggest is tonsillectomy. This used to be quite a common childhood operation, to reduce the frequency of sore throats, among other things, but it is done much less often today.

In one study, cited in *American Family Physician* (November 1991), children had significantly fewer and less severe strep throats after tonsillectomy, compared with a control group: 29 percent had three or more in the second year after surgery, compared with 79 percent in the control group. On the other hand, the procedure carries the risk of surgery and general anesthesia, and it causes a nasty sore throat in its own right. Children often find the experience traumatic.

And of course, many recurrent sore throats aren't caused by strep. Allergy, chronic sinusitis, or exposure to irritant dusts (at work or school, for example) may be to blame, and should be considered before you decide on surgery.

About 15 percent of the population carry the strep bacteria in their throat, in colonies too small to cause infection. This situation can persist for months, despite the usual antibiotics. According to the review in *Patient Care* (May 30, 1991), "carriers pose little risk to themselves or their associates." The organism apparently dwindles spontaneously and grows less virulent in such cases.

Rifampin, a powerful antibiotic that can have serious side effects, can usually eliminate the carrier state, but most experts feel this therapy isn't justified for adults and at least for most children.

✦ STROKE

Stroke—thrombosis (blood clot) or hemorrhage that destroys brain tissue—is the third leading cause of death in the United States and other Western nations. There are three to four nonfatal strokes for every fatal one, and up to one third of these cause long-term disability.

Stroke fatalities have declined substantially throughout the century (by 50 percent from 1960 to 1990, according to some surveys). The incidence of stroke has been declining since the early 1950s.

The reason for improved stroke survival is uncertain, since the reductions in incidence and fatalities began before the widespread use of antihypertensive drugs and the recommendations for lifestyle changes, such as a low-fat diet and smoking cessation.

The risk factors for stroke are well known, and putting this knowledge more widely into practice could vastly improve the outlook. Some suggest that half of the stroke deaths among people seventy years old or over could be prevented.

WILL LOWERING MY BLOOD PRESSURE REDUCE MY RISK OF STROKE?

There's been controversy about the connection between hypertension (at mild to moderate levels) and heart disease, but none about stroke. It's estimated that 40 percent of strokes can be attributed to systolic blood pressure above 140 mm Hg, the top number in a blood-pressure reading.

According to a review article in *Circulation* (November 1993), a meta-analysis* of fourteen trials found that hypertension treatment—for no more than five years—lowered the risk of stroke by 42 percent. "As a result of these trials, treatment of severe, moderate, and mild diastolic hypertension to prevent stroke and other complications has been widely

---

*Often studies exploring similar goals provide contradictory results. A meta-analysis is a method of pooling the results of the best-designed studies to come to one conclusion.

accepted for young and middle-aged patients," the author, Philip Wolf, M.D., wrote.

The reduction of 42 percent must be put in perspective, though, for the people with mild hypertension (140–159/90–99) because only a small fraction are likely to suffer a stroke or heart attack. Treatment doesn't eliminate the possibility of stroke; it reduces the incidence. The odds of a stroke in a person with mild hypertension is one in a thousand in the next fifteen years. Thus, treatment offers a 42 percent reduction of an infinitesimal risk.

Hypertension expert Michael Alderman, M.D., of Albert Einstein College of Medicine, Bronx, New York, advocates looking beyond high blood pressure to identify who is at risk for a stroke. "What's important is the totality: Does the patient have a family history of premature heart disease? Does the patient have high lipid [cholesterol] values, diabetes, evidence of kidney disease or peripheral vascular disease? Is the patient obese?"

SHOULD I WATCH MY DIET?

The connection between cholesterol and stroke is not as clear-cut as with heart disease. One reason is that stroke can take several forms: about 25 percent are caused by hemorrhage; 75 percent are not. About half of strokes are due to blood clots caused by atherosclerosis. In the Multiple Risk Factor Intervention Trial, which studied over 350,000 men, hemorrhagic stroke deaths were more likely in men with the *lowest* serum cholesterol, while deaths from nonhemorrhagic strokes rose along with cholesterol levels (*The New England Journal of Medicine*, April 6, 1989).

A meta-analysis of thirteen randomized, controlled studies, however, concluded that "lowering serum cholesterol through modified diets or medications does not reduce stroke mortality or morbidity in middle-aged men." And one cholesterol-lowering drug, clofibrate, appeared to increase the risk of fatal strokes (*Annals of Internal Medicine,* 1993, no. 119).

The connection between salt and blood pressure is a complex and controversial one: it would seem that the response to sodium intake varies from person to person. Reducing your consumption of salt will lower blood pressure only in a minority with hypertension (see High Blood Pressure for a fuller discussion of this issue).

There is evidence that other minerals also influence stroke risk. A good case can be made for potassium, in particular. A twelve-year study at the University of California, San Diego, found that people whose diets were low in potassium were almost twice as likely to suffer strokes, and to die of them.

The potassium contained in a daily extra serving of fresh fruit or vegetable cuts stroke risk by 40 percent, according to their figures. Bananas, oranges, cantaloupes, and avocados are particularly rich in the mineral; but supplements, which can be toxic, are dangerous to use without supervision.

CAN DRINKING PROTECT AGAINST STROKE?

Evidence that moderate alcohol consumption (two drinks or less daily) may reduce the risk of heart attack has attracted lots of attention in recent years. That case isn't proved, and the case for stroke reduction is a lot more complicated.

Again, the mixed bag of stroke is at issue, and racial complexities come into play as well. Among whites, nonhemorrhagic strokes decline with moderate alcohol consumption, but rise if drinking is heavier (what scientists call a "J-shaped curve"). Among Japanese, however, moderate drinking has no effect, and heavier drinking increases risk. In both groups, hemorrhagic strokes increase with any alcohol consumption.

If you have high blood pressure, as little as one or two drinks a day may make it higher, presumably cancelling out whatever risk reduction alcohol might otherwise confer.

WHAT ELSE CAN I DO TO PREVENT STROKE?

Cigarette smoking substantially increases the risk of stroke, as it does heart attack. It accelerates atherosclerosis and increases blood pressure, both of which make stroke more likely. Stroke rates are an estimated 40 percent higher in men and 60 percent higher in women who smoke, and the risk rises with the number of cigarettes. According to the Framingham Heart Study of four thousand men and women, those who averaged two packs or more daily had almost twice as many strokes as those who smoked ten or fewer cigarettes daily.

If you quit smoking, your stroke risk will decline to the level of a nonsmoker in five years.

Recreational drugs are a significant cause of strokes, particularly in young people who otherwise are unlikely to have them. In one series of 214 people, ages fifteen to forty-four, admitted to San Francisco General Hospital for stroke, one third were drug abusers: among those who were under thirty-five, drug abuse was a predisposing factor in nearly half. Cocaine was the drug most recently associated with stroke (*Annals of Internal Medicine*, December 1, 1990).

An OTC drug found in diet pills and cold remedies may also pose some risk. A paper in the *American Journal of Medicine* (April 1989) reported that in recent years, at least nineteen cases of cerebral hemorrhage have been associated with phenylpropanolamine, the fifth most widely used drug in the country. In a lab test, double the recommended dose of phenylpropanolamine sent blood pressures of healthy young men and women soaring; a smaller increase was seen when a standard dose was followed by a cup of coffee.

If you use a propanolamine-containing product (read the label), don't exceed the recommended dose, and avoid caffeine; if you have high blood pressure, check with the doctor first.

As for positive steps to reduce your risk, since atherosclerosis is responsible for most strokes, the same things that cut heart attacks are advisable here. Exercise appears to have a particular benefit—and the earlier you start it, the better.

In a comparison between 125 men and women who had just had their first stroke, and a group of matched controls, those who had exercised vigorously early in life (ages fifteen to twenty-five) had about a one-third risk of stroke of the others. Increasing the years of participation up to age fifty-five increased the protection. And for those who had been free of heart and circulatory problems, recent vigorous exercise or walking cut strokes by up to two thirds (*British Medical Journal*, July 24, 1993).

AM I A CANDIDATE FOR PROPHYLACTIC MEDICATION TO PROTECT AGAINST STROKE?

Anyone with coronary heart disease has an increased risk of stroke, which can be reduced by anticoagulant drugs or prophylactic aspirin. In one study, warfarin (an anticoagulant) halved the stroke rate among people who had suffered heart attacks.

Atrial fibrillation, a disturbance of the heart rhythm that becomes increasingly common with age, is a factor in 15 percent of stroke, according to the Framingham Heart Study. Warfarin appears extremely effective in protecting people with this disorder.

People who have had transient ischemic attacks (TIAs)—reversible reductions in blood flow to the brain that leave no permanent damage—appear at greatly increased risk for stroke. In one study, daily aspirin reduced that risk by 40 percent. Another trial found ticlopidine, a drug that prevents platelets from forming clots, was more protective than aspirin for people who had TIAs or previous strokes.

Atherosclerosis in the carotid artery leading to the brain is one of the most common causes of stroke. One large clinical trial found that an operation to widen the artery, cardiac endarterectomy, significantly reduced stroke risk when the narrowing was 70 percent or greater, and there were symptoms like TIAs. Another found medical treatment superior if the narrowing was under 30 percent. For the in-between group, and for people who have narrowing but no symptoms, results have been inconclusive.

Can healthy people cut their risk of stroke by taking a small amount of aspirin (a single tablet every other day)? This hypothesis is still being tested in large-scale trials. Although the doses recommended should have no side effects, the consequences of daily aspirin consumption over decades has never been studied.

WHAT CAN BE DONE AFTER A STROKE?

About one third of people who survive a stroke will be left with significant disability: they may have difficulty speaking, walking, or independently carrying out daily activities like bathing, dressing, and eating. About 10 percent will need long-term nursing care.

The immediate impairment after a stroke may not be permanent. Recovery from apparent damage takes place rapidly in the first few weeks, and continues for at least six months. During that time, and for a good deal longer, skillful rehabilitation, physical therapy, and hard work can make an enormous difference in restoring function and returning to a satisfying life.

Lately, researchers have been exploring the exciting possibility of limiting actual injury to the brain even after the stroke happens. Brain cells don't die within minutes of disrupted oxygen supply, it appears, and measures to restore circulation after a thrombotic stroke within four to six hours may prevent much damage.

Several small trials have used the same clot-dissolving drugs applied successfully during heart attacks to bring circulation back to the brain quickly. In France, twelve people who were judged unlikely to survive were treated with tissue plasminogen activator (TPA) to dissolve the clot. Seven died, but the other five recovered completely and were out of the hospital within ten days (*Journal of the American Medical Association*, January 13, 1993). Large, randomized, double-blind controlled trials of TPA are currently under way.

Other researchers have found that high blood levels of vitamin A at the time of stroke seemed to improve the chances that the event would be milder and less damaging. The vitamin, an antioxidant contained in green and yellow vegetables, might reduce the damage to vulnerable brain cells when the supply of oxygen is first cut off and then restored. If you resort to vitamin supplements, keep the dosage at the recommended dietary allowance of 4,000 IU for women and 5,000 IU for men. Vitamin A is fat soluble and can be toxic in excessive doses.

◆ SYSTEMIC LUPUS ERYTHEMATOSUS

When people talk about "lupus," they mean systemic lupus erythematosus (SLE), an autoimmune disease in which (like diabetes and rheumatoid arthritis) antibodies attack one's own tissues. What distinguishes lupus is the widespread scope of the attack, which can involve skin, joints, kidney, lungs, circulation, and nervous system. So diffuse are the symptoms of lupus that it's been called "the great mimic," and differentiating it from other diseases often requires considerable experience and skill.

Lupus is a serious, often *very* serious disease, and not to be taken lightly. But in recent decades, improvements in treatment have brightened the outlook dramatically. According to an article in the *Journal of the American Medical Association* (November 25, 1992), 90 percent of people with lupus now survive for fifteen years or longer. Forty years ago, another study reported, just half of those treated for lupus at Johns Hopkins School of Medicine survived for four years.

The majority of people with the disease live far longer than ten years, and many have a normal life span, according to an article in the *Maryland Medical Journal* (October 1991).

The number of cases of lupus has apparently increased, too: from 14.6 per 100,000 people in 1956–65, to 50.8 in 1967–73. This probably reflects earlier diagnosis and treatments that keep people alive longer. Women are nearly ten time more likely than men to get lupus, most often in the child-bearing years.

HOW CAN I BE SURE THAT WHAT I HAVE IS LUPUS?

How easily lupus is diagnosed depends on the severity and diversity of the symptoms. Some of its early manifestations—fatigue, fever, and weight loss—are extremely general. A characteristic rash, together with a combination of the disorder's varied symptoms, like arthritis, seizures, or pleurisy, make the diagnosis likely. Although there's no single foolproof lab test, a number of tests, which measure kidney function, blood cells, and antibodies, can point with some certainty toward lupus.

Lupus can also be caused by any number of drugs, including heart medications, antihypertensives, anticonvulsants, and sulfa drugs. There are fifteen thousand to twenty thousand cases of drug-induced lupus yearly in the United States, according to a 1993 textbook. The great majority is caused by a single medication: procainamide, a heart medication.

Drug-induced lupus generally goes away when the medication is withdrawn (although some treatment, including steroids, may be necessary for severe symptoms), so it's essential to make sure this possibility isn't overlooked.

HOW DO I DECIDE WHICH DRUGS TO USE?

The most effective drugs for lupus, and the treatment advance that has made the biggest difference in health and life expectancy for lupus sufferers, are corticosteroids. These are powerful medications; people with lupus must often use them over long periods of time, and their side effects can be severe. In fact, the long-term effects of steroids and other potent drugs (which include heart disease and osteoporosis) are now among the most frequent causes of death in lupus.

To get the most benefit with the least risk, experts advise matching the drug to the specific condition, symptom, or complication of lupus that needs treatment, and using the least potent and dangerous medication that's liable to be effective. The arthritis of lupus (one of the most common symptoms), for example, can often be treated effectively with nonsteroidal anti-inflammatories. More severe arthritis or pericarditis (an inflammation of the covering of the heart) may require relatively modest doses of steroids, while high doses are reserved for serious, life-threating complications like kidney disease and severe anemia.

Drugs more potent and potentially hazardous than steroids, like the immunosuppressant cyclophosphamide, are generally used for very severe aspects of lupus (such as kidney involvement), and only when steroids don't work or pose particular dangers. They often raise the risk of cancer (18 percent of people who are given cyclophosphamide for lupus kidney disease develop malignancies, for example). None have been approved by the FDA for the treatment of lupus.

HOW CAN I BE SURE THAT THE PROBLEM IS CAUSED BY LUPUS?

Because its effects throughout the body are so broad, what appear to be exacerbations or complications of lupus may just as well be caused by some other disease superimposed on it. It is vital to know the difference. If what seems like lupus lung disease is actually an infection, for example, treatment with high dose steroids would be worse than useless, even life-threatening.

Infection has become the most common cause of death from lupus, and high doses of steroids are major risk factors for such infections. "These facts again emphasize the importance of using the smallest effective dose of prednisone for the shortest possible time," the 1991 *Maryland Medical Journal* article said.

What seems to be a manifestation of lupus may also be a drug reaction. Nonsteroidal anti-inflammatories given for lupus arthritis, for example, may cause kidney disease resembling that of the disease itself.

WILL THE RESULTS OF THIS TEST MAKE BETTER TREATMENT POSSIBLE?

An unnecessary blood test does little harm (other than the added expense), but for any invasive test, you should know just why it's being done and what difference the outcome will make in treatment.

In lupus, this applies specifically to renal biopsy. Removal and microscopic examination of kidney tissue can help a doctor get a better idea of the chances that a particular person will maintain or lose kidney function. But no prospective study has determined whether this knowledge actually improves treatment and its outcome.

CAN YOU HELP ME LEARN TO USE NONDRUG TREATMENTS?

Lifestyle changes and nondrug treatments play a major role in living with the varied manifestations of lupus. The disease causes photosensitivity in about 73 percent of people—sunlight, or even fluorescent light, can produce a painful skin reaction, muscle pain, or fever. Over one third of people, in one study, said that sun sensitivity had a significant impact on the way they lived. You may need some help in learning to avoid sun exposure to the extreme that may be necessary.

People with lupus are often unusually susceptible to skin rashes from hair dyes, skin creams, and other cosmetics, or adverse reactions to OTC drugs. Ask your doctor how to minimize the risk.

There is no evidence that exercise can slow down the lupus disease process, but it has much to offer. As with any arthritic disease, the best exercises are those that strengthen muscles and keep you limber, without overly stressing joints: walking, swimming, and bicycling are often ideal. Exercising your way into better aerobic condition can reduce the fatigue that is often extreme in lupus.

If you have joint and muscle problems with lupus, a physical therapist can help you work out an exercise program that's best for your particular situation, and advise you about what recreational sports to avoid. He or she can also guide you in getting assistive devices to make activities of daily living easier and less fatiguing (see Rheumatoid Arthritis).

People receiving steroid therapy have even more to gain from exercise. Appropriate lower body exercise can prevent muscle wastage (steroid myopathy) common with these drugs.

Another frequent problem with steroids is osteopororis: about 40 percent of people using these drugs have significant bone loss, and fractures aren't infrequent when lupus is treated with steroids. Regular weight-bearing exercise can help the bone-building process, along with adequate vitamin D and perhaps a supplement of calcium. A study of 103 people starting long-term steroid therapy found that these two nutrients could prevent bone loss in the lower spine (*The New England Journal of Medicine,* June 17, 1993).

WHAT'S THE BEST DIET FOR LUPUS?

No particular diet has been shown to substantially affect the arthritis or other symptoms, or the disease process of lupus. (Fish oil doesn't appear to have the benefits suggested by studies of rheumatoid arthritis.)

Because lupus increases coronary heart disease risk, a low-fat, high-fiber diet is especially important, along with measures to correct other risk factors like high blood pressure. If you're taking steroids, your diet should be designed to limit salt and combat the high cholesterol that often comes with the treatment.

HOW CAN I BEST DEAL WITH EMOTIONAL DIFFICULTIES?

Most any chronic disease takes a lot of adjusting to, both for you and your family. Its fatigue and its erratic course of exacerbations and improvements, to name two aspects, make lupus particularly challenging. Counseling, therapy, or membership in a support group can ease the rough parts of the process.

Depression, anxiety, and other emotional turmoil can be a psychological reaction to lupus, and there's some reason to believe (although it hasn't been established) that the disease can also cause depression biologically. Whatever the cause, pronounced emotional pain needs help, whether by increased support, psychotherapy, or medication.

Psychological difficulties, including depression, are frequent side effects of steroids, particularly at the high doses often used in lupus, and this requires different treatment.

Keeping stress under control may ease the physical course of the disease. Studies have shown that a personal crisis often preceded the appearance of lupus, and suggest that stress can exacerbate the disease and cause it to flare. If your doctor can't give you useful advice about stress management, perhaps he or she can refer you to someone who can.

Resources

The Lupus Foundation of America (Maryland) will refer you to local support groups. Call (800) 558-0121.

◆ TUBERCULOSIS

Not long ago, it was easy to think of tuberculosis (TB) as a disease of the past. With the development of effective antimicrobial drugs, new cases in the United States dropped from 84,304 to 22,201 in the decades between 1953 and 1984, and some predicted the disease would be gone from this country early in the next century. Since then, however, the incidence of TB has risen: 26,673 new cases were reported in 1992. Twenty-two states reported increases in TB from 1991 to 1992, according to the Centers for Disease Control (*Journal of the American Medical Association,* October 6, 1993).

Worldwide, the picture is bleaker. There are an estimated 8 million active cases of TB, causing 2.9 million deaths each year.

What's worse, recent years have seen the emergence of strains of *Mycobacterium tuberculosis,* the TB organism, that are resistant to the drugs that had been effective for decades.

Tuberculosis is a public health problem as well as a personal health problem. Getting truly effective treatment is an act of social responsibility.

AM I LIKELY TO CATCH TB?

To a great extent, the rise in TB has targeted specific segments of the population. Rates are higher among African Americans, Hispanics, and Asians. The age-old connection between TB and poverty still holds true, according to an article in the *British Medical Journal* (September 25, 1993). In neighborhoods where poverty is high, TB may be far more common than elsewhere in the same city: from 1980 to 1991, rates in New York City increased by 143 percent, but in Central Harlem, they tripled.

Upon the whole, TB is not a very contagious disease. Close, prolonged contact, especially in a poorly ventilated area, is usually necessary for its transmission: getting coughed on by a fellow bus passenger isn't enough to do it.

This is probably one reason why rates are especially high in crowded institutional conditions, such as homeless shelters and jails. A study in the *Journal of the American Medical Association* (May 5, 1993) found that the length of time an inmate spent in jail significantly increased the chances he or she would get TB.

Some people contract TB while in the hospital or nursing home— either as patients or as health-care providers. The Centers for Disease Control recently issued revised guidelines and regulations to curb the spread of the disease in health-care facilities (*Journal of the American Medical Association,* October 27, 1993).

Poor health and undernutrition put you at risk of TB, as does anything that weakens the immune system, including aging. One fourth of people with TB in the United States are nursing home residents over sixty-five, and people with AIDS have been primary victims of rising rates, both here and all over the world.

SHOULD I BE TESTED FOR TB, EVEN THOUGH I HAVE NO SYMPTOMS?

Screening tests for TB are advised only for symptomless people who are at high risk of acquiring the disease. In addition to the above-mentioned groups, household members of persons with TB are also at risk for developing the disease.

IF I HAVE A POSITIVE SKIN TEST, DO I HAVE TB?

In the standard TB screening test, a small amount of tuberculin, a protein derivative of *Mycobacterium tuberculosis,* is injected under the skin. A swelling indicates that you have been exposed to the bacteria, but not that you have an active infection. In most healthy people, the organism may linger in the body, but never becomes strong enough to cause disease or contagion. An estimated ten million Americans have been infected by the TB bacteria, but only 10 percent will ever develop the active disease.

If you have a positive skin test, further evaluations, such as chest X ray and sputum (spit) culture, are necessary to determine whether you have a latent infection (no symptoms) or active TB.

The skin test is quite fallible. Infection with a related, but non-disease-causing, bacteria can cause a positive result. And if the immune response on which the test is based has been weakened, perhaps by disease or substance abuse, the results may be negative even in an infected person.

SHOULD I BE TREATED IF I HAVE POSITIVE TEST RESULTS BUT NO SYMPTOMS?

It is common practice to give the antituberculosis drug isoniazid prophylactically for six to twelve months to some people who have a positive skin test but who don't have the active disease. According to a review article in *Annals of Internal Medicine* (September 1, 1993), the decision should be based on the probability that you are truly infected and that there's a real risk of progression to a case of TB.

For this reason, doctors should consider how recently you appear to have been infected, whether you've been in close contact with someone who has TB, and what other medical conditions you have. The *Annals* review also recommended prophylaxis for those under thirty-five with a positive skin test, in view of the risk that the disease will develop over the course of a lifetime.

WHY IS IT NECESSARY TO TAKE SO MANY DRUGS FOR TB?

There are a number of bactericidal drugs that are effective against TB, but because bacteria that survive one drug will form a strain resistant to that drug, it has long been the practice to prescribe two or more drugs so each can prevent the emergence of a strain resistant to the other.

With the increase in resistant strains, however, it has become clear to many experts that two medications leaves too little margin for error; new guidelines from the Centers for Disease Control and the American Thoracic Society advocate initial treatment with four drugs. In communities where little drug resistance has been seen, two or three may be enough; in hospitals or jails with real outbreaks of resistant strains of TB, five or six may be necessary (*Journal of the American Medical Association,* August 11, 1993).

Susceptibility testing can reveal which drugs can kill the particular strain of TB, making it possible to adjust treatment with fewer, more precisely targeted drugs.

Anti-TB drugs can have adverse effects, including liver problems, allergic reactions, fever, and shooting pains in the arms and legs.

WHAT IS BEING DONE TO PREVENT DRUG RESISTANCE?

The most ominous thing about the current TB outbreak is the appearance of multidrug-resistant strains of *Mycobacterium tuberculosis*, which, according to an article in *The New England Journal of Medicine* (September 9, 1993), "has resulted in many cases of marginally treatable, often fatal disease." In the last three decades, the proportion of resistant strains has increased from 3 to 9 percent. Not only is the person with a resistant strain in danger, he or she is a danger to others.

Why the surge in resistance? One important factor is the failure of many people to take antituberculosis medications regularly or for as long as prescribed: in the future, the bacteria that have survived erratic or abbreviated therapy won't be susceptible to the drugs that were used.

But poor medicine is also to blame. A study of thirty-five people with multidrug-resistant TB found that the doctors of twenty-eight hadn't followed standards of practice defined by the American Thoracic Society, the Centers for Disease Control, and the American College of Chest Physicians—committing an average of almost four errors per person.

Most often, the doctors used only one drug at first, failed to change the treatment properly when it wasn't working, failed to identify preexisting resistance, failed to take steps when drugs weren't taken properly, or used prophylactic treatment when full-scale treatment was called for. "Aggressive professional education" is among the steps the authors of the study advocated to curtail the growing problem of resistance (*Journal of the American Medical Association,* July 7, 1993).

◆ ULCER

Ulcer isn't just a disease; it's part of the language (as in: "My boss is giving me an ulcer"). It's also a symbol for stress, as well as of an imprudent diet and indulgence in drink and tobacco. But the reality is something else. While stress, cigarettes, and alcohol can worsen ulcer and ulcer symptoms, the cause—in the majority of cases—appears to be a lot less colorful: a bacterial infection.

A bacterium was a suspected cause of peptic ulcers as long ago as the late nineteenth century, but it was not accepted to the satisfaction of many experts until 1982, when Australian researchers Barry Marshall and Robin Warren isolated *Helicobacter pylori* as the culprit. *H. pylori,* one of the rare bacteria able to survive in the acid environment of the stomach, appears to be the most common cause of ulcer in the stomach (gastric ulcer) or the first part of the small intestine (duodenal ulcer). Nonsteroidal anti-inflammatory drugs (NSAIDs) are responsible for most of the rest, and uncommon diseases that increase gastric secretion are a relatively rare factor.

An editorial in the *Journal of the National Cancer Institute* (August 18, 1993) suggested that the discovery of the role of *H. pylori* should result in "a second revolution" in the medical management of ulcer. But as often happens with medical revolutions, the word has been slow getting out from the research lab to the practicing physician.

HOW DO I KNOW IF MY ULCER IS CAUSED BY *H. PYLORI?*

Most people with gastric or duodenal ulcers are infected with *H. pylori.* But so are many healthy people. Evidence of a cause-and-effect relationship comes from studies showing that ulcers heal when the bacteria are eradicated by drugs that do not directly protect the stomach lining, and relapses afterward are uncommon.

The presence of *H. pylori* can be detected by biopsy of part of the stomach lining taken at the same time that the ulcer is diagnosed through an endoscope, a long, thin, hollow viewing instrument inserted into the stomach by way of the mouth. The simplest and cheapest noninvasive method is a blood test.

WHEN ARE ANTIBIOTICS USED?

It appears that adding antibiotics to drugs that reduce the stomach's acid output is the most effective approach to healing ulcers caused by *H. pylori*. A common combination includes tetracycline or amoxicillin, metronidazole, and bismuth subsalicylate (the active ingredient in Pepto-Bismol) added to ranitidine or cimetidine.

The barrage of drugs works well to heal ulcers. But then, so does the older approach of ranitidine or cimetidine alone (which is still the mainstay of most physicians in this country). The difference is in the frequency of relapse. After healing with conventional treatment, half of ulcers relapse within six months, and as many as 95 percent have come back after two years. Bactericidal therapy, on the other hand, is followed by relapse in less than 20 percent of people, according to an article in *Science* (April 9, 1993).

Those who have done much of the research into *H. pylori* and ulcer tend to advocate antibacterial therapy as the first treatment for ulcer when infection has been confirmed. "Eradication of *H. pylori* infection changes the natural history of gastric or duodenal ulcer," writes David Y. Graham, M.D., of the Veterans Administration Medical Center in Houston. "The disease is cured, and the risk of recurrence is virtually eliminated" (*The New England Journal of Medicine,* February 4, 1993).

IF ULCERS ARE CAUSED BY AN INFECTION, ARE THEY CONTAGIOUS?

Just how *H. pylori* is transmitted is uncertain. Epidemiological studies find that the infection rate is highest where sanitation is poor, suggesting that fecal contamination may play a role in spreading the bacteria in developing nations (as it does in the spread of hepatitis A and cholera).

This is not a likely explanation for the United States, however. Some research has shown that *H. pylori* infection tends to run in families. In a study of thirty-eight families reported at an annual meeting of the American College of Gastroenterology, where one parent was infected, so was the spouse, more than 75 percent of the time. In families where one parent was not infected, the spouse carried the organism only 9 percent of the time. Nearly half the children in families with an infected parent were also infected, compared with 5 percent in other families.

The pattern is good evidence that infection with *H. pylori* is transmitted from one person to another, or that whole households are infected by exposure to the same source. (That spouses tended to be both infected or uninfected suggests that heredity is not involved.)

This doesn't mean that *ulcers* are transmitted, however. The majority of people who carry *H. pylori* bacteria have no more difficulty than a mild stomach inflammation, if that. The families in the study just mentioned, in fact, were all free of symptoms. What additional factors combine with *H. pylori* to make an ulcer is not known.

A vaccine against *H. pylori* infection is currently in development.

CAN MEDICATION GIVE ME AN ULCER?

Among ulcers not related to *H. pylori,* the most common cause appears to be nonsteroidal anti-inflammatory drugs (NSAIDs) commonly prescribed in high doses for diseases like arthritis. These drugs counter inflammation by blocking the action of chemical messengers called prostaglandins. But prostaglandins also play a role in protecting the stomach lining.

There's no way around the fact that NSAIDs are hard on the gastrointestinal (GI) tract. One study found that over one third of people taking these drugs had digestive symptoms, and almost half of them had such symptoms daily. Another study found that among people sixty-five and older, NSAIDs were associated with a three- to fourfold increase in serious peptic ulcers.

You can minimize the risk of GI problems, including ulcer, by observing precautions with NSAIDs: take them with meals, stay away from alcohol while you're taking them, and don't take aspirin concurrently. There's less irritation when NSAIDs are started at the lowest effective dose.

One study found that the choice of NSAIDs made a major difference:

ulcers were far less common among people taking ibuprofen than other NSAIDs. Ibuprofen is the only NSAID available over the counter as well as by prescription. The OTC formulation is a much lower dose, which may reduce ulcer risk by making it possible to adjust the amount of drug to no more than is needed (*Annals of Internal Medicine,* February 15, 1991).

A synthetic prostaglandin, misoprostol, was recently approved by the FDA to prevent NSAID-induced ulcers in people at high risk. A review article in *The New England Journal of Medicine* (November 26, 1992) cited convincing evidence to confirm that misoprostol can "prevent the development of endoscopic gastric ulcers in patients receiving long-term NSAID therapy," but also noted that there were little data to support the assumption that the drug reduces complications like upper-gastrointestinal bleeding, perforation, or need for admission to the hospital. Routine use of the drug for people using NSAIDs "is not yet justified," the author concluded.

CAN STRESS OR DIET GIVE ME AN ULCER?

Lifestyle factors certainly don't play the role in ulcers that was once believed, but they may contribute to their development and make symptoms worse. The GI tract is particularly sensitive to the effects of stress, and increased stomach acid secretion is one consequence. People in stressful occupations or who experience their lives as stressful are significantly more likely to develop ulcers.

Excess alcohol consumption wreaks havoc all over the body, and the lining of the stomach and duodenum are not exempt. Cola and coffee, even the decaffeinated variety, stimulate acid secretion.

Other than alcohol and coffee, however, the role of diet in ulcer is unclear. Foods like milk, once prescribed for people with ulcer, are now known to increase stomach acid production, and spicy foods may have less effect than has been thought. Individual reactions to specific foods may differ substantially.

Cigarette smoking has long been associated with increased risk of duodenal ulcer, and of serious complications, including bleeding and death. Smoking also slows the healing process and makes recurrences more likely. A study reported in *Annals of Internal Medicine* (1993, no. 119) suggests that smoking inhibits secretion of bicarbonate by the lining of the duodenal, which normally protects against gastric acid.

IF I HAVE AN ULCER, AM I AT HIGH RISK OF STOMACH CANCER?

The connection between gastric ulcer and stomach cancer is uncertain. It has been shown, however, that *H. pylori* infection holds risk factors for both. In some people, the organism causes chronic lesions in the stomach lining that can progress to cancer. Who, among the many infected by *H. pylori,* are susceptible to this process, and whether these same people develop ulcers hasn't yet been clarified. Nor, for that matter, can much be said about the big question: whether eradication of *H. pylori* can reduce stomach cancer risk.

One thing that emerged from a number of large studies is that partial removal of the stomach—the most common surgery for very serious ulcer—increases the risk of gastric cancer. In the first twenty years after surgery, the risk of cancer is unchanged (if the surgery was for gastric ulcer) or goes down (if for duodenal ulcer), but then it goes to double or triple the rate in the general population for people who had duodenal or gastric ulcer, respectively, according to an article in the *Journal of the National Cancer Institute* (August 18, 1993).

Surgery is considered only in situations when bleeding or obstruction recur despite medical treatment, or when complications like perforation (the ulcer goes all the way through the stomach or duodenal wall) create an emergency. The rate of surgery has declined steadily since the 1960s, as medical treatment has improved, and the new approaches to *H. pylori* could eventually make the intervention extremely rare, the National Cancer Institute article suggests.

✦ URINARY TRACT INFECTION

Urinary tract infections (UTIs) affect some 10 to 20 percent of women in their lifetime. While uncommon in younger men, UTIs become more of a male problem after age fifty, usually because of prostate enlargement.

The urinary tract is the most common place for infections to develop in the hospital (generally connected with the use of a catheter). Among elderly people in nursing homes and other institutions, rates of infection (often without symptoms) run as high as 20 percent in men and 50 percent in women.

While the symptoms of bladder infection (cystitis)—difficulty and burning while urinating; abdominal pain—may be severe enough to interfere with sleep, work, and recreation, they usually respond quickly and well to antibiotics. Recurrent infections can be a frustrating problem, however; about one woman in five who has one episode of cystitis will have recurrences several months apart.

When the infection travels up beyond the bladder to the kidneys (pyelonephritis), it must be taken more seriously.

HOW DO I KNOW WHAT KIND OF INFECTION IS INVOLVED?

In women, painful urination is almost always due to cystitis, vaginitis, or a sexually transmitted disease. Other symptoms differentiate these conditions, and a urinalysis or culture can confirm that it's cystitis. According to a review article in *The New England Journal of Medicine* (October 28, 1993), an office dipstick test can detect pus in the urine (a sign of cystitis) with 75 to 96 percent accuracy. A microscopic examination or urine culture can pick up those cases missed by the dipstick test.

Since UTIs are rare in men under fifty, they've traditionally been assumed to indicate an anatomical abnormality of the urinary tract. It has recently become evident, however, that young men may get simple cystitis caused by the same organisms as women. Homosexual men are at increased risk.

A particularly virulent strain of bacteria can work its way up to the kidneys and cause pyelonephritis.

WHAT ANTIBIOTICS SHOULD BE USED AND FOR HOW LONG?

Since the vast majority of cystitis is caused by just a few organisms (80 percent by E. Coli and 5 to 15 percent by Staphylococcus saprophyticus), it's customary to use one of several antibiotics that are known to be effective: among them are trimethoprim-sulfamethoxazole (Bactrim; Septra), ampicillin, nitrofurantoin (Macrodantin), or a newer class of drugs called fluoroquinolones.

Bacterial resistance may be a factor in choosing an antibiotic: 33 percent of cystitis bacteria are resistant to ampicillin; 15 to 20 percent to nitrofurantoin; and 5 to 15 percent to trimethoprim-sulfamethoxazole.

The duration of therapy has been a matter of some dispute. According to The New England Journal of Medicine review, three days of antibiotics appears to be best: it works as well as seven days, but with lower cost and risk of side effects.

A single large dose of antibiotic has enjoyed popularity in recent years. This approach isn't quite as effective in curing cystitis, however, and is liable to fail when certain bacteria are involved. Most important, it carries a considerably higher risk of recurrence, apparently because the single dose is enough to kill the bacteria infecting the bladder, but leaves colonies lurking in the vagina and elsewhere, which can emerge as reinfection.

Young men with cystitis, and women who are pregnant, diabetic, over sixty-five, or diaphragm users are often given antibiotics for seven days. A bacterial culture to identify the organism responsible may also be indicated.

Pyelonephritis requires a longer course of antibiotics; if the illness is severe or accompanied by nausea or vomiting, it may need to start with intravenous therapy in the hospital.

WHAT CAN BE DONE FOR RECURRENT CYSTITIS?

It's uncertain why 20 percent of women who have cystitis suffer recurrent episodes, often just months apart. While recurrences sometimes can be traced to a continuing infection that's never fully eradicated, 90 percent of the time it's susceptibility to repeated new infections that causes recurrences. There's some evidence that a genetic vulnerability makes it easier for bacteria to adhere to cells lining the urinary tract of certain women, and to grow there.

Contraception is a risk factor you can change. Diaphragms and spermicides are associated with recurrent infections, probably because they change the chemical environment in the vagina in a way that allows *E. Coli* to flourish. In a study reported in the *Journal of the American Medical Association* (January 2, 1991), there were significantly more UTI-causing bacteria twenty-four hours after intercourse in the urine of women who had used diaphragm or condom and spermicide for contraception, but not in oral contraceptive users.

One strategy that prevents recurrences is prophylaxis: you take a low dose of antibiotics several times a week, indefinitely. In view of the role apparently played by sexual activity in initiating infections, some suggest scheduling prophylaxis around intercourse. In a randomized, double-blind, placebo-controlled trial, sixteen young women who were prone to UTIs took a low dose of antibiotic each time they had intercourse. In six months, two of them developed UTIs; during the same period, nine of eleven control women had infections.

For the placebo group, more frequent intercourse meant more infection; for the antibiotic group, it didn't (*Journal of the American Medical Association,* August 8, 1990).

Another approach puts you in charge: you keep a supply of antibiotics on hand to initiate treatment as soon as symptoms appear. *The New England Journal of Medicine* review article calls this "a convenient, safe, inexpensive, and effective management strategy."

Some self-help strategies are also said to minimize recurrences, such as urination soon after intercourse, to flush out bacteria. In general, urinate as often as you feel the need throughout the day.

The widespread belief that drinking cranberry juice will prevent or cure UTIs was confirmed in a preliminary study of 121 elderly women in a Boston long-term care facility. Half of the women drank ten ounces of cranberry juice daily for six months and half drank a placebo drink similar in taste to cranberry juice. The cranberry-juice drinkers had half the rate of bacteria in their urine compared to the placebo drinkers. Cranberry juice and blueberry juice contain chemicals that prevent E. Coli from attaching to the bladder wall (*Journal of the American Medical Association*, March 9, 1994).

WHAT CAN BE PRESCRIBED FOR OLDER WOMEN?

Recurrences often become more of a problem after menopause: about 10 to 15 percent of women over sixty have frequent UTIs. As the body's store of estrogen decreases, there is a thinning of the epithelial lining of the vagina, bladder, urethra, and the labia. The cells dry out, leaving the area susceptible to abrasions that can lead to inflammation. This is called vaginal atrophy.

Estrogen therapy will not only treat vaginal atrophy effectively but also re-create a healthy premenopausal condition in which the vagina is "colonized" with lactobacilli. In one trial, women who used topical estrogen had significantly fewer UTIs than those in a placebo control group; half as many women had vaginal colonies of infection-causing bacteria.

It appears that restoring estrogen allows harmless lactobacilli to flourish in the vagina, creating an acid environment where disease-causing bacteria can't survive (*The New England Journal of Medicine*, September 9, 1993).

WILL CIRCUMCISION LOWER THE RISK OF UTIs?

Although UTIs are relatively uncommon among young men, they seem more frequent among those who haven't been circumcised. A study reported in the *Journal of the American Medical Association* (February 5, 1992) suggested a significant association between UTI and the lack of circumcision. The organism involved was most often *E. coli,* which apparently finds a hospitable environment for growth in the foreskin.

WHAT CAN BE DONE ABOUT UTIs IN PREGNANT WOMEN?

UTIs are common in pregnant women, often without symptoms. They must be taken seriously, because they increase the risk of pregnancy complications, including premature labor. The American College of Obstetricians and Gynecologists recommends screening for infection, with or without symptoms, during pregnancy. In one recent study of more than a thousand pregnant women, 2.3 percent had urinalysis signs of infection (*Journal of the American Medical Association,* October 27, 1993).

During pregnancy, UTIs are generally treated with a longer course— one to two weeks—of a relatively nontoxic antibiotic such as ampicillin or cephalexin.

◆ VACCINATION

Childhood vaccination is a matter of law: in all fifty states. In order to attend school, a child must be immunized against pertussis (whooping cough), rubella, diphtheria, tetanus, measles, mumps, and polio. Two other vaccinations, against hepatitis B and *Haemophilus influenzae b* (a bacterium that causes respiratory infections and meningitis), also are recommended.

Mass vaccination programs are generally credited with making rare what were once common childhood diseases. Before the measles vaccine was introduced in the mid-1960s, there were a half-million to several million cases of measles yearly; in 1993, there were fewer than three hundred.

But not everyone is happy about the drive to more and more immunizations. Critics contend that at least some of the vaccinations are neither necessary nor absolutely safe. They cite side effects that range from unpleasant to dangerous, and suggest that sometimes vaccines actually cause the diseases they're supposed to prevent—or worse.

WHY NOT WAIT UNTIL MY CHILD STARTS SCHOOL WHEN VACCINATION IS MANDATORY?

The standard schedule, recommended by public health and medical groups, calls for immunization to be essentially complete within the first two years of life. It *must* be done before a child can enter school (or, in some states, certified day care programs). The delay in immunizing many young children, experts say, is a major public health problem, particularly in inner city communities, where, in a study of nine communities, just 12 to 46 percent of children had all the recommended shots by the age of two (*The New England Journal of Medicine*, December 17, 1992).

Exposure to disease can take place at any age, so public health people propose that infants should be protected as early as possible, especially because some childhood diseases, particularly pertussis (whooping cough) and measles, are most dangerous in the first years.

CAN VACCINATION CAUSE SERIOUS HARM?

Concern about adverse effects has made many parents reluctant to submit their children to immunization and has led to lawsuits that, for a time, put the continued availability of some vaccines in doubt.

The fact is, vaccines can cause serious reactions that may lead to permanent damage, even death. A 1993 report by the Institute of Medicine concluded that, among other things, there was evidence that diphtheria, tetanus, measles-mumps-rubella, and hepatitis B vaccines could cause the severe allergic reaction of anaphylaxis; that the measles vaccine could cause death from measles itself; and that the polio vaccine could cause polio.

Such reactions are extremely rare. The issue is the same as for drugs: do the benefits outweigh the risks? The consumer-led National Vaccine Information Center (see Resources) observed that the nation's reporting system for adverse reactions went into effect only in 1990 and is estimated to be catching only about 10 percent of the actual "adverse events."

Little is known about the consequences of vaccination many years later because of the lack of systematic follow-up studies. Some hints have emerged, though, about the measles vaccine. A measles epidemic occurred in the United States between 1989 and 1991, causing 132 deaths and illness serious enough to hospitalize about 20 percent of the fifty-five thousand infected. Ironically, the measles vaccine was introduced thirty years ago with the promise that it would provide lifelong immunity and eventually lead to the disease's demise. Prior to mass immunizations, measles was a disease largely confined to young children. Infants were protected by their mother's immunity (via the placenta) for the first year of life. The disease was uncommon in adults, because virtually everyone was exposed to the virus in childhood. Unfortunately, many of today's infants, born of vaccinated mothers, no longer show the immunity that traditionally protected babies. Critics of mass immunization programs say that instead of eliminating measles, it has merely shifted the disease to two groups—infants and adults—for whom it may be a far more serious and life-threatening disease.

IS THE WHOOPING COUGH VACCINE DANGEROUS?

Particular fear has surrounded vaccination for whooping cough (pertussis). It frequently causes an unpleasant reaction, including joint and muscle pain and fever. More alarming effects can include convulsions (in an estimated one infant in seventeen hundred and fifty), persistent crying, and fever over 105.

Some parent groups contend that pertussis vaccine causes much more serious harm that goes unrecognized, including more than eleven thousand cases of brain damage, and a thousand deaths each year.

Medical experts concede that a link between pertussis vaccine and serious neurological illness can't be entirely dismissed, but argue that it is so small as to be overwhelmed by the benefits in avoiding whooping cough (*Journal of the American Medical Association,* January 5, 1994). In a 1991 report, the Institute of Medicine concluded that the evidence is consistent with between zero and ten cases of acute brain disease per million immunizations.

The pertussis vaccine (actually, its share of the combined diphtheria-pertussis-tetanus vaccine) has been refined substantially in recent decades to reduce the amount of toxin in the product and presumably to reduce reactions accordingly.

A new "acellular" vaccine uses fragments of the pertussis bacterium to induce the immune response, rather than the whole organism, and causes far fewer reactions (3 to 4 percent compared with 15 percent). It has been approved for use as a booster shot in this country, and is expected to replace the old-fashioned vaccine entirely, if further studies confirm its effectiveness.

WHY SUBJECT MY CHILD TO VACCINATION RISK, HOWEVER SMALL, TO PROTECT AGAINST DISEASES NOBODY GETS ANYMORE?

It's true that diphtheria is virtually never seen in this country anymore (there were two cases in 1991, compared with 206,000 in 1921), and that whooping cough, mumps, and measles are now rare. Polio, once the summertime scourge of American parents, has vanished altogether—except for five to ten cases that are apparently caused each year by the vaccination itself.

So why take the chance? The reason vaccination is mandated by law is that it's as much a public health as a personal health issue. These diseases dwindled only when enough of the population was vaccinated to stop their spread: protection of each is necessary for protection of all.

In addition, none of these diseases is extinct everywhere. Diphtheria flourishes in Russia; measles in Africa; polio in Zaire and Nepal—all a jet flight away in our shrinking world. Imported cases do occur.

Polio is a case in point. The most recent outbreak in this country was in 1979 among Amish children (who are exempt from mandatory vaccination on religious grounds). It apparently had been brought back to the United States from an Amish wedding in Toronto attended by coreligionists from the Netherlands who had the disease.

CAN TOO MUCH VACCINATION WEAKEN THE IMMUNE SYSTEM OR CAUSE DISEASES LIKE ARTHRITIS OR DIABETES?

The theory that multiple vaccinations can overwhelm the infant immune system sounds plausible—so does the possibility that they can lead to autoimmune diseases. It must be recognized that our knowledge about vaccination and its long-term effects is surrounded by vast areas of ignorance. Many vaccines in use today (measles, mumps, and polio, for example) date back no more than forty years, and some—Hemophilus influenza type b(H16) and hepatitis B, have just a decade of experience. That they may someday turn out to have serious consequences later in life simply can't be ruled out.

A 1993 Institute of Medicine (IOM) report entitled "Adverse Effects of Pertussis and Rubella Vaccines" found a causal relationship between a currently used rubella vaccine strain and arthritis in adult women. (The rubella vaccine is often given again in adulthood to health workers.) The IOM concluded that long-term follow-up studies are needed.

IS MY CHILD'S RISK OF GETTING HEPATITIS ENOUGH TO JUSTIFY VACCINATION?

Hepatitis B is one of the more recent vaccines. Developed about a decade ago, it is currently recommended for all children at birth, but not required by most states for school attendance. In some countries, hepatitis B is widespread, but in the United States, it is rare among children—except those whose mothers are from countries in Asia and elsewhere where the disease still thrives.

The biggest danger of hepatitis B is the possibility that it will become chronic, which carries a significant risk of cirrhosis and liver cancer, sometimes decades later. Among adults with hepatitis B, only 5 to 10 percent become chronic; among infants and small children, the proportion is far higher (see Hepatitis).

When the vaccine was first developed, it was recommended at birth for children of mothers in high-risk groups (Asians, health-care workers, intravenous drug users, among others). The recommendation was made universal, according to a review article in *The New England Journal of Medicine* (December 17, 1993), in part because the selective approach was missing too many children who should get it.

What's more, public health officials contend, universal immunization in infancy is just about the only way to vaccinate large numbers before adolescence, when the risk of hepatitis transmission by sexual activity or drug use begins to rise. Will immunity start to wear off by then? There's a gap in the knowledge base; the vaccine hasn't been around long enough to find out. Significantly, *Pediatric News* reported in 1992 that a majority of pediatricians in the country are resisting the recommendation to immunize newborn infants for the hepatitis B vaccine. Most expressed reluctance to add three intramuscular injections (the amount needed for hepatitis B immunization) to the vaccination series normally given in the first twelve months of life. Other doctors question universal vaccination for a disease largely confined to high-risk groups, such as babies born to mothers known to be carriers, prostitutes, injecting drug users, receivers of blood transfusions, medical personnel exposed to blood, and those who have sexual relations with or household exposure to an infected person.

IF MY CHILD IS SICK, SHOULD I POSTPONE VACCINATION?

The American Academy of Pediatrics guidelines say that vaccination shouldn't be deferred because an infant has a cold, mild upper respiratory illness, diarrhea, or fever. There's no evidence that adverse effects will be worse, that the illness will be worse, or that the vaccine will be substantially less effective.

An ailing baby is unlikely to appreciate vaccination, however, and even mild side effects would aggravate discomfort. The effects of a vaccination, for that matter, could make it more difficult for a pediatrician to evaluate a sick child.

The rationale behind the no-delay rule is largely a public health one. Many children are rare clinic visitors, and an opportunity missed may not be recovered quickly. But there's no magic to a rigid vaccination timetable, and no harm in waiting a week or until the child is better.

Resources

The only nationally based vaccine consumer information source:

The National Vaccine Information Center
512 West Maple Avenue, Suite 206
Vienna, VA 22180
(703) 938-0342

Health Research Council
Box 75231
Washington, DC 20013
(202) 828-1947

◆ VARICOSE VEINS

A system of valves helps blood return from the lower body to the heart. If the valves don't work properly, or if the walls of the veins are too easily stretched, blood pools in the legs. The result: visibly bulging veins called varicose veins. Smaller veins that become engorged with blood form "spider veins" (also known as telangiectasia). The same process produces hemorrhoids, which are varicose veins in the area of the anus (see Hemorrhoids).

Varicose veins of the leg occur in an estimated 20 percent of American adults. They are twice as common in women as in men, and become increasingly frequent with age: 8 percent of women have them in their twenties, rising to 72 percent in their sixties (in men, they increase from 1 to 43 percent).

Heredity is a factor in the susceptibility to varicose veins. According to an article in *Family Physician* (September 1992), there's a family history in 43 to 90 percent of people with varicose or spider veins. The increased pressure in the abdomen during pregnancy often causes varicose veins to worsen.

WHEN SHOULD VARICOSE VEINS BE TREATED?

Not all varicose veins require treatment. Sometimes, the only effect is cosmetic. When they occur near the skin surface, they're unsightly, and what, if anything, to do about them is a matter of personal preference. Several self-care measures can be taken. Try staying off your feet as much as possible; lie or sit down with your legs raised above chest level; and try wearing support hose.

Not infrequently, however, they cause distressing symptoms; more than half of the people who seek medical advice are motivated by discomfort. Aching, a common complaint, may be more pronounced after long periods of standing. Some women suffer particular discomfort during menstruation or after intercourse. Leg cramps, heaviness, and swelling are equally common in men and women. Even relatively modest changes in the veins can be associated with significant distress.

More serious medical problems can develop from varicose veins. If pooling of blood is severe, there is the danger of leg ulcers—persistent sores that occur most commonly around the ankle. In certain situations, a blood clot can form in the vein (thrombophlebitis). If it breaks loose and lodges in the lung, the consequences can be serious, even fatal. Severe pain and swelling in a leg with varicose veins could mean a clot—and demands immediate medical attention.

WHAT TREATMENT IS BEST FOR ME?

The aim of treatment is to eliminate the affected veins; circulation is taken over readily by the remaining blood vessels. The basic methods are surgery to literally remove the veins, and sclerotherapy, in which they are injected with a solution that irritates the vein lining; they eventually turn into scar tissue and wither away. Laser and electrocautery are less common approaches, usually reserved for very small spider veins.

The choice of treatment depends, in large part, on the size of the affected veins and the degree to which they are damaged. Severely affected major veins are best removed surgically, while sclerotherapy may be preferable earlier in the disease process and is the treatment of choice for small, superficial spider veins. "One course of therapy will not fulfill all purposes for therapists or patients," according to an article in the *Journal of Dermatologic Surgery and Oncology* (1992, no. 18).

In the surgical procedure, also known as "stripping," the veins are removed with a flexible device, through an incision near the groin, and connections to deeper veins tied off. It requires anesthesia (usually local or regional), and carries a risk of wound infection and blood clots. Usually, it can be done as an outpatient procedure.

Sclerotherapy can be painful—the hypertonic saline (salt water) that is injected is likely to cause burning and cramping for several minutes—although the pain can be reduced by adding a local anesthetic to the solution. The use of other chemicals carries a risk of allergic reaction for some people. Permanent stains on the skin sometimes follow sclerotherapy. This approach usually requires several doctor visits.

Scarring and discoloration are also possible after laser and electrocautery.

According to a 1994 consumer pamphlet published by the Federal Trade Commission, the cost of both surgery and sclerotherapy typically varies from several hundred dollars to several thousand (depending on the number of veins treated, among other things). Surgery carries the additional cost of anesthesia and operating room facilities (and hospitalization, when required).

Some doctors do only surgery, others (like dermatologists) only sclerotherapy; some do both. The FTC advises consulting more than one doctor before choosing a treatment method, and inquiring about the doctor's experience with the approach you prefer.

ARE SURGERY AND SCLEROTHERAPY EQUALLY EFFECTIVE?

The effectiveness of either procedure depends in large part on how wisely it was chosen for the particular case, and the skill of the doctor administering it. They are comparable in outcome. Sclerotherapy relieves symptoms in up to 85 percent of both varicose and spider veins.

Recurrence, however, is likely after either surgery or sclerotherapy (or any other approach). Within five years, about 50 percent of varicose veins recur after surgery, and 90 percent after sclerotherapy (*Journal of Dermatologic Surgery and Oncology,* 1992, no. 18). In part, this simply reflects the fact that varicose veins are caused by an ongoing, progressive disease process.

If the varicose veins recur soon after surgery or sclerotherapy, it may mean that the procedure wasn't done completely, or that the extent of the disease wasn't fully recognized. The FTC stresses that no method has been shown to prevent recurrences. "Be wary of claims touting "major breakthroughs" or "permanent results," their pamphlet warns. "Always ask for specific documentation for claims made about particular recurrence rates or fewer health risks or cosmetic side effects."

IS IT POSSIBLE TO PREVENT VARICOSE VEINS?

Although varicose veins are quite common in the United States, they are "nonexistent to rare in whole populations of the developing world," according to an article in the *Southern Medical Journal* (September 1991). A survey of nine hospitals in five Asian countries found fewer than three reported cases of varicose veins, even among people over sixty, for example. The predominance of varicose veins in women, taken for granted in the Western world, has not been observed in India.

This is not, apparently, a matter of genetic differences: varicose veins are equally rare in blacks and whites in Nigeria, and common among blacks and whites in the United States.

There are many differences between life in developed and developing countries, such as diet, exercise patterns, and environmental exposures. One popular hypothesis links the increased risk of varicose veins to the lack of fiber in most Western diets. Less fiber means straining to pass stools, which raises pressure in the abdomen. According to the theory, this increased pressure, transmitted to the veins of the legs, causes the valves to fail.

Findings from the Framingham Heart Study, a large, ongoing population study, suggest that the same risk factors predispose to varicose veins and heart disease. It's another reason to follow a low-fat, high-fiber, calorie-controlled diet.

Resources

For a free FTC pamphlet called "Facts for Consumers: Varicose Vein Treatments":

Bureau of Consumer Protection
Office of Consumer and Business Education
Federal Trade Commission
Washington, DC 20580
(202) 326-3650

• YEAST INFECTION

Candida albicans, a species of yeast, normally grows on mucus membranes in various parts of the body, living in equilibrium with other organisms and causing no trouble. Sometimes, however, its growth accelerates, causing an infection.

Yeast infections (also called candidiasis) are most common in the vagina, causing a thick, white discharge, itching, and rash. Urination may be frequent or uncomfortable; sexual intercourse, painful.

Oral candidiasis, known as "thrush," is frequent in babies, much less so in otherwise healthy adults. Yeast infections also may cause itching, redness, and inflammation on the penis (particularly in uncircumcised men), or produce an itchy red rash with flaky white patches in folds of skin.

Localized yeast infections are pesky but generally limited and benign. More generalized infections, such as may occur in the hospital, can be dangerous, however, particularly in seriously ill or weakened people.

IF YEAST IS ALWAYS THERE, WHY DOES IT CAUSE AN INFECTION?

Something happens to disrupt the equilibrium that normally keeps the organism in check. Birth control pills or pregnancy, for example, can make infection more likely, possibly through hormonal changes that produce conditions in the vagina that are more conducive to the organism's growth.

It's not uncommon to have a yeast infection (usually vaginal, but sometimes oral) after taking antibiotics. These drugs kill harmless bacteria that normally live in balance with yeast; in their absence, the yeast proliferates in the vagina or mouth. Corticosteroids often prescribed for asthma or allergy suppress immune function and may lead to infection.

Anything that weakens the immune system may let yeast grow unchecked. Oral yeast infection, otherwise uncommon in adults, develops in people infected with HIV, often fairly early in the disease. Illnesses like diabetes or simply the debilitation associated with poor nutrition or old age can also be responsible.

CAN I TREAT A VAGINAL YEAST INFECTION MYSELF?

The basic treatment for yeast infections is antifungal drugs, and two of them, clotrimazole and miconazole, were approved for over-the-counter (OTC) use in 1991. These are topical drugs that have been prescribed by doctors for several decades, and they appear to work well.

If you're going to treat yourself, it's important to be sure that what you have actually is a yeast infection. Similar symptoms can be caused by a protozoan, *Trichomonas vaginalis* ("tric"), or bacteria. The labeling for OTC fungicides instructs women to use the product for recurrences of yeast infections, not for a first episode (presumably on the theory that you'll recognize it when it comes back).

If in doubt, it's best to check with your doctor. But it should be noted that the professional record in diagnosing yeast isn't spectacular either. In a study of yogurt for the treatment of recurrent yeast infections, one quarter of women recruited could not participate because what they had been told was a yeast infection was actually caused by other organisms.

Using an antifungal for something other than yeast probably won't do much harm, but it won't do much good, either, and it could allow a more serious problem to worsen. Abdominal pain, fever, or foul-smelling vaginal discharge indicates that you may have a more serious condition, and should get a prompt medical evaluation. Similarly, no improvement after three days of OTC treatment merits at least a phone call to your doctor. The same applies if symptoms recur within two months.

CAN ANYTHING BE DONE FOR RECURRENT VAGINAL YEAST INFECTIONS?

It is estimated that one woman in seven will develop at least one vaginal yeast infection during her reproductive years, and 10 to 25 percent will relapse within thirty days after treatment. Some women suffer infections as often as once a month.

The above factors (antibiotics, birth control pills, diabetes, etc.) may explain some of these cases, but for the most part, the reason for recurrence is a mystery. Theories include differences in immune response that may make some women less able to control yeast growth; persistent colonies of yeast elsewhere in the body; or interactions with other microorganisms.

While there is no foolproof way to end recurrent yeast infections, some measures can reduce vulnerability. Avoid feminine hygiene sprays, powders, or douches (unless they've been cleared by your doctor), as they can disrupt the body's natural chemistry. Nylon panties and panty hose trap moisture and create a climate in which yeast can thrive. Cotton panties and garter belts are good alternatives.

While yeast is not classically a sexually transmitted disease, you can be reinfected by your partner (even if he doesn't have symptoms). Recurrent episodes may end if he's treated, too.

CAN YOGURT HELP?

Eating yogurt is a folk remedy for vaginal yeast infections that has been favored for decades by alternative health practitioners. Several years ago, a small study supported this approach (*Annals of Internal Medicine,* March 1992).

Thirteen women who had recurrent yeast infections alternated between six months on a diet that included a cup of yogurt a day and six months on a yogurt-free diet. While they were eating yogurt, infections dropped to one third, compared with the control period.

The yogurt used in the study contained live *Lactobacillus acidophilus* cultures, and laboratory studies showed that colonies of these harmless bacteria increased in the vagina and rectum as *Candida* colonies decreased. *L. acidophilus,* the researchers suggested, inhibits the growth of *Candida,* perhaps by secreting acid that makes the vaginal environment less hospitable to yeast.

If you want to try this at home, make sure the yogurt you eat has *L. acidophilus;* not all "active culture" products do, and advertising can be misleading. If you make your own, start with acidophilus milk.

A variant of the yogurt approach—placing the product or acidophilus milk directly in the vagina—was not tested in this study.

CAN YEAST CAUSE SYMPTOMS THROUGHOUT THE BODY?

In recent years, yeast infection has been held responsible for headache, depression, impotence, constipation, diarrhea, fatigue, heartburn, and joint pain, among many other things. The theory is that susceptible people develop chronic, body-wide yeast infections, which provoke an allergic response and produce toxins capable of causing an extremely broad range of symptoms.

"The yeast connection" (as it is called in a popular book of that title) is treated not just by alternative healers but by some physicians as well.

The treatment for chronic yeast syndrome is rather extreme: a diet that eliminates yeast-containing and yeast-promoting foods (yeast breads, sugar, processed foods, cheeses, mushrooms, vinegar, alcohol, coffee, and tea). A physician may also prescribe oral antifungal drugs, like nystatin, for several months.

Although many people unquestionably feel better after treatment for chronic yeast infection, the theory has been subject to little scientific scrutiny, which means that the placebo response may well play a role. One randomized, double-blind study of forty-two women who met criteria for the syndrome found no difference in physical or psychological symptoms between those who received nystatin and placebo (*The New England Journal of Medicine,* December 20, 1990). The study has been criticized for not including diet therapy, such as restricting sugar intake, and for defining yeast sufferers inappropriately. "Additional scientifically sound studies will be needed to determine whether this syndrome does or does not exist, and if it does, what the optimal treatment is for patients," an editorial in the same *Journal* issue concluded.

If you do seek treatment for chronic yeast syndrome, make sure that your dietary changes leave you adequately nourished, and that long-term drug treatment, if any, is monitored by a physician.

INDEX

◆